INTRODUCTION to Surface Electromyography

Jeffrey R. Cram, PhD
Director, Sierra Health Institute
President, Clinical Resources
Nevada City, California

Glenn S. Kasman, MS, PT
Physical Medicine and Rehabilitation
Virginia Mason Medical Center
Seattle, Washington

with
Jonathan Holtz, MA, PT
Santa Cruz, California

AN ASPEN PUBLICATION®
Aspen Publishers, Inc.
Gaithersburg, Maryland
1998

The authors have made every effort to ensure the accuracy of the information herein. However, appropriate information sources should be consulted, especially for new or unfamiliar procedures. It is the responsibility of every practitioner to evaluate the appropriateness of a particular opinion in the context of actual clinical situations and with due considerations to new developments. Authors, editors, and the publisher cannot be held responsible for any typographical or other errors found in this book.

Library of Congress Cataloging-in-Publication Data

Cram, Jeffrey R.
Introduction to surface electromyography/
Jeffrey R. Cram, Glenn S. Kasman, with Jonathan Holtz.
p. cm.
Includes bibliographical references and index.
ISBN 0-8342-0751-6
1. Electromyography. I. Kasman, Glenn S.
II. Holtz, Jonathan. III. Title.
RC77.5.C73 1997
616.7′407547—dc21
97–21523
CIP

Orders: (800) 638-8437
Customer Service: (800) 234-1660

About Aspen Publishers • For more than 35 years, Aspen has been a leading professional publisher in a variety of disciplines. Aspen's vast information resources are available in both print and electronic formats. We are committed to providing the highest quality information available in the most appropriate format for our customers. Visit Aspen's Internet site for more information resources, directories, articles, and a searchable version of Aspen's full catalog, including the most recent publications: **http://www.aspenpub.com**
Aspen Publishers, Inc. • The hallmark of quality in publishing
Member of the worldwide Wolters Kluwer group

Editorial Resources: Jane Colilla

Library of Congress Catalog Card Number: 97-21523
ISBN: 0-8342-0751-6

Printed in the United States of America
1   2   3   4   5

Table of Contents

Foreword

The privilege of reading the manuscript of a book by distinguished authors before its publication is always a thrilling experience. When the material is as sparkling as in this book, one feels truly privileged and honored to be asked to write the foreword. This is a fine book that will meet the needs of many scientists and clinicians in a wide range of specialties. Both those who directly employ surface electromyography for any purpose and those who have to understand its consequences will be ever grateful to the authors.

This book is written in an astute style that clearly informs *all* readers, even such as this grizzled veteran. Only after a while will the novice reader awaken to the fact that, *mirabile diciu*, a profound learning experience has happened without the use of a computer or TV screen. Few scientific or clinical books today succeed in this game of seizing and holding the reader's interest in spite of the level of sophistication of either the reader or the subject matter.

Not only are the style and organization complete and well integrated, the choices of words and phrases are friendly and beckoning without annoying those readers who are more comfortable with scientific and clinical jargon. In this book, a spade is called a spade, but it is a shiny, well-used spade and not an "automated excavating system" used by over-anointed writers.

To summarize, it is simple and accurate to say this is a very fine book and I am happy to have read it before its birth. Moreover, I expect to refer to it *ad lib* after publication and to recommend it to others.

John V. Basmajian, OC, MD,
FRCP, FRCPS
Professor Emeritus
McMaster University
Hamilton, Canada

Preface

The cornerstone of this book is the electrode atlas found in Part II. Knowing the map of the territory—where to place the surface electromyography (sEMG) electrodes and what to expect to see during a given movement—will greatly assist the practitioner in understanding the energy that the muscle gives off. Indeed, many times during the collection of tracings for a particular set of muscles, I found myself and others asking "what happens if we do x?" Then we tried x and were either pleasantly surprised or confused and disappointed. Sometimes the system worked as we had been told by others. Sometimes it was far too complex to see what we expected to see, given the simple tools and procedures we were using. Capturing a valid sEMG tracing is sometimes associated with a subtle event. For example, I was duly impressed by the changes in recruitment patterns as we instituted small postural or positional requirements on the limbs or torso. To this day, I remember my amazement at how a simple sternal lift could facilitate the recruitment of lower trapezius. There are literally dozens of gems like this sprinkled throughout this book. The tracings in this book illustrate what can be seen using the sEMG technology. We hope that they stimulate the reader's curiosity and that readers explore the movement of their own patients while measuring muscle energy patterns.

The static and dynamic assessment chapters provide the background and protocols in detail for almost all of the current assessment procedures. This is a very interesting area in which to work, because the same end organ (the muscle) is under the command of three masters: gravity (posture), emotions, and movement. Muscle scanning is a method for assessing the neuromuscular aspects of posture; stress profiling is the method to quantify the emotional component; and dynamic sEMG procedures provide the basis for assessing movement. Practitioners need to think in this three-dimensional manner if they want to find successful solutions when something goes wrong.

Part I reviews the basic tenets of the treatment of musculoskeletal and pain-related disorders and provides a few examples of these approaches. Additional information is found in the companion book *Clinical Applications in Surface Electromyography: Chronic Musculoskeletal Pain*. I highly recommend that readers study this very scholarly, yet pragmatic review of what we know about the use of sEMG in treating a variety of conditions.

History, anatomy, physiology, and instrumentation are the foundations upon which the clinical practice of sEMG rests. Every practitioner who uses electromyography should have a sound understanding of what is behind the sEMG screen displays. Chapters 1 through 3 provide this information in an easy-to-understand fashion. For those who are new to the area of sEMG and are just learning the jargon, we have included a glossary (Appendix A) to provide definitions of some of the basic concepts.

Surface EMG is seen as an emerging technology. We have just begun to scratch the surface of its clinical potential. Chapter 11 provides some glimpses into where sEMG may be moving as it unfolds.

As is true for all manuscripts, literally hundreds of people have helped bring this book into print. The greatest contributors to this book were the many students in my workshops, whose curiosity and enthusiasm led me to seek out the "essence" of a given muscle, for a given movement, while exploring electrode placement strategies. Four of these students became dear friends, colleagues, and eventually my teachers. Will Taylor, Stu Donaldson, Jonathan Holtz, and Glenn Kasman helped to create the boundaries and channels into which this introductory volume on sEMG flowed. But it was Glenn Kasman's commitment to work on this book that set it in motion. And, once under way, it was the substantive editing of Steven Wolf that provided the basis for course corrections, and the buff and polish of Glenn Kasman, Blair Schular, Diana Huff, and Maya Cram that made it intelligible.

Many people made the tracings for the electrode atlas possible. With minds like those of Glenn Kasman and Jonathan Holtz, the power and beauty of sEMG recordings began to emerge as we intensively studied a few individuals. Some of those individuals, who spent hours or days with us and allowed us to place electrodes here and there while we asked them to move this way or that, deserve special recognition. Specifically, the efforts of David Rommen, Dennis Harmoo, Mark Woodburn, Carrie Hall, Paula Holtz, and Maya Cram helped to make the atlas possible. Finally, this book has hundreds of graphics contained within its pages. Many of these were created by Bella and Dave Bingham and Heidi Cram.

Jeffrey R. Cram, PhD

PART I

The Basics of Surface Electromyography

Jeffrey R. Cram and Glenn S. Kasman

CHAPTER 1

Introduction

"Electromyography is the study of muscle function through the inquiry of the electrical signal the muscle emanates."[1]

THE HISTORY OF SURFACE ELECTROMYOGRAPHY

The history of surface electromyography (sEMG) has to do with the discovery of electricity and the development of the ability to see things through the aid of instruments that cannot be seen, felt, or touched with the normal senses. It is also the story of the emergence of a new paradigm for assessing and treating the energy of the muscles—a form of "energy medicine," in which the emphasis is upon the energy of the body rather than its form. (In this paradigm, form is not unimportant, but it is only of a secondary interest.) As is true for all paradigm shifts, many individuals are reluctant to give up their investment in the old paradigm. For example, today, many practitioners still prefer clinical palpation and observation over measurement of the energy of the muscle, even though each technique may provide a different domain of information.

The theme of the development of sEMG can be traced back to the mid 1600s, when Francesco Redi[2,3] documented that a highly specialized muscle was the source of the electric ray fish's energy. By 1773, Walsh had been able to demonstrate clearly that the eel's muscle tissue could generate a spark of electricity. It was not until the 1790s that Galvani obtained direct evidence for a relationship between muscle contraction and electricity; he conducted a series of studies that demonstrated that muscle contractions could be evoked by the discharge of static electricity.[4] In 1792, Volta[5] initially agreed; he later concluded that the phenomenon Galvani had seen did not emanate from the tissue itself, but rather was an artifact from the dissimilar metals touching the muscle tissue. Galvani rebutted Volta's criticism and was able to demonstrate the firing of the muscle by contracting it with a severed nerve rather than metal. This finding, however, went unnoticed for four decades because of Volta's popularity. Volta had developed a powerful tool that could be used to generate electricity and also could be used to stimulate muscle. The technique of using electricity to stimulate muscles gained wide attention during the 19th century, and some people exploited this novel technique. In the 1860s, Duchenne[6] conducted the first systematic study of the dynamics and function of the intact muscle, using electrical stimulation to study muscle function.

It was not until the early 1800s that the galvanometer, a tool for measuring electrical currents and muscle activity, was invented. In 1838, Matteucci used the galvanometer to demonstrate an electrical potential between an excised frog's nerve and its damaged muscle.[1] By 1849, Du Bois-Reymond[7] provided the first evidence of electrical activity in human muscles during voluntary contraction. In his classic experiment, Du Bois-Reymond placed blotting cloth on each of his subject's hands or forearms and immersed them in separate vats of saline solution, while connecting the electrodes to the galvanometer.

He noted very minute but very consistent and predictable deflections whenever the subject flexed his hand or arm. He deduced that the magnitude of the current was diminished by the impedance of the skin. After removing a portion of the subject's skin, he replaced the electrodes and noted a dramatic increase in the magnitude of the signal during wrist flexion. By the early 1900s, Pratt[8] had begun to demonstrate that the magnitude of the energy associated with muscle contraction was due to the recruitment of individual muscle fibers, rather than the size of the neural impulse. In the 1920s, Gasser and Newcomer[9] used the newly invented cathode ray oscilloscope to show the signals from muscles. This feat won them the Nobel Prize in 1944.

As a result of continuing improvements in EMG instrumentation during the 1930s through the 1950s, researchers began to use sEMG more widely for the study of normal and abnormal muscle function. During the 1930s, Edmund Jacobson, the father of progressive relaxation, used sEMG extensively to study the effects of imagination and emotion on a variety of muscles.[10] He also used sEMG to study systematically the effects of his relaxation training protocol on muscle activity.[11] In the 1940s, researchers began to use sEMG to study dynamic movement. For example, Inman and his colleagues conducted a highly regarded study on the movements of the shoulder.[12] In the late 1940s, Price and her colleagues[13] studied clinical populations of back pain patients and noted that the sEMG activation patterns began to migrate away from the site of original injury. This represents the first documentation on antalgic (painful) postures or protective guarding muscle patterns. Floyd and Silver,[14] in the early 1950s, presented an exceptionally strong study of EMG and the erector spinae muscles. They clearly demonstrated that as the person goes through forward flexion of the trunk, the back muscles shut off as the trunk goes out onto ligamental support. During the late 1950s and the 1960s, George Whatmore,[15] a student of Jacobson, used sEMG to study and treat emotional and functional disorders. His work was summarized in a

very unusual book, *The Physiopathology and Treatment of Functional Disorders*,[15] in which he used sEMG to augment the basic progressive relaxation technique he had learned from Jacobson. In addition, he coined the term *dysponesis* to describe bad muscle energy patterns that can be observed using sEMG instrumentation.

During the 1960s, the technique of biofeedback was born. Basmajian's[16] work on single motor unit training provided some of the impetus for research on biofeedback. Although this type of training entailed the use of fine-wire electrodes rather than surface electrodes, it clearly demonstrated that the neuromuscular system could be trained using EMG biofeedback, down to its most basic element—the single motor unit. Elmer Green[17] first used sEMG with biofeedback at the Menninger Clinic, where he modified Basmajian's single motor unit training paradigm for general relaxation training. A few years later, Budzynski and colleagues[18] began using sEMG feedback to treat muscle contraction headaches. From there, the biofeedback arena began to expand rapidly.

Clinical use of sEMG for the treatment of more specific disorders began in the 1960s. Hardyck and colleagues[19] were among the first practitioners to use sEMG. They used sEMG to teach students not to subvocalize during silent reading, which accelerated students' reading development. Booker and colleagues[20] demonstrated retraining methods for patients with various neuromuscular conditions, and Johnson and Garton[21] used sEMG to assist in the restoration of function of hemiplegic patients. Wolf et al[22,23] were among the first to use sEMG biofeedback techniques in the assessment and treatment of low back pain. For a comprehensive review of the history of sEMG and low back pain through the early 1990s, see Sherman and Arena[24] or an earlier review article by Dolce and Raczynski.[25]

In the early 1980s, Cram and Steger[26] introduced a clinical method for scanning a variety of muscles using a handheld sEMG sensing device; a few years later, Cram and Engstrom[27] presented a normative database on 104 normal subjects, which they used to guide their clinical work. Using the scanning tool, they rapidly sampled the right and left aspects of up to 15 muscle sites for patients in both the sitting and standing postures. This level of analysis of the postural elements of muscle led to the differentiation of three clinical concepts: (1) site of activity, (2) impact of posture, and (3) degree of symmetry. Donaldson and Donaldson[28] took the concept of symmetry and made it dynamic. They studied the degree of symmetrical recruitment during symmetrical and asymmetrical movement patterns in both normal subjects and patients. From this work, they concluded that 20% asymmetry is acceptable during symmetrical movements, while levels greater than this are considered pathognomonic. On the other hand, asymmetrical movements should bring about asymmetrical recruitment patterns. Donaldson popularized the concept of *cocontractions* as an abnormal finding in asymmetrical movements. During the 1980s, Will Taylor[29] introduced the concept of measuring synergy patterns in the upper and lower trapezius during abduction. Following the work of Karol Lewit,[30] Taylor noted that myalgias in the upper quarter were commonly associated with postural muscles doing the work of their phasic counterparts. Here, the upper trapezius dominated the stabilizing muscular action associated with abduction to 90 degrees, even though the lower trapezius should have been doing the stabilizing role. Thus, Taylor saw the hyperactivity of the upper trapezius as being facilitated by the inhibition of the lower trapezius. Susan Middaugh and colleagues[31] have also clearly delineated the role of a hyperactive upper trapezius in headache, neck, and shoulder pain. They concluded that almost all of the dysfunctional patterns in the upper back involve hyperactivity of upper trapezius.

Scholarly research on sEMG has also flourished. During the early 1960s Basmajian conceived of an international forum to share information on sEMG, and in 1965 the International Society of Electrophysiological Kinesiology (ISEK) was formed. The organization still exists today, publishing one of the only journals that specifically addresses issues pertaining to sEMG (*The Journal of Electromyography and Kinesiology*). The American and European academic communities (especially the Scandinavians) have provided a strong fundamental basis for understanding EMG in general and sEMG in particular. Space limits the ability to acknowledge the many contributors to this field, but the influence of Carlo deLuca and his colleagues at the Neuromuscular Research Institute in Boston cannot be overlooked. Much of their work on spectral analysis and muscle fatigue[32] has shed light on the physiology of muscle and methods of measuring it. The work of Scandinavian researchers on tension myalgia in the workplace is very impressive,[33–38] and has clearly added to our understanding of dysfunctions in the workplace. In addition, an excellent summary of the use of sEMG in the occupational setting may be found in a book by Soderberg.[39]

THE ADVANTAGES AND DISADVANTAGES OF SURFACE ELECTROMYOGRAPHY

The use of sEMG has many advantages. Surface EMG recordings provide a safe, easy, and noninvasive method that allows objective quantification of the energy of the muscle. It is not necessary to penetrate the skin and record from single motor units in order to obtain useful and meaningful information regarding muscles. One can "see" synergies in the energy patterns that cannot be seen with the naked eye. The technique allows the observer to see the muscle energy at rest and changing continuously over the course of a movement. And, with multiple sensor arrays, it is possible to differentiate how different aspects of muscles do different things. Although palpation skills, muscle testing, and visual observation of posture and movement should never be discarded, they have their limitations. By adding sEMG recording information to the practitioner's fund of knowledge about the muscle function of a particular patient, the practitioner begins to blend valuable information concerning how the nervous system participates in the orchestration of the muscle function. By using sEMG, practitioners may be able to answer the following questions: Is the resting tone congruent with the palpation exam? Do the muscles fire early or late in a recruitment pattern? Does a particular exercise actually activate the muscle it is intended to, or is there a substitution pattern present? Does the muscle turn off following a given movement, or does it show irritability following movement?

The tracings and numerical printouts associated with sEMG provide information to clinicians and researchers regarding mechanisms of muscle function and dysfunction; they also suggest methods to improve treatment approaches. The objective tracings and data from sEMG recordings allow clinicians to communicate with one another and to insurance carriers about their findings, and in the Western world, objective findings are essential. Finally, the biological information obtained via sEMG methods can be fed back to the patient, providing a basis for neuromuscular reeducation and for self-regulation. Such information can fine-tune the response of the patient's nervous system to the therapist's verbal instructions. When the therapist asks the patient to relax the muscle between movements, the patient can actually see whether he or she has "let go" of the recruitment pattern or if it is necessary to "let go" again. As the patient learns to recruit a particular muscle, the initial attempts may be compared to the current attempts. This type of information provides feedback and motivation for the patient's therapeutic efforts. It may also become an important source to demonstrate to third-party payers that the prescribed treatment is having the desired effect.

The weakness of sEMG is inherent in the anatomy we study, the instruments we use to study it, and the methods or procedures we choose. It is important that clinicians acknowledge and understand these limitations. One limitation is our ability to monitor only a few muscle sites. The neuromuscular system is very rich and complex, and to reduce it to one or two channels of sEMG information is very limiting. At a minimum, a four-channel sEMG instrument allows one to study the right and left aspects of two opposing groups. At this level, the information becomes much more meaningful and practical. Scanning multiple sets of muscles in their resting state may help the practitioner to decide which regions of the musculature might be of further interest. A possible shortcoming of sEMG recordings has to do with muscle substitution patterns. The neuromuscular system may express the same movement using different muscle groups. When this occurs, the naive practitioner may believe that sEMG recordings are either inconsistent or unreliable. Thus, it is important for practitioners to understand what the "normal" case is, so that they can interpret recordings with greater confidence. To that end, this book contains an atlas of tracings for many movement patterns (see Part II).

Another difficulty with sEMG is the possibility of "cross-talk," a phenomenon where energy from one muscle group travels over into the recording field of another muscle group. When this happens, there may be problems in specificity of sEMG recordings. It may make it difficult or even impossible to isolate the sEMG recordings from a specific muscle. Some electrode placement sites have greater specificity than others. The electrode atlas grades the electrode sites according to their specificity. Three grades are used: general, quasi-specific, and specific. An additional limitation to sEMG is that, to date, there are only a few published guides to electrode placement[35,40–42] and two video presentations.[43,44] Unfortunately, none of these guides has become the standard. Thus, an upper trapezius recording from one clinic or study may not represent the same energy pattern from another clinic, because of differences in electrode placement. The atlas in this volume should be complete and comprehensive enough to encourage a more standardized method for sEMG electrode placement. Use of a standardized method strengthens the interpretation of EMG recordings at a given muscle site.

The practitioner should remember that sEMG is not a measure of force. Nor is it a measure of strength, or of the amount of effort given, or of muscle resting length. It is simply a measure of the electrical activity given off by the muscle as it contracts and does work. Practitioners must be cautious about how they interpret the sEMG findings, being careful not to overinterpret them. For example, under normal circumstances, one should not compare the sEMG amplitudes recorded from one muscle (eg, upper trapezius) with that of another muscle (eg, lower trapezius). Differences in the sEMG amplitudes during dynamic procedures may simply be due to differences in the amount of muscle mass present for each muscle, rather than to differences in how hard the muscles are working. In order to compare across muscle groups, one must normalize the sEMG data first (see Chapter 3). Thus, clinicians might normalize the activity of the upper trapezius to lower trapezius as a ra-

tio. Or clinicians might reference muscle groups to a maximum voluntary isometric contraction (MVIC) and work with the percentage of MVIC.

A final shortcoming is that sEMG electrodes are not totally unobtrusive. The electrodes and leads can potentially encumber a movement pattern or make the patient feel self-conscious abut a posture or movement. Thus, the sEMG recordings may not perfectly reflect the customary patterns of use for the patient. Practitioners are encouraged to have several different kinds of electrodes on hand so that they can choose the correct type of electrode for the muscle and movement pattern they wish to study.

Readers are encouraged to keep the above strengths and limitations of sEMG in mind as they read this book. By learning what sEMG can and cannot do, clinicians will be able to serve their patients better.

REFERENCES

1. Basmajian JV, DeLuca C. *Muscles Alive.* 5th ed. Baltimore: Williams & Wilkins; 1985.

2. Redi F. *Esperienze intorno a diverse cose naturali e particolarmente a quelle che ci sono portate dalle Indie.* Florence, Italy: 1617:47–51.

3. Wu CH. Electric fish and the discovery of animal electricity. *Am Scientist.* 1984;72:598–607.

4. Galvani L; Green RM, trans. *Commentary on the Effect of Electricity on Muscular Motion.* Cambridge, MA; 1953.

5. Volta A. Mommoria prima sull' elettricita animatle. In *Collezione dell'Opere, II.* Florence, Italy: G. Piatti; 1792.

6. Duchenne GB; Kaplan EB, trans. *Physiology of Movement.* Philadelphia: WB Saunders; 1949.

7. Du Bois-Reymond E. *Untersuchungen ueber thiersiche electricitae* (vol 2, second part). Berlin: Teimer-verlag; 1849.

8. Pratt FH. The all or none principle in graded response of skeletal muscle. *Am J Physiol.* 1917;44:517–542.

9. Gasser HS, Newcomer HS. Physiological action currents in the phrenic nerve. An application of the thermionic vacuum tube to nerve physiology. *Am J Physiol.* 1921;57:1–26.

10. Jacobson E. Electrical measurement concerning muscular contraction (tonus) and the cultivation of relaxation in man: relaxation times of individuals. *Am J Physiol.* 1934;108:573–580.

11. Jacobson E. *You Must Relax.* New York: McGraw-Hill; 1976.

12. Inman VT, Saunders JB, Abbott LC. Observations on the function of the shoulder joint. *J Bone and Joint Surg.* 1944;26:1–30.

13. Price JP, Clare MH, Ewerhardt RH. Studies in low backache with persistent spasm. *Achiev Phys Med.* 1948; 29:703–709.

14. Floyd WF, Silver P. The function of the erector spinae muscles in certain movements and postures in man. *J Physiol.* 1955;129:184–203.

15. Whatmore G, Kohli D. *The Physiopathology and Treatment of Functional Disorders.* New York: Grune & Stratton; 1974.

16. Basmajian JV. Control and training of individual motor units. *Science.* 1963;141:440–441.

17. Green EE, Walters ED, Green A, Murphy G. Feedback techniques for deep relaxation. *Psychophysiology.* 1969;6:371–377.

18. Budzynski T, Stoyva J, Adler C, Mullaney DJ. EMG biofeedback and tension study. *Psychosomatic Med.* 1973;35:484–496.

19. Hardyck CD, Petrincovich LV, Ellsworth DW. Feedback of speech muscle activity during silent reading: rapid extension. *Science.* 1966;154:1467–1468.

20. Booker HE, Rubow RT, Coleman PJ. Simplified feedback in neuromuscular retraining: an automated ap-

proach using EMG signals. *Arch Phys Med.* 1969; 50:621–625.

21. Johnson HE, Garton WH. Muscle re-education in hemiplegia by use of electromyographic device. *Arch Phys Med.* 1973;54:320–322.

22. Wolf S, Basmajian JV. Assessment of paraspinal electromyographic activity in normal subjects and chronic back pain patients using a muscle biofeedback device. In: Asmussen E, Jorgensen K, eds. *International Series on Biomechanics, VI-B.* Baltimore: University Press; 1978.

23. Wolf S, Nacht M, Kelly J. EMG feedback training during dynamic movement for low back pain patients. *Behav Ther.* 1982;13:395–406.

24. Sherman R, Arena J. Biofeedback for assessment and treatment of low back pain. In: Basmajian JV, Wolf S, eds. *Rational Manual Therapies.* Baltimore: Williams & Wilkins; 1994:177–197.

25. Dolce JJ, Raczynski JM. Neuromuscular activity and electromyography in painful backs: psychological and biomechanical models in assessment and treatment. *Psychological Bull.* 1985;97:502–520.

26. Cram JR, Steger JC. Muscle scanning and the diagnosis of chronic pain. *Biofeedback and Self-Regulation.* 1983;8:229–241.

27. Cram JR, Engstrom D. Patterns of neuromuscular activity in pain and non-pain patients. *Clin Biofeedback and Health.* 1986;9:106–116.

28. Donaldson S, Donaldson M. Multi-channel EMG assessment and treatment techniques. In: Cram JR, ed. *Clinical EMG for Surface Recordings, II.* Nevada City, CA: Clinical Resources; 1990:143–174.

29. Taylor W. Dynamic EMG biofeedback in assessment and treatment using a neuromuscular re-education model. In: Cram, JR, ed. *Clinical EMG for Surface Recordings, II.* Nevada City, CA: Clinical Resources; 1990:175–196.

30. Lewit K. *Manipulative Therapy in Rehabilitation of the Locomotor System.* Boston: Butterworth Heinemann; 1991.

31. Middaugh SJ, Kee WG, Nicholson JA. Muscle overuse and posture as factors in the development and maintenance of chronic musculoskeletal pain. In: Grzesiak RC, Ciccone DS, eds. *Psychological Vulnerability to Chronic Pain.* New York: Springer Publishing Co; 1994:55–89.

32. DeLuca C. Myoelectric manifestations of localized muscular fatigue in humans. *CRC Crit Rev Biomed Eng.* 1984;11:251.

33. Hagberg M. Occupational musculoskeletal stress disorders of the neck and shoulder: a review of possible pathophysiology. *Int Arch Occup and Environ Health.* 1984;53:269–278.

34. Hagberg M. Muscular endurance and surface EMG in isometric and dynamic exercise. *Arch Phys Med.* 1981;60:111–121.

35. Jonsson B. Kinesiology. With special reference to electromyographic kinesiology. *Cont Clin Neurophysiol EEG Suppl.* 1978;34:417–428.

36. Mathiassen SE, Winkel J, Hagg GM. Normalization of surface EMG amplitude from the upper trapezius muscle in ergonomic studies: a review. *J Electromyogr and Kinesiol.* 1995;5:199–226.

37. Veiersted KB, Westgaard RH, Andersen P. Electromyographic evaluation of muscular work pattern as a predictor of trapezius myalgia. *Scand J Work Environ Health.* 1993;19:284–290.

38. Winkel J, Mathiassen SE, Haag GM. Normalization of upper trapezius EMG amplitude in ergonomic studies. *J Electromyogr and Kinesiol.* 1995;5:195–198.

39. Soderberg GL, ed. *Selected Topics in Surface Electromyography for Use in the Occupational Setting: Expert Perspective.* Washington, DC: US Dept of Health and Human Services; 1992. US Dept of Health and Human Services publication NIOSH 91-100.

40. Basmajian JV, Blumenstein R. Electrode placement in electromyographic biofeedback. In: Basmajian JV, ed. *Biofeedback: Principles and Practice for Clinicians.* Baltimore: Williams & Wilkins; 1989:363–377.

41. Cram JR. *Clinical EMG for Surface Recordings, I.* Poulsbo, WA: J&J Engineering; 1986.

42. Fridlund AJ, Cacioppo JT. Guidelines for human electromyographic research. *Psychophysiology.* 1986; 23:567–598.

43. Cram JR, Holtz J. *Introduction to Electrode Placement* [videotape]. Nevada City, CA: Clinical Resources; 1995.

44. Wolf S. *Anatomy and Electrode Placement: Upper Extremities; Face and Back; Lower Extremities* [videotape]. Nevada City, CA: Clinical Resources; 1991.

CHAPTER 2

Anatomy and Physiology

BASIC OVERVIEW OF THE NEUROMUSCULAR SYSTEM

To consider the human musculature outside the context of a complex and interdependent system such as the human body is probably not fair. Without the connective tissue providing the "sacks" for the muscle fibers, the muscles would neither be organized into meaningful directions of pull, nor would they be anchored to the bones, and their actions would not produce movement of the body. Without a digestive system, there would be no glucose available for the body to burn. Without the lungs, there would be no oxygen to fan the flames of cellular respiration and produce the gasoline for the muscle—ATP (adenosine triphosphate). Without a circulatory system, these vital substances would neither find their way to each and every cell, nor would the waste products of muscular metabolism (lactic acid) be carried away. And finally, without the nervous system, the muscle cells would not know when to fire or how to orchestrate their firings with other muscle cells.

Huxley states that the muscle is truly the primary organ of the human body, the dominant tissue of animal life.[1] After all, 70% to 85% of gross body weight is typically that of muscle. Exceptions to this occur with extreme obesity. Muscle is the largest consumer of energy in the body. The metabolic needs of muscle increase radically as a function of work, while the needs of the other organ systems increase to only a small degree. In the human body there are literally millions of tiny muscle cells called myofibrils. These muscle cells do their work through shortening their resting length via a process of ratcheting myosin fibers against the actin fiber. And without an adequate supply of oxygen and glucose to form APT, along with the removal of lactic acid, muscle fatigue sets in and the muscle ceases to function.

It is essential to understand the connective tissue and bones to understand muscle function. Connective tissue is found throughout the human body and is essentially responsible for "gluing" it all together. For muscles, it provides the sacks or fasciae that house and organize the muscles. There are over 600 of these muscle compartments, each of them systematically placed under the direction of the genetic code. Not only does connective tissue form the boundaries of each and every muscle, but also the connective tissue known as tendons connects the muscles to the bones, and provides a series of anchors or pulleys through which the forces of muscle action work. When there are tears, shortenings, or other irregularities in this connective tissue, the organization of the muscles in the immediate area may become disordered.

The bones provide the rigidity needed for erect posture and movement of the extremities. Without the bones, our muscles would pool as a quivering mass on the floor, unable to do any work. Muscles are affected by asymmetrical growth patterns in the bones. Leg length discrepancies of more than a half inch, for example, cause faulty posture. Ligaments, another type of connective tissue, secure bone to bone. They also provide the needed limitations in range of motion, while adding stability to the bones themselves. In fact, all of the bones in the body are knit together with ligaments. This lends a certain coherence to the support that the bones provide. The spine and pelvis are very clear examples of this.

Mother Nature would much prefer that we rest on our bones and ligaments as the means of holding ourselves erect in the neutral posture against the gravitational field, thus sparing the metabolic consequences of using muscle to do the same task. But what happens to our muscles when we habitually defy the well-aligned posture? In essence, they overwork and often eventually ache. It is as if Mother Nature is using the ache to beckon us back into stacking our weight on our bones and ligaments. What happens if we fall or otherwise tear the connective tissue from around the bones? Such microtears are not uncommon in spinal flexion/extension injuries associated with motor vehicle accidents. This ligament laxity may create disorder in associated muscles. The muscles tend to increase their tonus around the injured joint, as if to provide an internal splint to the bones. Although this splinting may provide an effective short-term solution to a weakened joint, the long-term consequence is usually pain. If there is asymmetry in the nature of connective tissue associated with a particular joint, this usually leads to an asymmetrical recruitment of the muscles associated with that joint. For example, if the left temporomandibular joint (TMJ) has ligament laxity while the right aspect of the joint has normal ligamental support, an asymmetrical recruitment of motor units will be seen in surface electromyography (sEMG) recordings from homologous muscles during a symmetrical movement (eg, opening the mouth). Surface EMG monitoring can help clinicians interpret information about the joints (end range of motion or joint play) and can help manual therapists demonstrate the effects of mo-

bilization of the joint. The postmanipulation effects on sEMG should yield normalized recruitment patterns ($\pm$20%) during symmetrical dynamic movements. In addition, feedback and retraining of the newly mobilized joint may help prevent the movements and postures of life from creating the same limitation in the future.

If the fasciae provide the sacks for the muscles, and the bones provide the rigidity needed for an erect posture, then it is the muscle bulk (along with other connective tissue) that gives the body its final shape. In addition, muscles provide stability to the bones. The skeleton cannot stand erect by itself. It is the muscles that give us our posture—our stance toward life. This stance has both mechanical (gravitational) and emotional contributions. And it is the muscles that give us the dynamic movement we associate with life itself.

The recruitment of muscle would not happen were it not for the nervous system. The *motor unit* is the final common pathway of the alpha motor system's outflow to the end plates located on the muscle fibers. The lower motor neuron associated with the motor unit resides in the dorsal horn of the spinal cord. Hundreds or even thousands of interneuronal connections converge upon that motor neuron (see Figure 2–1). There is a segmental interplay of the spinal reflexes driven by excitatory and inhibitory potentials. The stretch receptors of the muscle spindle place an excitatory valence on the lower motor neuron, while the Golgi tendon organs provide the reflex-driven inhibitory potentials. These two inputs function as sensory motor integrators that deal with gravity, the mass of everyday life and our efforts to interact with the world. They keep us up and moving and inform the rest of the nervous system of the instantaneous length of each muscle and the force it is exerting. The lower motor neuron is also regulated by upper motor neurons. Some of these come directly from the cortex, carrying out fine motor intentions. The thought behind a movement originates in the frontal lobes. It then passes through the prefrontal cortex to pick up the general body

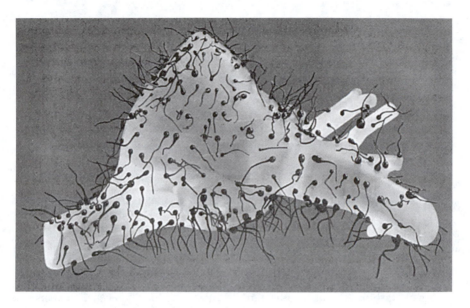

Figure 2–1 A reconstructed model of a spinal motor neuron showing the large number of small presynaptic knobs from other neurons terminating on it. *Source:* Reprinted with permission from Haggar and Barr, Quantitative Data on the Size of Synaptic End Bulbs in the Cat's Spinal Cord, *Journal of Comparative Neurology*, Vol 93, pp 17–35, © 1950, John Wiley & Sons, Inc.

position in space needed for the movement. Then it goes through the motor strip to pick up the final details of any fine motor aspects of the movement. Some of the cortical outflow goes directly to the lower motor neuron via the pyramidal tracts. Some travel via the extrapyramidal tract, which synapses with lower centers of the brain. Here the intended movement is integrated with the internal (kinesthetic) and external senses, and is blended with motor patterns associated with given and acquired reflexes. The cerebellum monitors the whole affair, fine-tuning the final act.

When examining muscles, clinicians tend to study each compartment for its own function. Manual muscle testing is routinely taught as a method to isolate the strength of a given muscle. In order to test muscles correctly, one must know how to position the limb, where to resist it, how to coach the subject to exert effort, and finally how to grade the strength of the resulting effort. These tests are far from natural movement patterns. They are more like slices of

unique movement patterns, taken out of a normal muscle contraction context and frozen in time. They are relevant only to the extent that the information gained can be placed into a more functional context.

A single, discrete muscle rarely works on its own in a real and varied life situation. The nervous system has more than 600 muscles to choose from and an area as large as the human form to work with. Many muscles need to serve the three functions of posture, emotions, and motions. To think of testing one muscle is entirely too simplistic. The only way in which muscle testing works is to have a theory of dysfunction that involves areas of effort up and down the kinetic chain of movement. Then, in the process of determining which muscles are weak or strong in that chain, all or part of the chain might be tested.

When testing muscles, the clinician should assess muscle grouping such as agonists (prime movers), synergists (helpers), and antagonists (opposing muscle groups). In addition, as the tests move toward real and varied life activities, it is necessary to address issues of timing. Surface EMG as an assessment tool, like muscle testing, begins to make sense only when viewed in a much broader perspective. Along with muscle testing, sEMG can be used to monitor the muscles involved or suspected. In this way, clinicians can assess not only the muscles' strength, but also their synergy with other muscles.

This type of thinking is illustrated by simple abduction of the left arm. Imagine that the subject is standing with arms at his or her sides. The intention is to raise the left arm out from the side to a horizontal 90-degree posture. The muscle fibers of middle deltoid act as the primary mover. The anterior and posterior aspects of deltoid assist in a synergistic fashion. The upper fibers of trapezius, along with the deeper supraspinatus, also assist. The middle and lower fibers of trapezius, serratus anterior, and others stabilize the scapula to anchor the weight of the 15-pound arm against the chest wall. Because this is an asymmetrical action, the erector spinae muscles on the contralateral (right) side begin to activate to stabilize the cantilevered effect of gravity's pull on the torso. This places a strain on the pelvis, which is stabilized by the gluteus medius and tensor fasciae latae. The left leg bears a greater weight, and muscles are slightly activated in various aspects of the thigh, calf, and foot. In addition, it is necessary to superimpose the waves of respiration in the abdominal and intercostal area upon this holding pattern. Place a little bit of emotional arousal into the situation, and the overall tone is increased by, say, 10%. Place a 10-pound weight in the outstretched hand, and the recruitment pattern along the entire kinetic chain increases dramatically. Such a weight can be held at this height for only a short period of time, because the more distal muscles begin to fatigue much faster than the more proximal postural muscles. Within the first minute, the volley of activity to the middle deltoid has increased and synchronized to counter the fatigue factor, but within 4 minutes the failure point is reached, the arm gives way to the gravitational pull, and the posture is recalibrated.

MUSCLE FIBERS AND HOW THEY WORK

To understand how muscles work, it is helpful to examine the muscle from a macroscopic to a microscopic level. On a macroscopic level, muscle fibers are grouped together and traditionally identified by their line of action, their direction of pull, and their origins and insertions. But a closer examination of this arrangement reveals that the muscle is really comprised of compartments. Rather than being one massive muscle, some muscles are really a series of smaller compartments that run in the same direction or slightly different directions. Each compartment provides a subtly different pull on the lever arm. Researchers have demonstrated "compartmentalization" for the biceps,[2,3] extensor and flexor carpi radialis,[4,5] soleus,[6] and gastrocnemius.[7] Researchers are beginning to understand the compartmentalization of muscles better, and compartmentalization may soon come to replace the more macroscopic view of origins and insertions that is presently taught in educational programs as the primary level for understanding muscle function.

Each muscle compartment contains muscle fibers (see Figure 2–2). These fibers may be clustered together into narrow subcompartments separated by a thin septa of connective tissue that holds the muscle cells together in their parallel arrangements. These individual fibers may be broken down into clusters of individual *myofibrils*, which are tiny hairlike strands. Under a microscope, myofibrils appear to be braided in light and dark bands. Each myofibril consists of aggregates of *myosin* and *actin* filaments. The basic anatomical structure from which all muscles are made is called a *sarcomere*. This is defined as a single unit of overlapping myosin and actin filaments from one *Z* line to the next *Z* line in the muscle. These dark lines reflect the attachment of actin fibers. Within the sarcomere, there are areas where only actin resides (*I* bands), areas where only myosin resides (*H* bands), and areas where myosin overlaps the actin fibers (*A* bands). The *A* band is where all of the work of the cross-bridging takes place.

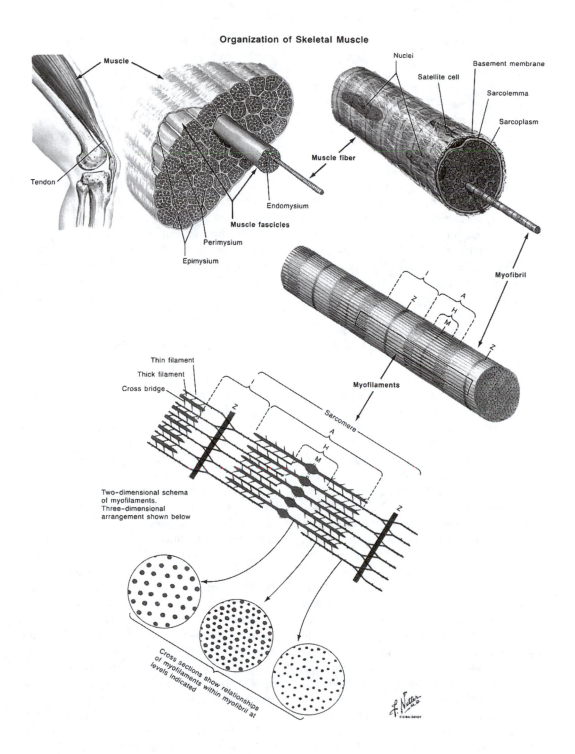

Figure 2–2 The composition of muscle cells, muscle fascicles, muscle fiber, myofibril, myofilaments, sarcomere, thick and thin filaments. *Source:* Copyright 1987. Novartis. Reprinted with permission from *The Ciba Collection of Medical Illustrations*, illustrated by Frank H Netter, MD. All rights reserved.

The actin filament is a thin fiber with two negatively charged molecules that spiral around each other. The myosin filament is a much thicker filament, made up of molecules with "globular heads" on it. These filaments are also negatively charged. In the resting state, these two filaments lie next to each other, mutually repelled by their negative charges. In the 1950s, Huxley[8] proposed a "ratchet" or sliding filament model that describes the generation of active tension. In this model, each globular head of the myosin fiber has one ATP molecule attached to it, which is negatively charged.

The nerve action potential from the lower motor neuron causes a release of acetylcholine (ACh) at the neuromuscular junction. This sends a charge through the transverse tubules (Figure 2–3) that, when it reaches the sarcoplasmic reticulum, allows pores to be opened and calcium to flood the space where the myosin and actin fibers are located. The calcium has a very strong positive charge to it, and it bonds instantly with the actin filament. At this point, the negatively charged myosin filament with its ATP molecule is strongly attracted to the now positively charged actin filament (Figure 2–4). As these two filaments are pressed against each other by the chemically induced electromagnetic attraction, the globular heads are forced to flatten out; this provides the ratchet effect, and forces the two filaments to move past each other. The force of the bending of the globular heads, however, causes the ATP molecule to be released. The energy associated with this release provides the energy needed to free the calcium from the actin fiber and pumps it back to the sarcoplasmic reticulum. Simultaneously, the myosin and actin filaments separate, being held slightly apart by the two negative charges. Immediately, another ATP molecule attaches to the globular head on the myosin filament and the cycle is ready to begin all over again. Thus, the globular heads of the myosin act as crossbridges for the actin chains. Through successive activations and cross-bridging, the muscle twitches while it shortens and work is done.

The metabolized ATP molecule, now known as ADP (adenosine diphosphate), is reconstituted in the mitochondria. Using the Krebs cycle, the mitochondria rebuilds the ADP back into ATP, using the glucose and oxygen provided by the circulation system. The by-products of this action include lactic acid, free hydrogen ions, and carbon dioxide. These by-products need to be removed and transported away from the muscle cell via the circulatory system.

The strength of the contraction is greater when the muscle is elongated to about its midpoint of the filament sliding range. This phenomenon has to do with the structure of the myosin and actin fibers. Figure 2–5 illustrates the relationship of strength (percentage of maximum tension) to the degree of myosin-actin overlap. Strength is lost when there is very little overlap of the two fiber types and when the overlap is complete. Strength is found in the middle range, where a number of myosin-actin crossbridges can be formed.

Muscle fibers can be divided into three broad categories based on appearance, speed of contraction, and fatigability: (1) Slow-twitch muscles take more than 35 milliseconds to complete a depolarization/repolarization cycle and are reddish in appearance. These muscles twitch at less than 25 twitches per second, usually around 10 to 20 hertz (Hz—a unit of frequency equal to one cycle per second). (2) Fast-twitch, fatigue-resistant muscles are pale in appearance and, like the slow-twitch muscles, have a considerable ability for aerobic metabolism. These are classified as Type I, fast-twitch fibers. (3) Fast-twitch, fatigable muscles take less than 35 milliseconds to complete a contraction or twitch cycle and are whitish in appearance. These are classified as Type II, fast-twitch fibers. Fast-twitch fibers twitch at a rate faster than 25 twitches per second, which is typically between 30 and 50 Hz. A classic example in the human body of fast- and slow-twitch muscles is found in the calf of the leg. The soleus consists of predominantly slow-twitch fibers and is reddish in color, while the gastrocnemius consists prima-

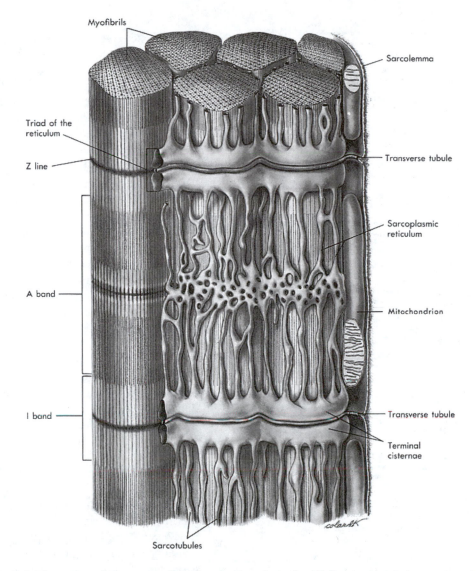

Myofibrils

Sarcolemma

Triad of the reticulum

Z line

Transverse tubule

Sarcoplasmic reticulum

A band

Mitochondrion

I band

Transverse tubule

Terminal cisternae

Sarcotubules

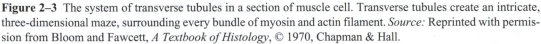

Figure 2–3 The system of transverse tubules in a section of muscle cell. Transverse tubules create an intricate, three-dimensional maze, surrounding every bundle of myosin and actin filament. *Source:* Reprinted with permission from Bloom and Fawcett, *A Textbook of Histology*, © 1970, Chapman & Hall.

rily of fast-twitch fibers and is a paler color. The morphological differentiation of the fiber type is determined by the type of motor nerve that activates the fibers. Small, slow nerve fibers develop slow-twitch muscles; large, fast nerve fibers develop fast-twitch muscles. Most muscles contain a mixture of fast- and slow-twitch fibers.

Characteristics of two of the muscle fiber types are listed in Table 2–1. These distinctions, slow, fatigue-resistant versus fast, fatigable, represent a gross oversimplification; in reality, a gradation along a continuum for the attributes given below would better represent the types of muscle fiber. In general, however, Type I fibers are smaller in size and produce less tension.

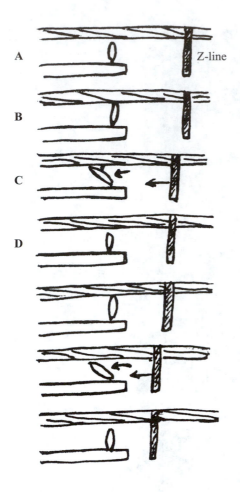

Figure 2–4 The ratchet effect. (**A**) Prior to the calcium bonding, the myosin heads with their negative ATP molecule are held away from the negative actin filament. (**B**) After calcium bonding, the negative ATP myosin heads attach to the now positive actin. This positive bond is also attracted to the negative myosin shaft. (**C**) The myosin head folds downward pulling the actin chain forward one notch. (**D**) The ATP myosin bond breaks under the stress of the folding and releases the myosin filament from the actin chain, allowing the globular head to stand upright again. Immediately, another ATP molecule attaches to it. As the muscle fibers depolarize, ratchet themselves to a shorter resting length, and repolarize, they undergo one motor unit action potential (MUAP) or twitch.

They are innervated by small, slow-moving neuronal axons. They are fairly resilient to fatigue and are more amenable to anaerobic glucolysis. They have a low reflex threshold from the muscle spindle and Golgi tendon organ and generally tend to maintain a tonic repetitive discharge. On the other hand, Type II fibers have a low reflex threshold and respond reflexively with short burst patterns. In general terms, the Type I fibers appear ideal for postural activities and the Type II fibers seem best suited for phasic movement.

Not only do different fiber types do different types of work, but the same muscle fiber types can do work in different ways. There are three clearly identifiable types of muscle contractions: isometric, concentric, and eccentric. The sEMG patterns observed during dynamic protocols may differ, depending upon which type of contraction one is studying.

1. *Isometric contractions* are muscle contractions in which a constant muscle length is maintained. Technically, the contractile force does not exceed the force of resistance and, therefore, there is no change in muscle length. These contractions are used in postural control and while stabilizing axial body parts during extreme movements. They are also used during manual muscle testing. Surface EMG recordings are typically greatest under isometric testing conditions.

2. *Concentric contractions* occur when the muscle shortens during the contraction. Technically, it is defined as a contraction with enough force to overcome the external resistance, thus allowing the muscle to shorten. During concentric contractions, the moving body part usually accelerates. It is the action taken by a prime mover during the active phase of a movement pattern. A classic example of concentric contractions is biceps activity during elbow flexion associated with lifting a weight. The amount of muscular energy available is greater during an iso-

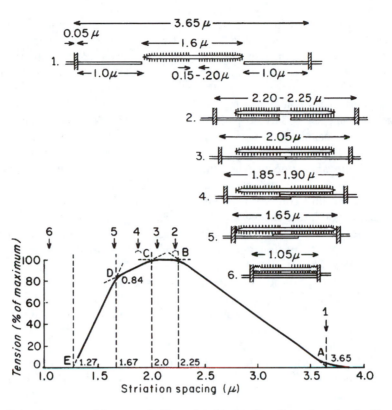

Figure 2–5 Length-tension curve of frog muscle fiber related to overlap of myosin and actin filaments. *Source:* Reprinted with permission from the *Journal of Physiology*, Vol 184, pp 170–192, © 1966, The Physiological Society.

Table 2–1 Properties of Fast, Fatigable and Slow, Fatigue-Resistant Motor Units

Type I—Slow, Fatigue-Resistant	*Type II—Fast, Fatigable*
High oxidative metabolism	Low oxidative metabolism
Low lipid metabolism	Low lipid metabolism
Low glycogen stores	High glycogen stores
Low ATP activity	High ATP activity
Slow contraction time (>35 ms)	Fast contraction time (<35 ms)
Small size, low tension	Large size, high tension
Rich capillary supply	Sparse capillary supply
Innervation by small motor neurons with slow-conducting axons	Innervation by large motor neurons with fast-conducting fibers
Low reflex discharge	High reflex threshold
Tonic reflex discharge	Phasic reflex discharge
Minimal fatigability	Great fatigability

Source: Reprinted with permission from Patton, *Introduction to Basic Neurology*, p 85, © 1976 WB Saunders Company.

metric contraction than during a concentric contraction. This is because 20% of the energy efficiency of the movement is lost during concentric contraction due to the shortening of the muscle. Thus, the greatest load that a concentric muscle contraction can carry is only 80% of the load carried by maximum isometric contraction.

3. *Eccentric contractions* occur when the muscle lengthens during a contraction. Technically, eccentric contractions occur in an already shortened muscle where the external force is greater than the tension created by the muscle contraction. Here, the muscle acts as a braking agent as a load is manipulated. The classic example of eccentric contraction is biceps activity as the weight is slowly lowered during elbow extension. Eccentric contractions are extremely common. Every movement in the direction of gravity is controlled by an eccentric contraction. Other examples include sitting, squatting, lying down, bending forward or sideways, and going down stairs. The amount of energy expended during an eccentric contraction is always less than that observed during a concentric contraction for the same muscle. The amount of metabolic work associated with eccentric contractions is one third to one thirteenth of the work of concentric contractions. In sEMG recordings, the microvolt amplitude of a concentric contraction is always larger than for the eccentric contraction, given the same amount of weight. For example, the erector spinae of the low back work harder and show higher levels of recruitment when returning from a flexed position than when going down into forward flexion from the neutral position. Researchers believe that the eccentric contractions require less sEMG activity because much of the work has to do with "breaking" the already existing cross-bridges rather than building new cross-bridges.

Another form of contraction is isotonic contraction, a subset or special class of the concentric and eccentric contractions. Isotonic contractions occur when there is a constant muscle force observed as the muscle either shortens or lengthens. This type of force is studied most commonly on instruments in which the force is controlled over the range of motion.

Surface EMG recruitment patterns may differ when they are observed in an open versus closed kinetic chain. In an *open kinetic chain*, the distal segment is free to move—as in the case where one is not bearing weight in the lower extremities. The open kinetic chain entails a movement that is not resisted manually or through weight bearing. Movement of one joint does not necessarily cause movement in other joints. In a *closed kinetic chain*, the distal segment is fixed as in weight bearing for the lower extremities. Movement at one joint induces movement at another joint. For example, in sitting with the leg hanging over the edge of the table (open kinetic chain), a person can move the ankle without moving the knee or hip. But when the person stands (closed kinetic chain), he or she cannot move the ankle without affecting other joints. Surface EMG recruitment patterns are typically greater under the conditions of a closed kinetic chain compared to those observed under the conditions of an open kinetic chain. For example, the level of sEMG activity from rectus femoris during a squat (closed kinetic chain) is greater than when the muscle is contracted from the seated position and the knee extends without resistance (open kinetic chain).

SENSORY MOTOR INTEGRATION

Initially, researchers thought that the muscle was a relatively insensitive structure. They derived this conclusion from the observation that a surgeon could cut and probe the muscle tissue with the patient experiencing little or no pain. However, researchers have discovered that muscle is actually quite rich and sophisticated in its sensory apparatus. Of the sensory organs found within the muscle, the two major sensory systems are the *muscle spindle* and *Golgi tendon organ.*

The muscle spindle is the stretch receptor. It has specialized nerve endings that provide the nervous system with information concerning the instantaneous resting length of the muscle and velocity (or rate) of change. The output of the muscle spindle is transmitted to the cord and terminates on excitatory interneurons. This assists in the fine calibration of alpha motor output and the resulting muscle contraction at a local or spinal level. If the output from the muscle spindle is strong or sharp enough, it may result in alpha motor output, causing the extrafusal fibers that surround the muscle spindle to contract, thus causing the muscle in which it is located to shorten (see Figure 2–6). In addition, the muscle spindle simultaneously transmits information to the reticular core and basal ganglia to help modulate the descending motor pathways. However, spindle activity is not projected to the cortex and, thus, is not consciously perceived.

These tiny stretch receptors are associated with *intrafusal muscle fibers,* which are scattered among and run parallel to the large extrafusal muscle fibers in which they are housed (see Figure 2–7). The intrafusal muscles are much smaller (5 to 10 fibers) and shorter (4 to 10 mm) than the extrafusal muscle fibers. The extrafusal fibers are innervated by the *alpha motor system* and are designed to do the work of moving bones, and the intrafusal fibers are innervated by the *gamma motor system* and are designed to adjust the calibration of the stretch receptor. Because muscles are constantly changing their length as they do work, and because the stretch receptors inform the central nervous system (CNS) of the instantaneous length and velocity of the muscle fibers, it is vitally important to continually adjust the tonus on the stretch receptor. Perhaps that is why nearly one third of the descending efferent motor nerve fibers are associated with the gamma motor system. These gamma motor nerves are smaller and have slower conduction velocities than the alpha motor nerves. The gamma motor system primarily emerges from the lower centers of the brain, while the alpha motor system originates primarily from the cortex. There is commonly a CNS linkage or coactivation of the alpha and gamma motor systems. This was first observed by Hunt and Kuffler[9] in the 1950s, and elaborated upon by Vallbo[10] in the 1980s.

The primary purpose of the muscle spindle, then, is to regulate the muscle length, make postural adjustments, and maintain a predicted muscle length and velocity. An artificial example of this is the knee jerk. When the patella tendon is delivered a swift blow, the quadriceps muscle is unpredictably and suddenly elongated, and the muscle spindle is stretched. This leads to excitatory outflow to the motor neuron, which results in the contraction of the quadriceps muscle. This, in turn, quiets the muscle spindle. The briskness of this response is commonly graded in neurological examinations. On a functional level, the briskness of the response is determined by the output of the gamma motor system. Edmund Jacobson[11] ran studies on progressive relaxation procedures, in which he was able to demonstrate a substantial diminution (if not frank absence) in the knee jerk in patients who were deeply relaxed. Thus, one can learn to alter and control the sensitivity of the stretch receptor through alterations in the level of gamma motor activity through deep relaxation. In real-life situations, the muscle spindle monitors the effects of the gravitational field upon a person's posture and helps keep the person erect. For example, when a person walks along an uneven surface, the muscle spindle constantly adjusts the tone of the muscle (excitatory input to the alpha motor neuron) to compensate for the unpredicted stretches upon the muscle. The resting tone of the gamma motor system is especially important for an athlete. If the muscle tone is too high or too low, the timing and effort of the athletic performance can be thrown off. Researchers have recently found that the muscle spindle responds to emotional arousal.[4] Perhaps this is why professional and Olympic athletes work on their emotions and attitudes toward their performances just as much as their motor coordination skills.

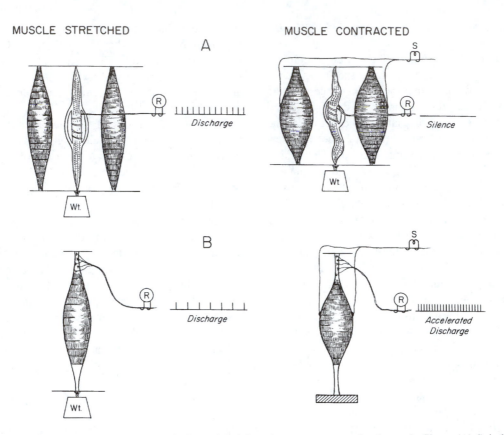

Figure 2–6 Relationship of muscle spindle and Golgi tendon organ to extrafusal muscle fibers. (**A**) Spindle is parallel to the muscle fibers so that the muscle contraction slackens tension on the spindle. (**B**) Golgi tendon organ is in series with the muscle fibers (resides between the muscle fibers and their bony attachments) so that both passive and active contractions of the muscle cause the receptor to become active. *Source:* Reprinted with permission from Ruch and Patton, *Physiology and Biophysics,* © 1965, WB Saunders Company.

Recently, the muscle spindle has been suggested as a potential site for the *trigger point*.[12] Trigger points are anatomical locations that, when activated by pressure or movement, refer pain to the immediate area or a distant site.[13] Dynamic sEMG studies[14] have reported that during a symmetrical movement (ie, forward flexion of the head), muscles that have an active trigger point tend to contract at a higher level of activation than to the contralateral muscle without a trigger point. This finding suggests that an active trigger point in a muscle tends to alter the sensitivity of muscle spindles for the involved muscle, making it more sensitive to changes in its length.

Another important sensory organ within the muscle is the *Golgi tendon organ* (see Figures 2–6 and 2–7). It is found at the muscle tendon junction and runs in series with the muscle. It is exquisitely sensitive to the tension placed on the tendon, and it perceives the effort given out by the muscle. On its most basic level, the output from the Golgi tendon organ loops through the cord and inhibits the alpha motor neuron for the 5 to 10 motor units that are pulling on it. In essence, the inhibitory influence of the Golgi tendon organ protects the muscle from tearing itself loose from its attachments. On a more subtle level, the Golgi tendon organ informs the central nervous system of the effort that is under way

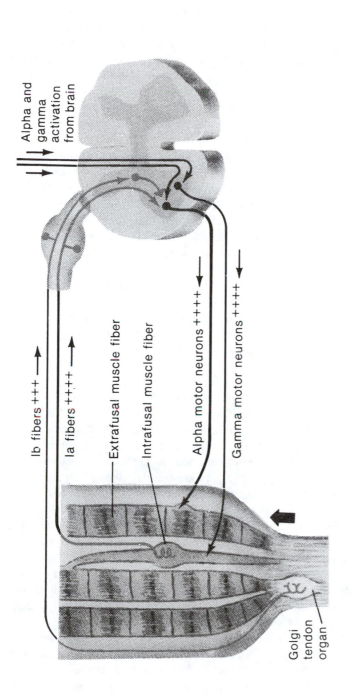
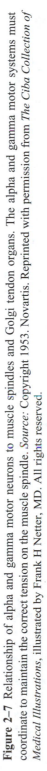

Figure 2–7 Relationship of alpha and gamma motor neurons to muscle spindles and Golgi tendon organs. The alpha and gamma motor systems must coordinate to maintain the correct tension on the muscle spindle. *Source:* Copyright 1953. Novartis. Reprinted with permission from *The Ciba Collection of Medical Illustrations*, illustrated by Frank H Netter, MD. All rights reserved.

and facilitates the necessary inhibition needed for learning. For example, when a piano student is learning to distinguish between playing the piano softly and playing it loudly, the student must learn to press on the keys in soft and hard fashion. While the ear can readily hear the difference, the Golgi tendon organ can feel the difference; it provides the proprioceptive basis for knowing when the key has been pressed just hard enough. The output of the Golgi tendon organ terminates in the lower centers of the brain (ie, basal ganglia). This output does not reach the cortex, and we are therefore unconscious of its presence. Yet it is through the interaction of the information supplied by the Golgi tendon organ with that of higher centers that we acquire basic and refined motor skills. Like the spindle apparatus, the Golgi tendon organ makes our muscular efforts more efficient.

There are two other sense organs to consider inside the muscle itself. One is the *pacinian corpuscle*, which is capable of measuring the deep, internal pressure within the muscle. The second is a *free nerve ending*, which is sensitive to nociception or pain. The afferent pain travels via the lateral spinothalamic tract, reaches the cortex, and is consciously perceived. This pain receptor is activated by a change in the acidity of muscle or by chemical changes associated with swelling, edema, and inflammation. When the muscle does work, the metabolic by-product is a substance called *lactic acid*. When this acid is retained in the muscle due to the lack of adequate circulation (associated with a sustained muscle contraction), the free nerve ending is activated. For example, when a person makes a very tight fist and holds it for several minutes, he or she begins to feel a dull ache in the forearm muscles. This dull ache emanates from the free nerve ending and is associated with the disturbance of the microcirculation in the muscle itself and the resultant buildup of lactic acid. Usually this type of pain follows a prolonged activation pattern in fairly close temporal sequence. Pain associated with inflammation usually lags behind the activating event by several hours. Inflammation can be brought about by the overuse

of muscles, but because of fluid transport issues, it simply takes longer to develop. For example, a person who is out of shape and goes skiing for the first time of the season will probably tire from time to time but might not experience pain during the skiing because of adequate perfusion of the tissue associated with the rhythmic use of the muscles. However, on the ride home or the next day, that person might feel the muscle soreness associated with the overuse of the muscles. This overuse may be associated with microtears in the muscle tissue and is accompanied by inflammation. The afferent from the free nerve endings (nociception) loops through the cord, placing an excitatory bias on the lower motor neuron, forming the basis for the withdrawal reflex. In addition, this afferent interfaces with the gamma motor system, potentially providing the basis for muscle *splinting*—Mother Nature's way of providing a muscular "cast" for an injured area.

Another source of information about muscle function is found in the *joint receptors* (eg, Ruffini nucleus). Such apparatus is found in each and every joint. It is sensitive to one degree of arc, and never habituates (turns off). It continuously provides the nervous system with information concerning joint angle and position. One of the important aspects of this sensory system is that we are conscious of it. Although we are not conscious of the level of tension in our muscles, we are readily aware of our limb and joint position. For example, it may make more sense to talk to a patient about how high the shoulders are than to talk about how tense the upper trapezius muscles might be. It is easier for patients to respond to the request to lower the shoulders than to relax them. It simply makes more sense to patients, because they can be consciously aware of joint movements yet consciously blind to their tension levels.

The sensory network of the muscles provides a wealth of information to the central nervous system concerning muscle function. Some of these influences are excitatory, some are inhibitory, some reach the cortex and are conscious, and some terminate in the lower brain and are not consciously perceived. All pass through the cord and influence the segmental intelligence of the total system. Figure 2–8 illustrates one piece of this puzzle, the afferent control of the alpha motor neuron at the segmental level.

NERVOUS SYSTEM CONTROL

The nervous system's control of the neuromuscular system can be roughly broken into three levels, which are organized both hierarchically and in parallel. The lowest level is the spinal reflex, with its segmental and suprasegmental organization and intelligence. This level is primarily associated with survival and the mechanical work humans do against gravity. The middle level is represented by the lower brain. This level includes some of the prewired reflexes, some of the acquired reflexes, postural reflexes aided by the semicircular canals, the fine-tuning of movements by the cerebellum, and the limbic system that controls the emotional aspect of muscle. At the highest level is the cortex, where three quarters of all of the nerve cells reside. It is here that intentionality of movement occurs, along with learning, associations, and thought.

If a person wants to touch a finger to the nose, the following events will more than likely take place. At a cortical level, the frontal lobes create the plan; the plan passes through the premotor cortex to organize how the body, as a whole, will fit into the plan; and the motor strip integrates the fine movements of pointing the finger. Some of this information passes directly on to the motor units associated with the fine motor control of the upper extremity. Other aspects of the cortical information connect with the basal ganglia to pick up the reflexes (acquired) needed to assist in this movement and to integrate the other senses, such as the eyes, into the movement. As the plan for the postural tone necessary to conduct the movement is initiated, the gamma motor system is engaged. It is important for the person not to be thrown off balance as he or she moves off the center of gravity to conduct the movement. The cerebellum becomes engaged to monitor the movement and assist in the final touchdown, so that the person does not stop short or move the hand too far and break the nose. At a spinal level, the alpha motor neurons for the prime movers and stabilizers are activated, along with the gamma motor neurons to set the right muscle tone. As the act of touching the nose is placed into motion, the muscle spindles inform the nervous system about the instantaneous length of muscle and its velocity of change; the Golgi tendon organs inform the nervous system about the amount of effort they perceive; the joint receptors inform the nervous system about the movements at the joint; and the cerebellum monitors the whole affair and orchestrates a perfect touchdown. With all this complexity, it is no wonder that the police use this test to determine whether alcohol has affected a driver's neuromuscular system.

The Spinal Reflexes

The spine controls simple reflexes. Simple reflexes are hard wired and obligatory movements. Three of these reflexes—stretch reflex, flexion and cross-extension reflex, and scratch reflex—are shown in Figure 2–9. Another basic reflex is the *withdrawal reflex*. Here, the muscle moves the body part away from the source of pain. If a person touches something hot, the hand is reflexively moved away before the person is even aware of the sensation. If this stimulation is strong enough, it can create a *flexion/cross-extension reflex*. This is a polysynaptic reflex that excites the flexor group and inhibits the extensor group on the ipsilateral side of pain, while simultaneously exciting the extensor group and inhibiting the flexor group on the contralateral side. The *scratch reflex* is an example of a polysynaptic suprasegmental reflex, where the stimulus evokes a motor response several vertebral segments away that has an action directed toward eradicating the stimulation of the original segment.

During the early stages of human development, one can observe a number of primitive and very predictable reflexes in the infant. One set of

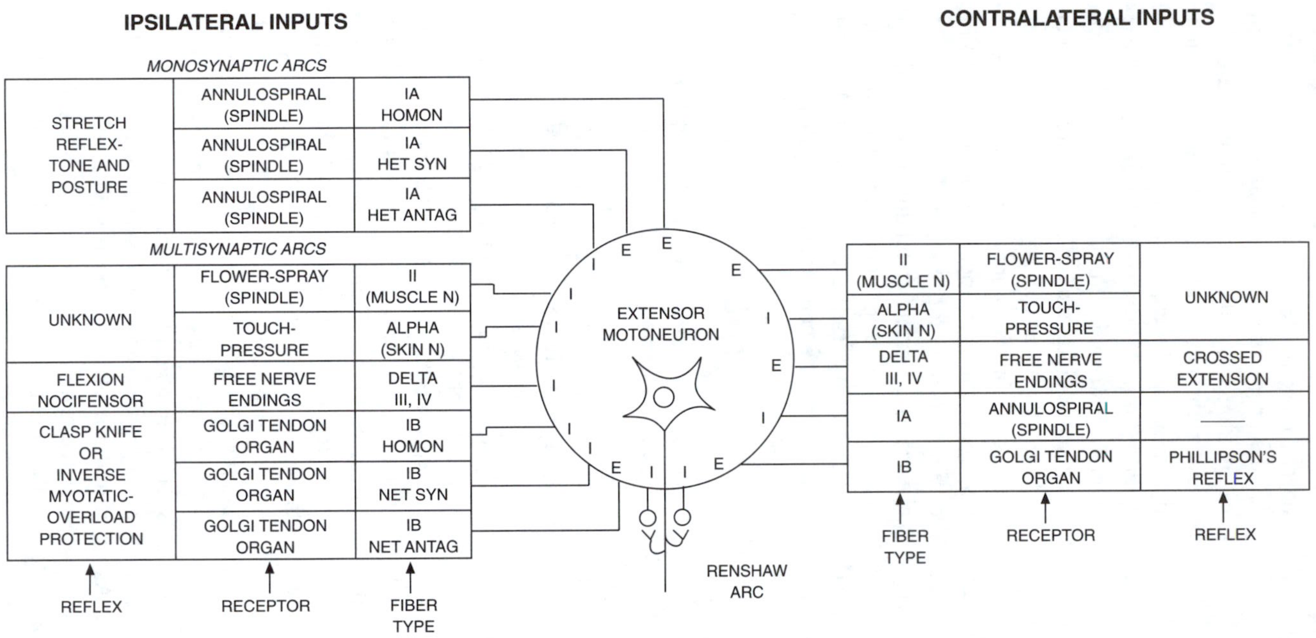

Figure 2–8 Segmental afferent inputs converging on a typical motor neuron supplying an extensor muscle. The influence of each input is indicated as excitatory (*E*) or inhibitory (*I*). *Source:* Reprinted with permission from Ruch and Patton, *Physiology and Biophysics,* © 1965, WB Saunders Company.

reflexes is called the *tonic labyrinthine reflexes.* These reflexes are stimulated by the effects of body or head position on the labyrinthine receptor (part of the semicircular canals). Below is a description of these reflexes:

- *Labyrinthine righting reflex:* Stimulation of the labyrinthine receptor evokes contractions of the neck muscles that orient the head in relationship to the gravitational force.
- *Body-on-head reflex:* Asymmetrical stimulation of the skin receptors from the supporting surface leads to contraction of the trunk, limb, and neck muscles that lift the head into an upright position.
- *Neck righting reflex:* Proprioception from the joints of the neck bring about contractions of the trunk and limbs to bring the head in alignment with the body.
- *Body-on-body righting reflex:* Asymmetrical stimulation of the skin receptors causes contraction of the trunk muscles, which raises the body toward the upright position.
- *Visual righting reflex:* Visual feedback is used to orient the head and body correctly with the environment.

Neck reflexes result from stimulation of the joint receptors in the cervical spine, particularly when the head is inclined forward, backward, or rotated. These *tonic neck reflexes*, described below and illustrated in Figure 2–10, are present from birth and are present until approximately the age of 6 to 8 weeks.

- *Head ventriflexed (flexion):* Evokes upper extremity flexion and lower extremity extension.
- *Head dorsiflexed (extension):* Evokes extension of the upper extremities while lower extremities are flexed.
- *Head rotation:* When the head is rotated to the left, it evokes extension and abduction of left upper and lower extremities, while the right upper and lower extremities are adducted and flexed. The reverse pattern is true when the head is rotated to the right.

As humans mature, they begin to integrate these reflexes into new patterns of behavior. Learning, then, is essentially the integration of reflexes. However, this does not mean that these reflexes go away. Consider the person who spills a water-filled ice tray as a result of these reflexes. The tray is full of water; the person is ready to slip it into the freezer, momentarily looks away, and spills a small amount. The tonic neck reflexes more than likely caused a slight flexion or extension of the upper extremity as the person rotated the head one way or the other. Or consider a youngster who is learning how to dive into a swimming pool for the first time. The labyrinthine righting reflex can cause the young diver to belly flop because he or she raises the head due to the loss of balance. When the nervous system is compromised, these primitive reflexes may return. This is clearly seen in stroke patients. In a more subtle way, it has also been seen in patients with carpal tunnel syndrome. Using sEMG to study carpal tunnel syndrome, researchers have demonstrated that in a majority of these patients, head rotation is associated with recruitment in the forearm musculature.[15] Researchers believe that this reflexively driven activation of the forearm muscles leads to the inflammation of the synovial lining of the carpal tunnel. In addition, it has been demonstrated that when the tonic neck reflexes are integrated again, the forearm firing subsides and the conduction velocities at the carpal tunnel improve.

The Midbrain

The lower centers of the brain are where the cell bodies of the gamma motor system are most densely organized. The midbrain is both phylogenetically and ontogenetically the oldest part of the brain, and it is commonly referred to as the "reptilian" brain. It controls arousal levels and consciousness. It is responsible for regulating the heart, breath, body temperature, body weight, libido, thirst, and hunger. It contains all of the ancient knowledge contained in the obligatory reflexes mentioned in the prior sec-

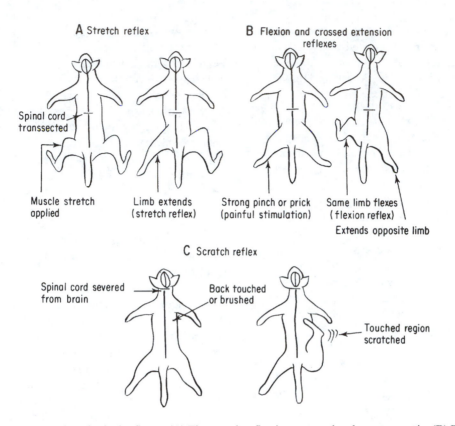

Figure 2–9 Examples of spinal reflexes. (**A**) The stretch reflex is segmental and monosynaptic. (**B**) Flexion and cross-extension reflexes are polysynaptic and involve several segments. (**C**) The scratch reflex is suprasegmental and polysynaptic. *Source:* From *Foundations of Physiological Psychology* by Richard F Thompson and Timothy J Taylor. Copyright © 1967 by Richard F Thompson and Timothy J Taylor. Reprinted by permission of Addison Wesley Educational Publishers, Inc.

tion. It helps to integrate the senses by allowing eye movements to precede the head turn, allowing head position to follow sound, extending an upper extremity in the direction of the head turn, and so forth. These actions are accomplished by the integrated action of the reticular formation, the basal ganglia, the thalamus, the limbic system, and the cerebellum.

The *reticular formation* is responsible for our level of arousal. It wakes us up in the morning and turns off so we can drift off to sleep. It is the seat of human consciousness. It alerts the cortex of incoming information. The *thalamus* acts as a relay station between the reticular formation and specific areas of the cortex. It signals the cortex,

preparing it to receive the upcoming sensory-based information. From a muscular point of view, the reticular formation regulates whether movements are calm, trembling, or sluggish.

The *basal ganglia* help to orchestrate the neuromuscular system's response to sensory stimulation. They contain some of the reflexes described above and regulate the sequence and timing of muscle contraction. Basal ganglia are comprised of multiple parts, each of which addresses a different aspect of movement. The *substantia nigra* is particularly responsible for the interpretation and coordination of the overall sensory information coming from the muscle spindles and Golgi tendon organs. When this

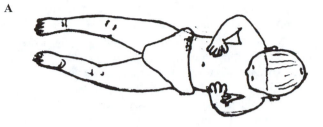

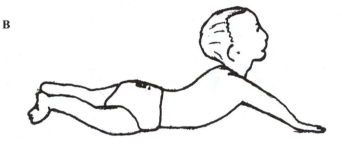

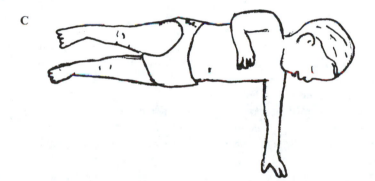

Figure 2–10 Tonic neck reflexes in a 7-month-old child. (**A**) Head ventriflexed evokes upper extremities flexed and lower extremities extended. (**B**) Head dorsiflexed evokes upper extremities extended with lower extremities flexed. (**C**) Head rotation to the left evokes left upper and lower extremities to be abducted and extended, while the right upper and lower extremities are adducted and flexed.

part of the basal ganglia is damaged, coordination is seriously affected. The classic example is Parkinson's disease, which grossly affects the substantia nigra. The *globus pallidus* interprets the incoming sensory information so that humans can appropriately brace certain parts of the body in order to support the prime movers. It fixes body parts into position to facilitate movement. For example, the lower trapezius and serratus anterior must be activated to support the anterior, middle, and posterior deltoid's movement of the arm up into abduction or forward flexion. The *striate body* initiates and monitors a wide range of stereotyped movement patterns—

from individual movements that have common utility, to movements that are the synchronized background motions necessary for limb movements, to movements that communicate emotional intentions (eg, sexual arousal, docility, fear, anger, sadness, disgust, and joy).

Although these lower centers of the brain are imbued with the ancient knowledge of human reflexes, they are also open to the acquisition of new habits. The learning associated with the integration of reflexes is partially stored here. Through hundreds or thousands of repetitions, the ancient and acquired reflexes begin to blend. And, it is in the lower brain that some of the human's unique, individual stances toward life are recorded and stored. Because the basal ganglia are heavily populated with gamma motor neurons, this stance is readily passed on to the end organ, the muscle.

In addition to all of the motor control directed toward movement and postural tone, one needs to factor in the *limbic system*, the seat of the emotions. This system communicates with the frontal lobes concerning the emotional valence of perception. When one sees a bear, for example, the limbic system recognizes the danger of the situation and alerts the frontal lobes of the condition of fear. The frontal lobes then lay down the plan of response (eg, run, climb a tree, shoot a gun, etc), which is then carried out through the total orchestration of the neuromuscular system. It is the limbic system that is responsible for the lines on our faces. The emotional displays that humans give to and receive from the faces of others are directed by the limbic system. Negative emotions tend to affect the upper face more than the lower face, and the left side of the face more than the right side of the face.[16] Notice how common it is for the lines on the left side of people's faces to be much more developed than those on the right side. The limbic system also plays a major role in setting the overall muscular tone. One of the channels of outflow of the limbic system goes to the hypothalamus and then onto the ascending reticular system. Whatmore and Kohli[17] have described a situation in which the incoming afferent of mus-

cular bracing may also play a role in activating the limbic system.

In addition to the basal ganglia and limbic system, the centers of muscular organization in the midbrain include the *cerebellum*, where the fine-tuning of sensory motor integration occurs. The cerebellum processes neural information 10 times faster than cortical processing. It receives sensory input from all of the senses (visual, auditory, vestibular, proprioceptive, etc). It receives input from all of the muscle spindles and Golgi tendon organs. It receives a large portion of the extrapyramidal output from the cortex, and gamma motor output from the basal ganglia. No alpha or gamma motor responses originate from the cerebellum, but almost all of them pass through its influence. It is highly organized and mapped, just like the cortex, with its own sensory and motor homunculus. It sends out information to the reticular formation, the basal ganglia, the thalamus, the motor cortex, and the spine. Its basic job is to take the cortical plan for movement and compare the incoming sensory information with the descending alpha and gamma motor information and fine-tune the final output so that the movement is smooth and coordinated.

The Cortex

Control of the neuromuscular system is quite complex and involves three major divisions—cortex, brainstem, and spinal cord—which operate in a hierarchical arrangement as well as in parallel. Figure 2–11 illustrates a dynamic systems approach, in which there is a very strong interrelation between the various levels. Thus, the motor areas of the cortex can influence the spinal cord both directly or through systems descending through the brainstem. All three levels of the motor system receive sensory information and are under the influence of two independent subcortical systems: the basal ganglia and the cerebellum. Both the basal ganglia and cerebellum act on the cerebral cortex through the relay nucleus of the thalamus.

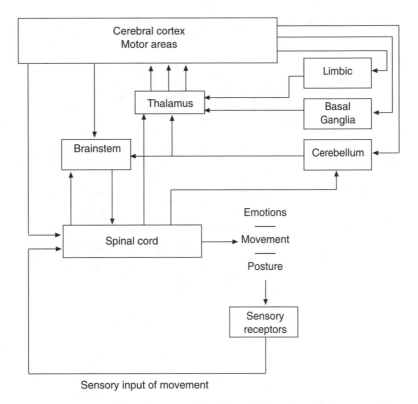

Figure 2–11 A highly schematized flow diagram of the hierarchical and parallel aspects of the motor system.

The cortex plays an important role in neuro-muscular control. The cortex is the location where all new learning takes place. Its surface area is highly differentiated, with different parts taking on different functions. Figure 2–12 shows the basic cortical layout. The premotor (or supplemental) and motor areas are most important for muscle control. The premotor (or supplemental) area is just anterior to the motor area. It is here that the gross motor plan for movement is formed. This information is then passed onto the motor area, where fine motor co-ordination is set forth. The motor area is laid out in a highly differentiated fashion, as seen in the anatomical map shown in Figure 2–13. In this figure, the size of the icon for a particular body part represents the amount of cortical space allo-cated to that region. It is clear that the face and hand consume most of the neurons. From the motor area, nearly 60% of the fibers travel in a finely differentiated fashion directly to the lower motor neurons via the pyramidal tracts. The other 40% synapse along the way in the basal ganglia and the stem to receive fine-tuning from the cerebellum and to integrate some of the higher order reflexes. The extrapyramidal sys-tem has three distinct descending tracts, each with its own function: (1) the vestibulospinal tract primarily has to do with righting reflexes, postural stabilization, and the facilitation of ex-tensors and inhibition of flexors that assist in maintaining the upright posture; (2) the reticulospinal tract primarily mediates the facili-tation or inhibition of the gamma motor system; and (3) the rubrospinal tract carries the fine-tun-ing information coming out of the cerebellum.

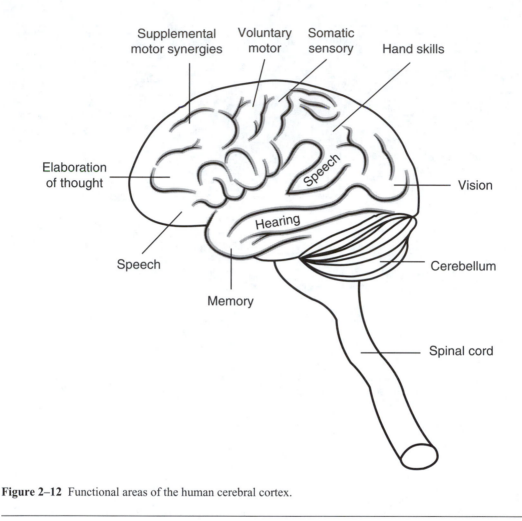

Figure 2–12 Functional areas of the human cerebral cortex.

All of these tracts carry information that ultimately modifies the inherited reflexes, usually by inhibiting the obligatory responses in favor of some learned pattern.

It would appear that we have two very different sensorimotor systems: the alpha and gamma motor systems. Each has its own muscles, motor neurons, and principles of organization. The *gamma motor system*, with its origins primarily in the basal ganglia, carries out the "ancient knowledge." It controls the resting length of the stretch receptors and thus passes on our species-specific postures and behaviors through control of our reflexes. These reflexes have been selected and passed down through thousands of generations; they are fixed and obligatory and

there is no danger of forgetting them. Yet, they are modifiable with enough repetitions of a new posture or movement. The *alpha motor system*, on the other hand, with its origins in the cortex, provides us with the opportunity to acquire and use new knowledge. It primarily modulates or inhibits the obligatory reflexes we inherited. While the gamma motor system provides us with the wisdom of our ancestors, the alpha motor system allows us to adapt to the ever-changing aspects of our world. Together, these two systems provide us with the best of both worlds.

It is important to recognize that the neuromuscular system is extremely complex and that it involves more than these two motor systems. The neuromuscular system is, in fact, a very interac-

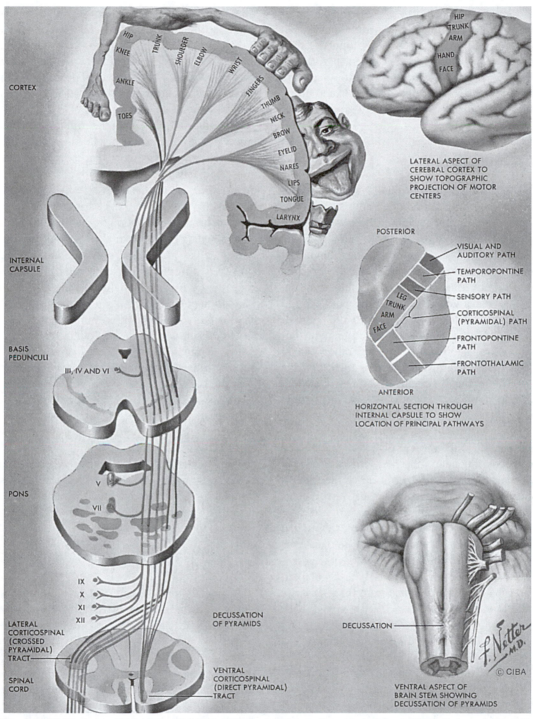

Figure 2–13 The pyramidal system is highly differentiated from the cortex through the spinal cord. Note the degree of cortical representation of the various body parts. *Source:* Copyright 1983. Novartis. Reprinted with permission from *The Ciba Collection of Medical Illustrations*, illustrated by Frank H Netter, MD. All rights reserved.

tive and dynamic, multilayered system that operates in both hierarchical and parallel modes. No one part of the system is more important than any other. In fact, for the system to survive successfully as a whole, all of the various parts are linked together through feedback and feedforward loops that must be integrated at any given movement.

THE MOTOR UNIT

The basic level of nervous system organization of the muscle is the motor unit, and its associated alpha motor system. This is represented by the lower motor neuron, its axon, and the muscle fibers it innervates. The number of muscle fibers per motor unit varies greatly in the human body. The muscles of the face represent the highest level of innervation, with the extraocular muscles having an innervation ratio of 3 to 1, the highest level of innervation in the human body. The lowest innervation ratio (2000 to 1) is found in the gastrocnemius muscle of the leg. The higher innervation ratios are excellent for fine motor tasks, while the lower innervation ratios are ideal for strength production.

The lower motor axon branches so that it can attach itself to the muscle fiber at the motor end plate, creating neuromuscular synapses. When a nerve action potential travels down the axon, it reaches the neuromuscular synapse and releases ACh, which causes the breakdown of the ionic barrier of the muscle tissue and sends the signal throughout the entire system via the transverse tubules. This creates the motor unit action potential, and the muscle contracts. The depolarization runs in both directions from the motor end plate to the tendinous attachments at both ends (see Figure 2–14).

Extracellular recording of the energy exchange described above provides the basis for electromyography. For specific details concerning the genesis of action potentials, consult a basic physiology text.[18] Action potentials are associated with a sudden increase in the cell's membrane permeability to sodium (Na+). This causes a sudden influx of Na+ into the muscle fiber that is associated with a measurable change in the resting potential of the cell. Near the peak of this influx, a rapid efflux of potassium (K+) causes a rapid repolarization of the cell. This may be seen in Figure 2–15. Depolarization of muscle cells conforms to that of the squid cell noted in tracing B.

The motor unit has a number of branches and innervates a number of muscle fibers. Because the branching nerve fibers that extend to each muscle fiber vary in their length and diameter, the time at which the nerve action potential reaches the motor end plate varies, resulting in an asynchronous activation of the muscle fibers belonging to a given motor unit. A single muscle fiber receives input from only one motor unit. However, different motor units tend to overlap their fiber territories spatially (see Figure 2–16). The action potentials from each of the muscle fibers spatially and temporally summate to form a *motor unit action potential*. When motor unit action potentials are recorded using an indwelling electrode, the magnitude of energy recorded is in the millivolt range. With surface sensors, clinicians tend to record from populations of motor units (rather than single motor units) and the magnitude of energy recorded is in the microvolt range. This reduced amplitude is due to the loss of energy associated with the impedance of the body tissue. In essence, the tissue absorbs some of the electrical potential from the muscle as it makes its way to the surface of the skin.

MOTOR UNIT RECRUITMENT PATTERNS

Muscle tone represents a state of low-level contraction that is characteristic of muscles at rest. This represents the resting volley of central nervous system activity sent down the motor units to the muscle. Its function is to stabilize the skeletal structure and to keep the joints from slipping apart. Muscle tone provides the basis for resistance to gravity's pull, emotional tone, and movement. The pull of gravity is ubiquitous, and the muscles must respond to this call. This is, in fact, a normal part of muscle function.

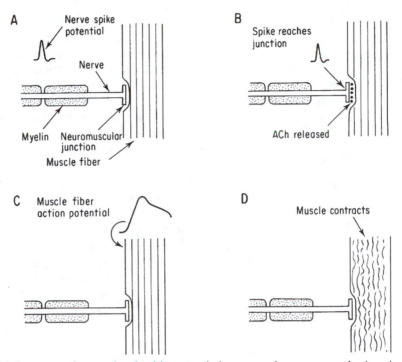

Figure 2–14 Sequence of events involved in transmission across the neuromuscular junction or synapse. (**A**) Nerve action potential approaches the junction. (**B**) The spike reaches the junction and triggers the release of ACh. (**C**) ACh acts on the muscle fibers to produce the muscle action potential. (**D**) The muscle contracts. *Source:* From *Foundations of Physiological Psychology* by Richard F Thompson and Timothy J Taylor. Copyright © 1967 by Richard F Thompson and Timothy J Taylor. Reprinted by permission of Addison Wesley Educational Publishers, Inc.

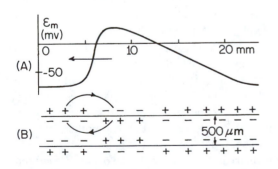

Figure 2–15 Mechanisms of conduction in unmyelinated squid axon (**B**). (**A**) shows the action potential propagating from right to left. The arrow shows the direction of the current flow in front of the action potential. *Source:* Adapted with permission from Ruch and Patton, *Physiology and Biophysics,* © 1965, WB Saunders Company.

Without it, the muscle cells would not thrive (for example, this is why astronauts who return from extended stays in outer space experience muscle atrophy). On the other hand, if muscle fibers fired continuously in order to counter this force, they would soon become exhausted. This predicament is handled by asynchronous stimulation of the motor units. This means that the central nervous system rotates which motor units are firing within a given muscle group. In this way, the postural load of a muscle is transferred from one motor unit to another in a smooth and continuous fashion. In addition to its mechanical work, muscle tone provides the basis for emotional tone. Anxiety or fear tends to take up the general slack of the neuromuscular network. George Whatmore[17] called this "bracing." In layman's terms, this is referred to as "being uptight." And finally, movements are superim-

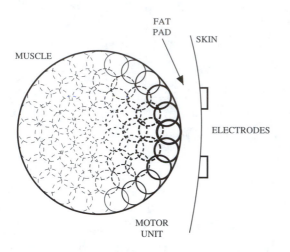

FAT PAD   SKIN

MUSCLE

ELECTRODES

MOTOR UNIT

Figure 2–16 Motor unit territories relative to surface EMG electrodes. The motor unit recruitment territories are represented by the small, overlapping circles. Only the heavy, dark motor unit pools contribute substantially to the sEMG recordings.

posed upon the resting tone of muscle. In our daily lives, as well as in athletic competitions, it is important to have the correct tone for the task at hand. Too much or too little tone, and the timing of actions becomes distorted.

When a muscle contraction occurs, motor unit recruitment is based upon the size principle. Here, the smallest muscle fibers/motor units are recruited first, with larger muscle fibers/motor units being called into play as the synaptic drive continues to increase. The firing rate of muscle fibers is usually in the range of 8 to 50 Hz. As the exertional demands increase, the firing rate moves from slower to higher frequencies. In addition, the motor unit recruitment strategy can move from an asynchronous to a synchronous pattern. All of these mechanisms result in higher sEMG readings.

FACTORS THAT AFFECT MUSCLE TENSION OR FORCE

Fatigue

If the contraction of a muscle is sustained with enough force for a long enough period of time, the conduction velocities of the action potentials along the muscle fibers begin to slow down and the muscle begins to discharge or twitch less frequently. This can be seen in 1 to 5 minutes of continuous muscle contraction at 11% of maximum voluntary contraction.[19] The effects of this muscle fatigue are associated with inadequate perfusion of the tissue, the depletion of energy sources, and the buildup of metabolites (excessive hydrogen ions) in the muscular tissue.[20] Researchers believe that it is the buildup of excessive hydrogen ions that slows down the wave form of the motor unit action potential. This phenomenon can be regarded as intracellular "rush hour" traffic, in which the ion channels simply get jammed up. Thus, it is not uncommon to see two electrophysiological events associated with fatigue prior to the failure point: (1) increased amplitude associated with synchronization of the motor unit pools, and (2) a reduction of the median frequency of the muscle energy.

During a muscular contraction, an internal pressure develops that is associated with the shortening of the muscle fibers. At 10% to 50% of the maximum voluntary contraction, the amount of internal pressure developed is substantial enough to collapse the small arteriole walls of the vessels that are feeding the muscle.[21,22] During rhythmic muscular contractions, the pressure waves of the contraction actually assist the muscle in distributing the metabolic resources and removing the resulting metabolites. However, during a sustained contraction, the muscle is deprived of its nutrients and sustains the buildup of toxic wastes. Perhaps this is why it is essential for the muscle to have interspersed or "micromomentary" (less than 0.5 second) rest periods as part of its activity cycle. Researchers have reported that workers who do not demonstrate "sEMG gaps" or micromomentary rest periods in their work activities tend to develop tension myalgias.[23]

Force-Amplitude Relationships

In general, sEMG amplitude does not equal force. But, how well does sEMG activity reflect the amount of force developed by a muscle? This topic has been studied extensively, and an excellent review of this topic can be found in Basmajian and DeLuca.[20] A synopsis of the findings is as follows. First, there appears to be a high level of individual variability in the findings. In a population of subjects, the contraction force has a dispersion equal to approximately 25% of the mean value. This may reflect different levels of muscle conditioning across the subjects studied. Deconditioned individuals may display higher levels of sEMG activity to exert the same amount of force exerted by someone with a well-conditioned muscle. Second, the force curve relationship varies, according to the muscle studied. This can be seen in Figure 2–17, where multiple isometric contractions are normalized to the maximum voluntary contraction and plotted as a percentage of maximum voluntary contraction. During isometric contractions of the smaller, first dorsal interosseous muscle, there is a quasi-linear relationship between force and sEMG. The larger muscles such as the biceps, however, take on a curvilinear relationship. The differences between the large and small muscles may possibly reflect the differences in the firing rates of the muscles (slow versus fast), their recruitment properties (which fibers recruit as a function of the strength of the contraction), as well as other anatomical and electrical considerations. In general, muscles that are comprised of predominantly one fiber type tend to have a more linear relationship between force exerted and sEMG. In muscles of a mixed fiber type (fast- and slow-twitch), the relationship appears to be more curvilinear, with the breaking point at approximately 50% of maximum voluntary contraction.

Length-Tension Relationships

The amount of effort or force that a muscle can put forth depends upon the resting length of the muscle. As was noted in an earlier section of this chapter, the length-tension relationship is mediated by the degree of overlap of the sarcomeres (see Figure 2–5). In essence, when there is too little or too much overlap of the actin and myosin fibers, the number of potential crossbridging sites diminishes, causing the strength of the contraction to diminish. Figure 2–18 illustrates the relationship between muscle tension

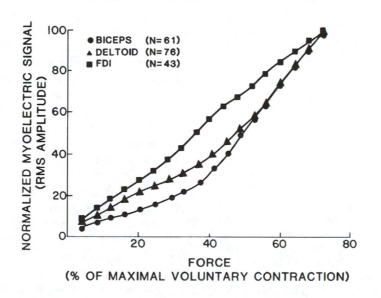

Figure 2–17 Effects of muscle on sEMG signal-force relationship. FDI = first dorsal interosseous muscle. N = average number of isometric contractions for each muscle group. *Source:* Reprinted with permission from JH Lawrence and C DeLuca, *Journal of Applied Physiology,* © 1983, The American Physiological Society.

and percentage of resting length in an isolated muscle. Both the passive elastic properties of the muscle while being stretched (curve 1) and the total tension exerted by the actively contracting muscle (curve 2) are presented. Curve 2 represents the sum of both the elastic force contribution as well as that due to the contraction of the muscle. Curve 3 subtracts the force exerted by the elastic properties of the muscle, thus representing the amount of tension generated by the contraction itself. Several facts can be discerned from this graph. First, the muscle is unable to exert any tension whatsoever when it is at less than 50% of its normal resting length. In general, most muscles have the capacity to shorten 50% of their muscle length, and the ability of a muscle to exert force is reduced as it is placed in a shortened position. At its normal resting length, the amount of tension produced by the contraction of the muscle (curve 3) is greatest. However, the total tension of the muscle is augmented by the elastic properties of muscle when it is stretched (curve 2). Thus at 120% of its rest-

ing length, the total tension possible (contraction + elastic properties) reaches its peak. This length coincides with the length of the muscle when the joint is in the relaxed position.[24] Beyond that point, the force attributable to muscle contraction begins to fall off rapidly. By 200% of its resting length, all of the tension in the muscle has transferred exclusively to the elastic properties of the muscle itself.

Force-Velocity Relationships

The contraction velocity of a muscle also affects the amount of tension or force that a muscle produces.[25] This is clearly seen in Figure 2–19. The speed at which a muscle can contract is primarily limited by the rate at which the cross-bridging can be manifested at the sarcomere level. Under conditions in which there is no change in the velocity of the contraction (ie, an isometric contraction), cross-bridges are built more rapidly when the resistance to the contraction is low. Therefore, the amount of time it takes to reach a given tension level is determined solely by the amount of tension to be developed. Lower tension levels are reached more quickly than higher tension levels. In the case of concentric contractions, however, the amount of tension generated is moderated by the velocity of the contraction. In situations where different velocities of contractions are conducted using the same amount of resistance, contractions that require higher speeds build fewer cross-bridges than those conducted at slower speeds. This results in the generation force of less during faster concentric contractions than during slower concentric contractions. In the case of eccentric contractions, however, the amount of force or tension created by the muscle actually increases as the velocity of the eccentric contraction increases.

Surface EMG amplitudes do not equal muscle tension or force. The relationships described above refer only to force and tension, not sEMG amplitudes. For example, the sEMG amplitudes of a concentric contraction are greater than those of an eccentric contraction when lifting or letting down the same weight.

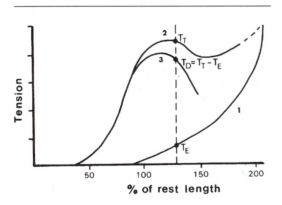

Figure 2–18 Tension-length curves for isolated muscle. Curve 1 = passive elastic tension T_E in a muscle passively stretched to increasing lengths. Curve 2 = total tension T_T exerted by muscle contracting actively from increasing initial lengths. Curve 3 = developed tension T_D calculated by subtracting elastic tension values on curve 1 from the total tension values at equivalent lengths on curve 2 ($T_D = T_T - T_E$). *Source:* Reprinted with permission from B Gowitzke and M Milner, *Scientific Bases of Human Movement*, 3rd Edition, © 1988, Williams and Wilkins.

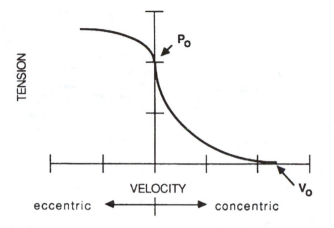

Figure 2–19 Velocity-active tension relationship for muscle. *Source:* Reprinted from G Soderberg, *Selected Topics in Surface Electromyography for Use in the Occupational Setting: Expert Perspective.* DHHS (NIOSH), Publication No. 91-100, Washington DC, NIOSH, 1992.

REFERENCES

1. Huxley HE. The mechanism of muscular contraction. *Sci Am.* December 1965.

2. Brown JMM, Solomon C, Paton M. Further evidence of functional differentiation within biceps brachii. *Electromyogr Clin Neurophysiol.* 1933;33:301–309.

3. Haar Romeny BMT, Denier van der Gon JJ, Gielen CCAM. Relation between location of the motor unit in the human biceps brachii and its critical firing levels for different tasks. *Exp Neurol.* 1984;85:631–650.

4. McNutty W, Gevertz R, Berkoff G, Hubbard D. Needle electromyographic evaluation of a trigger point response to a psychological stressor. *Psychophysiology.* 1994;31:313–316.

5. Riek S, Bawa P. Recruitment of motor units in human forearm extensors. *J Neurophysiol.* 1992;68:100–108.

6. Jorgensen K, Winkel J. On the function of the human soleus muscle. In: Jonsson B, ed. *Biomechanics, X.* Champaign, IL: Human Kinetics; 1987:259–264.

7. Wolf S, LeCraw D, Barton L. Comparison of motor copy and targeted biofeedback training techniques for restitution of upper extremity function among patients with neurologic disorders. *Phys Ther.* 1988;69:719–735.

8. Huxley AF. Muscle-structure and theories of contraction. *Prog Biophys.* 1957;7:255–318.

9. Hunt CC, Kuffler SW. Stretch receptor discharges during muscle contraction. *J Physiol (Lond).* 1951; 113:298–315.

10. Vallbo AB. Basic patterns of muscle spindle discharge in man. In: Taylor A, Prochazka A, eds. *Muscle Receptors and Movement.* London: MacMillan; 1981.

11. Jacobson E. Electrical measurement concerning muscular contraction (tonus) and the cultivation of relaxation in man: relaxation times of individuals. *Am J Physiol.* 1934;108:573–580.

12. Hubbard D, Berkoff G. Myofascial trigger points show spontaneous needle EMG activity. *Spine.* 1993; 18:1803–1807.

13. Travell J, Simons D. *Myofascial Pain and Dysfunction: A Trigger Point Manual, I and II.* Baltimore: Williams & Wilkins; 1983.

14. Donaldson S, Skubick D, Clasby R, Cram J. The evaluation of trigger-point activity using dynamic EMG techniques. *Am J Pain Manage.* 1994;4:118–122.

15. Skubick D, Clasby R, Donaldson CCS, Marshall W. Carpal tunnel syndrome as an expression of muscular dysfunction in the neck. *J Occup Rehab.* 1993;3:31–43.

16. Sackeim HA, Gur RC, Saucy MC. Emotions are expressed more intensely on the left side of the face. *Science.* 1978;202:434–436.

17. Whatmore G, Kohli D. *The Physiopathology and Treatment of Functional Disorders.* New York: Grune & Stratton; 1974.

18. Guyton AC. *Textbook of Medical Physiology.* 6th ed. Philadelphia: WB Saunders; 1981.

19. Chaffin DB. Localized muscle fatigue—dimension and measurement. *J Occup Med.* 1973;15:346–354.

20. Basmajian JV, DeLuca C. *Muscles Alive.* 5th ed. Baltimore: Williams & Wilkins; 1985.

21. Hagberg M. Occupational musculoskeletal stress disorders of the neck and shoulder: a review of possible pathophysiology. *Int Arch Occup Environ Health.* 1984; 53:269–278.

22. Mortimer JT, Kerstein MD, Magnusson R, Petersen H. Muscle blood flow in the human biceps as a function of developed muscle force. *Arch Surg.* 1971;103:376–377.

23. Veiersted KB, Westgaard RH, Andersen P. Electromyographic evaluation of muscular work pattern as a predictor of trapezius myalgia. *Scand J Work Environ Health.* 1993;19:284–290.

24. Butchthal F, Guld C, Rosenfalch P. Multi-electrode study of the territory of a motor unit. *Acta Physiol Scand.* 1978;39:83–103.

25. Hill AV. The heat of shortening and the dynamic constants of muscle. *Proc R Soc London (Biol).* 1938; 243:136–195.

Chapter Questions

1. The connective tissue associated with muscle is known as:
   a. fascia
   b. tendons
   c. ligaments
   d. all of the above

2. Without muscles, would the bones and ligaments provide enough stability to allow the skeleton to stand on its own against gravity?
   a. yes
   b. no

3. How many muscles are in the human body?
   a. 200
   b. 400
   c. 500
   d. 600+

4. The two main molecules that make up a muscle fiber are:
   a. myosin and Golgi
   b. Golgi and spindle
   c. actin and myosin
   d. spindle and Ruffini

5. A sarcomere is made up of which of the following bands?
   a. A, Z, G, I
   b. A, Z, I, H
   c. H, G, I, J
   d. A, I, K, Z

6. The sarcoplasmic reticulum stores:
   a. glucose
   b. calcium
   c. potassium
   d. myosin

7. It is proposed that muscles do their work through a process that involves:
   a. cross-bridging
   b. hatcheting
   c. the Krebs cycle
   d. minicontractions

8. How large of a voluntary contraction does it take to create a disturbance in the microcirculation of muscle?
   a. 5–10% maximum voluntary contraction
   b. 10–50% maximum voluntary contraction
   c. 70–80% maximum voluntary contraction
   d. 90+% maximum voluntary contraction

9. Which of the following does not describe the fast-twitch muscle fiber type?
   a. great fatigability
   b. large size, high tension
   c. rich capillary supply
   d. high glucose stores

10. Which of the following is not an element of the motor unit?
    a. upper motor neuron
    b. lower motor neuron
    c. axon
    d. muscle fibers

11. Which muscle tends to have the highest innervation ratio (3 to 1) of muscle fibers to motor units?
    a. the trapezius
    b. the extraocular muscles
    c. the biceps
    d. the quadriceps

12. Which of the following sensory mechanisms runs parallel to the muscle fibers?
    a. muscle spindle
    b. Golgi tendon organ
    c. Ruffini nucleus
    d. free nerve ending

13. Which of the following sensory mechanisms runs in series to the muscle fibers?
    a. muscle spindle
    b. Golgi tendon organ
    c. Ruffini nucleus
    d. free nerve ending

14. The gamma motor system controls the:
    a. extrafusal fibers
    b. intrafusal fibers
    c. motor unit
    d. none of the above

15. When the muscle spindle is activated by a stretch, it causes the muscle that it is located within to:
    a. relax
    b. become inhibited
    c. contract
    d. undergo flexion/cross-extension

16. It is speculated that trigger points are located in the:
    a. extrafusal fibers
    b. intrafusal fibers
    c. muscle spindle
    d. dermatome

17. The Golgi tendon organ is sensitive to:
    a. the amount of muscle tension or effort
    b. joint position
    c. instantaneous muscle length
    d. velocity of muscle

18. The gamma motor system regulates:
    a. movement
    b. posture
    c. coordination
    d. all of the above

19. Free nerve endings are sensitive to:
    a. nocioception
    b. too much lactic acid retention
    c. inflammation and swelling
    d. all of the above

20. The Ruffini nucleus senses:
    a. muscle tension
    b. joint position
    c. velocity of contraction
    d. pain

21. Which of the following muscle sense organs is consciously perceived?
    a. muscle spindle
    b. stretch receptor
    c. Golgi tendon organ
    d. joint receptors

22. Which of the following reflexes is suprasegmental?
    a. stretch reflex
    b. withdrawal reflex
    c. flexion/cross-extension reflex
    d. scratch reflex

23. Which part of the brain controls arousal?
    a. ascending reticular formation
    b. basal ganglia
    c. cerebellum
    d. cortex

24. The basal ganglia stores:
    a. primitive reflexes
    b. acquired reflexes
    c. postures
    d. all of the above

25. Which part of the brain conducts/processes information the fastest?
    a. cortex
    b. cerebellum
    c. spinal cord
    d. pyramidal tract

26. Which part of the brain has as its primary purpose the final execution and refinement of each and every movement?
    a. cortex
    b. cerebellum
    c. spinal cord
    d. extrapyramidal tract

27. What percentage of the motor neurons exiting the motor strip stop off in the lower brain before going down to the lower motor neuron?
    a. 10%
    b. 20%
    c. 40%
    d. 60%

28. When a muscle shortens during a contraction, this is called a:
    a. concentric contraction
    b. eccentric contraction
    c. isometric contraction
    d. mesocentric contraction

29. When from a standing position a person squats down and comes back up, this is called:
    a. an open kinetic chain
    b. a closed kinetic chain
    c. an isometric contraction
    d. an ergonomic chain

30. In sEMG, which of the following can be expected to show the largest recruitment pattern?
    a. eccentric contraction
    b. concentric contraction
    c. isometric contraction
    d. flexion relaxation

31. What type of contraction do we primarily use when we go down stairs?
    a. eccentric contraction
    b. concentric contraction
    c. isometric contraction
    d. reflexive contraction

32. Which muscles tend to show a quasi-linear relationship between force and sEMG amplitudes?
    a. small fine motor
    b. large gross motor
    c. soleus muscle
    d. erector spinae

33. At which point of muscle resting length would one expect to see the greatest strength?
    a. 50%
    b. 75%
    c. 90%
    d. 125%

34. What is the relationship between force and velocity?
    a. the faster the contraction, the greater the force
    b. the slower the contraction, the greater the force
    c. force and velocity are independent of each other
    d. none of the above

35. In general, is it reasonable to think that sEMG amplitude equals the amount of muscle force generated?
    a. yes
    b. no

CHAPTER 3

Instrumentation

INTRODUCTION

The energy that is generated by the muscle has a very small value and is measured in millionths of a volt (microvolts). It is necessary to use very sophisticated and sensitive instruments to amplify this signal so that it can be seen and heard. In essence, a surface electromyography (sEMG) is nothing but a very sensitive voltmeter.

In the early days of sEMG, the amplifiers that were used were easily contaminated by other electromagnetic energy in the recording environment. Thus, sEMG recordings were commonly conducted in a "copper room." These rooms were sometimes merely copper screens, as seen in Figure 3–1. The copper screen caught the electrical noise in the room and sent it to "ground," thus eliminating it from the recording environment.

During the 1950s, biomedical engineering introduced the differential amplifier. This amplifier essentially eliminated the need for the copper rooms, and sEMG recordings moved out of the realm of researchers to the realm of clinicians. Because of the advances in instrumentation, clinical sEMG began to flourish. Clinical sEMG was initially used by psychologists for biofeedback, and later sEMG began to spread to such other specialties as chiropractic, physical therapy, physical medicine, neurology, and urology.

The purpose of this chapter is to familiarize the practitioner with the basic concepts behind

the instrumentation of sEMG. It covers the fundamentals of the electronics behind what is seen on the screen; the different types of sEMG displays and the ways in which the sEMG signal can be processed; how to identify noise and artifact; and how to set specifications for an sEMG instrument. Figure 3–2 shows a block diagram of the various components of sEMG instrumentation. Each of the elements in this diagram will be addressed in this chapter. For more in-depth reading on this topic, consider Peek's excellent chapter for clinicians,[1] Basmajian and DeLuca's more technical discussion in *Muscles Alive*,[2] or an edited book by Soderberg.[3] For a broader view of the topic, see Cacioppo et al.[4]

THE SOURCE OF THE ELECTROMYOGRAPHIC SIGNAL

Let us begin with the first element of the diagram in Figure 3–2, the source of the sEMG signal, and work through the subelements leading up to differential amplification. The tissue and electrode elements are depicted in Figure 3–3. The source of the sEMG signal is the motor unit action potential (MUAP). Action potentials are given off by each of the motor units activated during a given contraction. In any given recruitment pattern, populations of motor units are activated in an asynchronous pattern. This asynchronous pattern of activation provides the possibility of smooth movement. Figure 3–4 shows the activity from all of the active motor

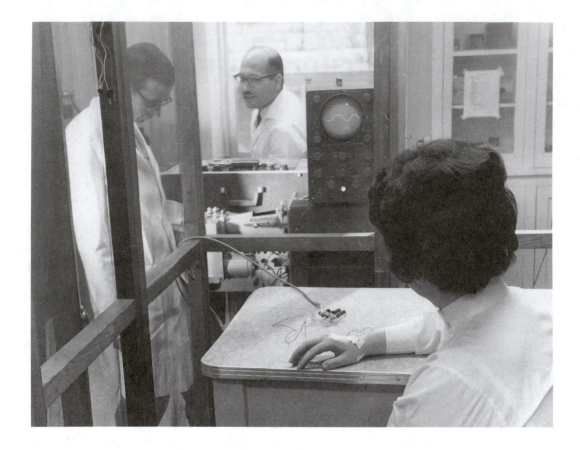

Figure 3–1 Surface EMG recording of first dorsal interossi conducted in a copper-screened room. John Basmajian, the father of sEMG, is shown in the middle. Courtesy of John Basmajian.

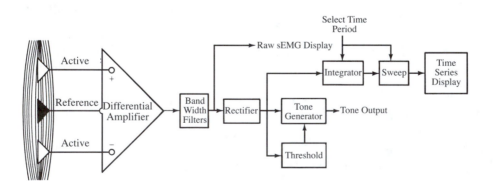

Figure 3–2 Block diagram of sEMG instrument with several options.

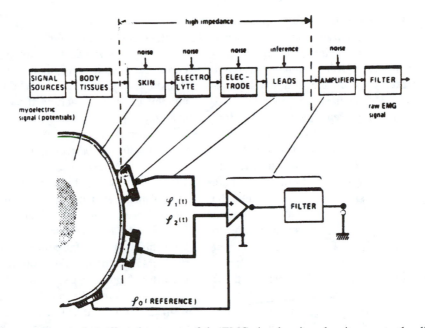

Figure 3–3 The components that affect the source of the EMG signal as it makes its way to the differential amplifiers. *Source:* Reprinted from G Soderberg, *Selected Topics in Surface Electromyography for Use in the Occupational Setting: Expert Perspective.* DHHS (NIOSH), Publication No. 91-100, Washington DC, NIOSH, 1992.

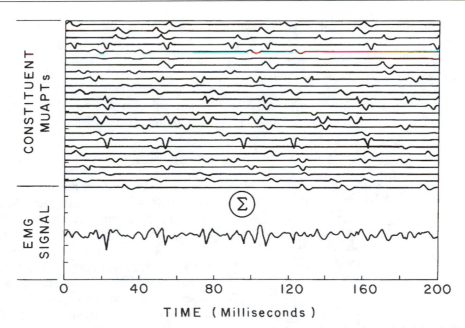

Figure 3–4 An sEMG signal is formed by adding the constituent motor unit action potential trains (MUAPTs). *Source:* Reprinted with permission from JV Basmajian and C DeLuca, *Muscles Alive,* © 1985, Williams and Wilkins.

units recruited for the given contraction, along with the sum of their activity, which is shown at the bottom of the graph. It is the sum of the activity that constitutes the volume conducted signal, which is picked up at the electrodes and amplified by the sEMG instrument. In Figure 3–5, each small circle represents the fiber's territory associated with one motor unit recruitment area. Note how they slightly overlap. The solid circles closest to the surface of the skin and therefore closest to the recording electrodes contribute most heavily to the sEMG signal. The fainter the circle, the farther away it is from the recording electrodes and the less likely it is to contribute to the sEMG recording. The farther the signal needs to travel through body tissue before reaching the recording electrodes, the more resistance it encounters. This resistance absorbs the energy, and thus less of the original energy reaches the surface electrode. In addition, the body tissues tend to absorb higher-frequency components of the signal, allowing slower frequencies to pass through more readily. Thus, the body tissue is considered to provide a low pass filter for the signal.

In addition, if there is adipose tissue between the muscle and the recording electrodes, more of the signal gets absorbed. The fatty layer acts like an imperfect electrical insulator between the muscle and the recording electrodes. An insulator stops the flow of electrical current, much like the plastic coverings that surround extension cords. Because it is an imperfect insulator, the thicker the layer of adipose, the smaller the amount of signal reaching the electrodes. For example, given the same movement and electrode placement strategy (eg, monitoring upper trapezius during abduction), it is not uncommon to see higher resting and peak amplitudes of sEMG activity in a thin person than in a person with a thick layer of fat beneath the recording electrodes. Even within an individual, the amplitude of sEMG is likely to be greater over areas with thin layers of fat compared to areas with thicker layers of fat. For example, amplitudes recorded from the extensors of the forearm muscles are typically much greater than those from the gluteal muscles. Because the gluteus maximus has a much larger muscle mass than the forearm extensors, one might expect to see much larger sEMG amplitudes. But this is not the case. The attenuating effects of adipose tissue cannot be overlooked. We have observed that the correlation between skin-fold thickness at the electrode site (an indication of adipose thickness) and sEMG amplitude values are higher ($r \sim -0.5$) in the resting state than during an active recruitment pattern ($r \sim -0.25$). Thus, it appears that the fatty layer plays a larger role in the interpretation of resting sEMG values than in dynamic sEMG recordings.

IMPEDANCE

Once the energy from the muscle reaches the skin, it is sensed by the electrodes. The interface between the sensing electrode and the skin is a delicate matter. For example, the impedance of the skin (also referred to as resistance in a direct current, or DC, circuit) may vary as a function of the moisture of the skin; the superficial skin oil content; and the density of the horny, dead-cell layer. In addition, some sort of electrolytic medium is commonly used to provide a cushion between the surface of the electrode and the surface of the skin. This is usually hypersalinic and

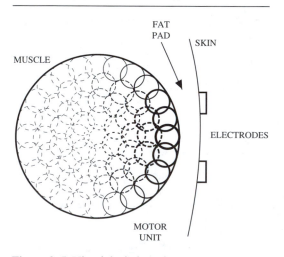

Figure 3–5 Visual depiction of motor unit activity in relation to the recording electrodes.

potentiates the sEMG from the skin to the electrode. If no electrolyte is used (a dry electrode), the skin senses the presence of the foreign object (the electrode) and eventually begins to produce sweat, thus providing its own electrolytic medium. In sEMG, it is important to keep the impedance of the skin at the electrode site as low as possible and balanced for the two recording electrodes. This is commonly accomplished by abrading the skin vigorously with an alcohol pad. For research purposes, the impedance at the electrode site should be below 5,000 to 10,000 ohms. In some research settings, the experimenter may actually puncture the skin at the site of the electrode to ensure a low impedance at the site. This is too rigorous for most clinical purposes. Yet the practitioner needs to get the impedance low enough to provide a clean signal. When the impedance at the electrode skin interface is too high or too imbalanced, the common mode rejection of the sEMG amplifier is defeated, and thus the amplification process is affected by the 60-cycle interference from the energy in the room. This is explained in greater detail in a later section.

How low should the impedance at the skin be to allow a valid and meaningful clinical recording? The answer to this question depends upon the sEMG instrument. One attribute of the sEMG amplifier is its input impedance. The interface of skin impedance and input impedance must be matched in certain ways, and this is schematically represented in Figure 3–6. The input impedance of the preamplifier (represented as I_i) essentially absorbs the muscle energy that has reached the electrode-skin interface, and thus provides a basis for amplifying the small signal. Oscillating voltages can be measured only as a function of impedance. This is based on Ohm's law: $E = IR$ (voltage = current × impedance). So, the sEMG amplification system puts out a known input impedance to absorb the energy that it wishes to quantify. For this fancy voltmeter to work, it is important that the impedance of the skin (I_s) is less than that of the input impedance of the preamplifier (I_i). *The input impedance of the sEMG preamplifier should be 10 to 100 times*

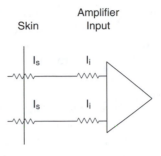

Figure 3–6 The interface of skin impedance and input of sEMG preamplifier. I_i represents input impedance of the preamplifier. I_s represents impedance of the skin. Courtesy of Will Taylor, Blue Hills, Maine.

greater than the impedance at the electrode-skin interface. Thus, if an sEMG instrument has an input impedance of 1 megohm (1 million ohms), then it will tolerate impedance at the electrode-skin interface of up to 10,000 ohms. However, if the sEMG instrument has an input impedance of 1 gigaohm (1 billion ohms), the preamplifier can tolerate impedance at the electrode-skin interface of 10 million ohms (or 10 megohms). As a general rule, the greater the input impedance of the sEMG preamplifier, the better. This is because higher input impedance makes the sEMG more robust to poor electrode skin connections. The latter amplifier certainly will provide a nice basis for clinical work. However, one should not be seduced into thinking that because the sEMG will allow resistance at the electrode-skin interface of 10 megohms, it is not necessary to abrade or otherwise prepare the skin for the electrode; dry, horny skin or oily skin can easily exceed an impedance of 10 megohms.

Surface EMG amplifiers, regardless of their input impedance, are still sensitive to imbalances in the impedance at the two recording electrode sites. Differences in impedance may occur when one electrode is on a slightly hairy portion of the body, while the other electrode is not. One should avoid placement on hairy areas whenever possible. In addition, imbalances may occur when one electrode loses good adhesion to the skin during a dynamic evaluation or treatment session. In any event, sEMG amplifiers can usually tolerate up to a 20% discrepancy in the impedance between the two sites. Differences greater than 20% lead to faulty elevations in the signal amplitude. Figure 3–7 shows what can happen to an sEMG recording when one electrode temporarily comes loose during a dynamic study. The rhythmic quality of the poor recording reflects the ringing of the amplifier as it attempts to compensate electronically for the imbalance in the impedance between the two electrodes. This may be seen in both raw and processed sEMG recordings.

Two other elements can moderate the impedance of the signal. The first is the electrode itself. This is explained in greater detail in Chapter 4. In general, the size of the electrode and the material it is made of can make a difference. Today, most electrodes are made up of silver chloride. The second element is the cable that exists between the electrode and the amplifier itself. This is actually one of the most vulnerable parts of the sEMG system; it usually breaks and must be re-

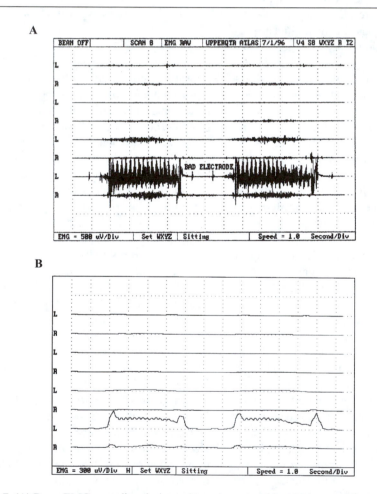

Figure 3–7 (**A**) Raw sEMG recording during a dynamic protocol in which one of the recording electrodes periodically comes loose. (**B**) Processed root mean square (RMS) tracing of (**A**). The "ringing" of the circuit is associated with excessive 60-Hz noise. *Source:* Copyright © Clinical Resources, Inc.

placed at some point during the lifetime of the instrument. If a lead does break, this causes an infinite resistance and thus totally saturates the amplifier. It is best to keep these cables as short as possible and to inspect them from time to time.

DIFFERENTIAL AMPLIFICATION AND COMMON MODE REJECTION

Once the action potential from the muscle has crossed the electrode-skin interface, it passes through the process of differential amplification and common mode rejection. During amplification, the size of the biological signal is "boosted" or made larger. This is referred to as *gain*. The amount of gain or amplification determines how large or how small the sEMG appears on the visual display.

The development of *differential amplification* and *common mode rejection* brought sEMG out from behind the copper cage and into the clinic. In differential amplification, three electrodes are necessary: two recording electrodes and one reference electrode. The recording electrodes are placed over the muscles with the reference electrode simply making good contact somewhere on the body. The biological energy that reaches both recording electrodes is then compared to the reference electrode, and only the energy that

is unique to each recording electrode is passed on for further signal conditioning and display. This works because the energy given off by a muscle follows the course of the muscle fibers from the motor end plate to the tendinous insertions at both ends. When the recording electrodes are placed parallel to the muscle fibers and slightly off the center of the muscle belly where the highest density of motor end plates can be found, the action potential given off from the fiber travels to and reaches the two recording electrodes at different times. Thus, this energy is unique to each electrode and is passed on for further amplification. It is the energy that is common to both recording electrodes—the common mode—that is eliminated by this process. The common mode signal typically comes from external electromagnetic noise, such as the 60-cycle current that powers lights and computers.

Sometimes the use of an analogy helps to clarify a concept. Peek[1] uses a sound metaphor with some clarity—monitoring the amplitude of bird songs in the field (see Figure 3–8). Using the differential amplifier model, two large microphones are set up to record the bird songs. As the birds fly toward the two microphones, each microphone receives a slightly different sound, since the birds are closer to one microphone than the other. The differential amplifier simply subtracts the level of song on one microphone from

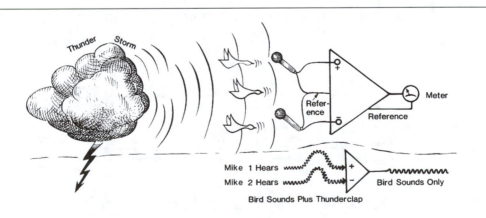

Figure 3–8 Analogy using bird songs to illustrate noise subtraction in a differential amplifier. *Source:* Reprinted with permission from Schwartz, *Biofeedback*, p. 55, © 1987, Guilford Publications, Inc.

that of the other, presenting the difference as the index of loudness. The louder the birds sing, the larger the difference and the higher the loudness meter. Now suppose that a thunderstorm in the area produces a roll of thunder. The thunder moves out in all directions, eventually reaching the microphones. Because the thunder comes from a distant source, it reaches the microphones at nearly the same time and the same intensity. The microphones pass on the thunder roll and the bird songs to the differential amplifier. Because of common mode rejection, the thunder roll that is common to both microphones is subtracted out of the signal, leaving only the bird songs to be passed on to the loudness meter.

The degree to which a differential amplifier is successful at common mode rejection is described by the common mode rejection ratio (CMRR). This is calculated by dividing the amplification of the common mode signal (A) by the amplification of the differential mode signal (B), and finally multiplying this quotient by 20 $\log_{10}$ to achieve a value termed dB. Mathematically, this would look like this:

$$20 \log_{10} (A/B) = CMRR\ dB$$

The higher the CMRR dB, the better. It is typically between 90 and 140 dB.

FILTERING THE ELECTROMYOGRAPHIC SIGNAL

Once the sEMG signal has been boosted by the differential amplifiers, it is then processed in some way. The first level of processing is known as filtering. Most sEMG instruments contain a 60-Hz notch filter. This filter may be found in the electronic circuitry of the sEMG instrument (an analog filter) or in the software it uses (a digital filter). A *notch filter* is a band reject filter that is typically very narrow in width (59 to 61 Hz) and has a very steep slope to the filter. The purpose of this notch filter is to eliminate any of the electrical noise (60 Hz) from the recording environment that exceeds the capabilities of the common mode rejection scheme. In other words, it rejects or does not let through any energy that is between 59 and 61 Hz. Unfortunately, these filters are not perfect; if the noise levels are too great, they readily saturate out the filter. Figure 3–9 represents such a phenomenon. The rhythmic beats seen in the third and seventh tracings represent the ringing of the amplifying circuits due to the presence of too much 60-Hz noise.

The next essential filter for sEMG is the *band pass filter*. This filter passes only a certain frequency range of energy on for further quantification and display. For example, a typical band

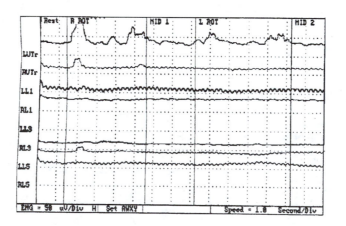

Figure 3–9 Surface EMG example of the ringing of the amplifiers due to the presence of too much 60-cycle noise. This ringing can be seen in the third and seventh channels. *Source:* Copyright © Clinical Resources, Inc.

pass filter might let all of the energy above 20 Hz through and then close the gate at 300 Hz. The lower cutoff point assists the practitioner by eliminating much of the electrical noise associated with wire sway and miscellaneous biological artifacts associated with slow-moving DC potential shifts. The upper cutoff point eliminates the tissue noise at the electrode site.

Selecting the filters for sEMG recordings is somewhat of an art, because certain filters are better for some applications than others. For example, for sEMG recordings from the face, a 25-to-500–Hz band pass filter is preferable because the muscles of the face readily emit frequencies up into the 500-Hz range. This has to do with the innervation ratio of the muscles of the face, along with their repetitive firing patterns. The 100-to-200–Hz or 100-to-500–Hz filter is effective for eliminating heart rate artifact. However, it may be insensitive to fatigued muscles, because the frequency spectrum of muscles shifts to the slower range during fatigue. Figure 3–10 illustrates the difference in processed sEMG recordings from the upper trapezius site using a 100-to-200–Hz filter (left side) and a 20-to-1000–Hz filter (right side). The 100-to-200–Hz filter essentially eliminates the electrocardiogram (ECG) artifact. In addition to changing the visual presentation of the tracing, these filters also alter the values yielded during the quantification of the sEMG. The wider band pass sample has the large ECG spikes and yields an amplitude of approximately 30 microvolts RMS (root mean square), while the narrower band pass filter yields a much smaller signal with a much smaller amplitude of approximately 15 microvolts RMS.

SPECTRAL ANALYSIS, FATIGUE, AND BAND PASS FILTERS

The energy from muscles has a frequency spectrum. Much like the rainbow colors seen with light refracted through a prism, the sEMG signal can be displayed so as to see its range of frequencies. "Power spectral density" curves plot the frequency components of the sEMG signal as a function of the probability of their occurrence. To do this, spectral analysis uses a mathematical technique called *fast fourrie transformations* (FFT) to decompose the signal into its various frequency components. As illustrated in Figure 3–4, the sEMG signal that reaches the differential amplifier consists of the sum of many motor units firing. Consider a case in which there are only three sources of energy that simultaneously reach the preamplifier. Figure 3–11A shows the three independent signals whose frequencies are 0.5, 1.0, and 1.5 Hz. Figure 3–11B shows a composite of the three signals. In sEMG recordings, the amplifiers always see the composite. Were an FFT spectral analysis to be conducted on this composite signal, it would decompose the energy into the spectral graph shown in Figure 3–12, which illustrates that the composite signal is composed of three frequencies at 0.5, 1.0, and 1.5 Hz.

Figure 3–13 illustrates the power spectral density of the sEMG for a muscle. The height of the curve at any given frequency indicates how prevalent the muscle energy is at that frequency. In this case, the 20-to-300–Hz filter (single hatch) represents nearly all of the energy in the spectrum of the muscle. If one were using a 100-to-200–Hz band pass filter (double hatched),

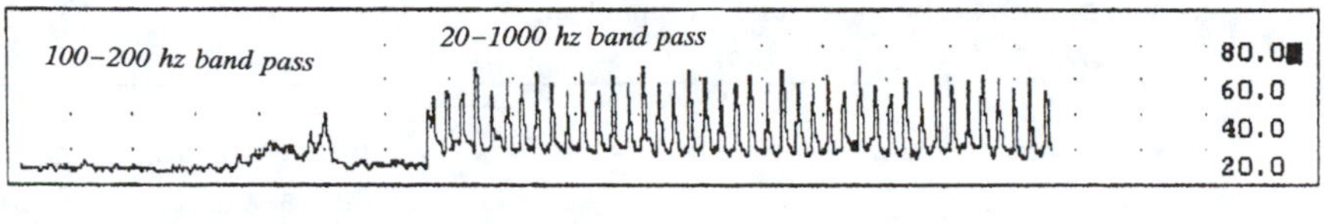

Figure 3–10 Elimination of ECG artifact from upper trapezius lead by using a narrow 100-to-200–Hz filter (left side) and a 20-to-1000–Hz filter (right side).

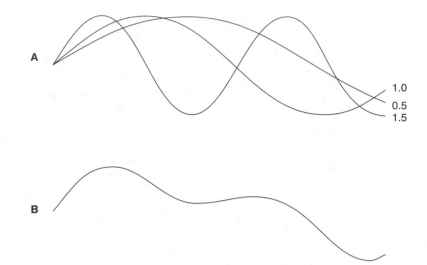

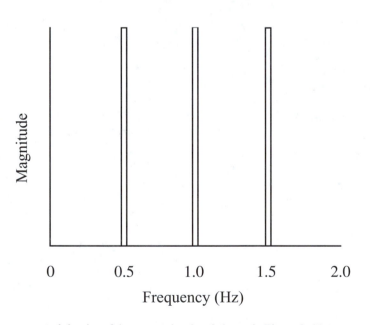

Figure 3–11 (**A**) Three independent signals of 0.5, 1.0, and 1.5 Hz and (**B**) their composite signal.

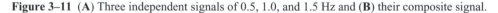

Figure 3–12 Power spectral density of the composite signal shown in Figure 3–11.

however, only a portion of the energy of the muscle would be observed.

The relationship of muscle energy represented by the two filters described above could shift under various conditions. For illustrative purposes, consider work versus fatigue. Figure 3–14A shows the raw and processed sEMG of the first dorsal interosseous muscle once it has been passed through a 20-to-300–Hz band pass filter. The top line of the graph represents the

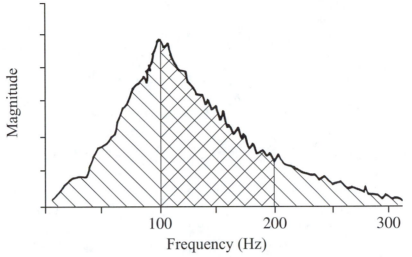

Figure 3–13 Power spectral density of the EMG signal with two band pass filters represented. *Source:* Reprinted with permission from JV Basmajian and C DeLuca, *Muscles Alive*, © 1985, Williams and Wilkins.

amount of force exerted over time. The amount of force eventually declines, and this is referred to as the *failure point* (point b). Just prior to that point, the RMS amplitude increases briefly. Figure 3–14B shows the power spectral density curves computed at the beginning of the contraction (point a) and just before the failure point (point b). During the initial part of the contraction, the median frequency of the spectrum (the 50th percentile) resides slightly above 100 Hz. During the muscle fatigue observed in this case, there is a downward shift in the shape of the power density such that the median frequency now resides around 55 Hz. In fatigued muscles, the shape of the frequency spectrum changes such that there is a diminution of the higher frequencies and an augmentation of the slower frequencies (see curve labeled (b)). This shift or fall in the median frequency could be attributed to the synchronization of motor unit recruitment patterns, a slowing of the conduction velocities of the muscle fibers, a shift in dominance from fast-twitch fiber to slow-twitch fiber as a result of the fatigability of the fast-twitch fibers, or a combination of all of the above.

In order to quantify the spectral shift secondary to fatigue, however, one must ask the patient to exert a steady isometric contraction at approximately 80% of maximum voluntary con-

traction (MVC) for a period of 1 minute. Such an analysis can be quite powerful. Researchers who studied the back muscles in this way in control subjects and pack pain patients reported that the initial shift in the median frequency and its course of recovery after 1 minute showed a sensitivity and specificity of 88% to 100%.[5] This type of specificity and sensitivity may be useful in distinguishing patients with true back pain from malingering patients. The work of DeLuca[6] and Roy et al[7,8] provides more information on this topic.

An understanding of spectral analysis and band pass filters will help practitioners interpret their clinical findings. The spectral analysis presented in Figure 3–15 is from a recording from a normal latissimus dorsi at 75% MVC for a 6-second epoch. A 1.7-second sample is taken from the middle of the contraction (marked by the vertical lines) and submitted for analysis. There are two spectral analyses, one for the right and one for the left aspect of the muscle. The 60-Hz notch filter is seen in each, with the power of the spectrum dropping sharply at the 60-Hz point. The median frequency of the spectrum is 92.2 Hz for the left aspect and 92.7 for the right aspect.

Figure 3–16 shows a raw sEMG tracing using a 20-to-450–Hz band pass filter, along with the power spectral density curve observed during a

A

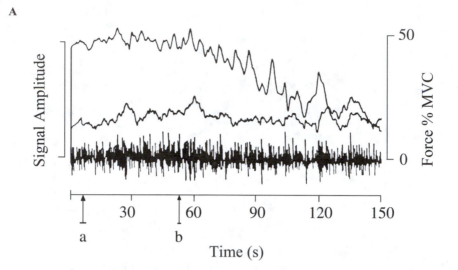

B

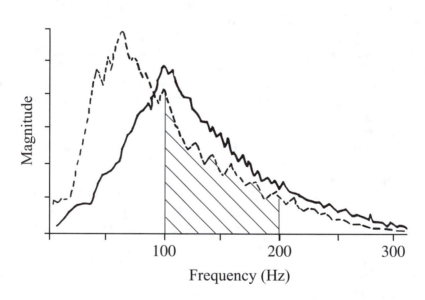

Figure 3–14 **(A)** Raw and RMS display of sEMG activity along with force exerted. **(B)** Power density display of the EMG signal during work (first peak) and fatigue (second peak). *Source:* Reprinted with permission from JV Basmajian and C DeLuca, *Muscles Alive*, © 1985, Williams and Wilkins.

resting baseline on a 17-year-old woman during an intense headache. The RMS microvolt level for the 15-second recording was 74.7 microvolts. Upon examining the power density curve, one can easily see that almost all of that energy resided below 40 Hz. Perhaps this is an indication of chronic muscle fatigue. Had the practitioner selected a 100-to-200–Hz filter during this examination (note the amount of energy present between 100 and 200 Hz on the spectral

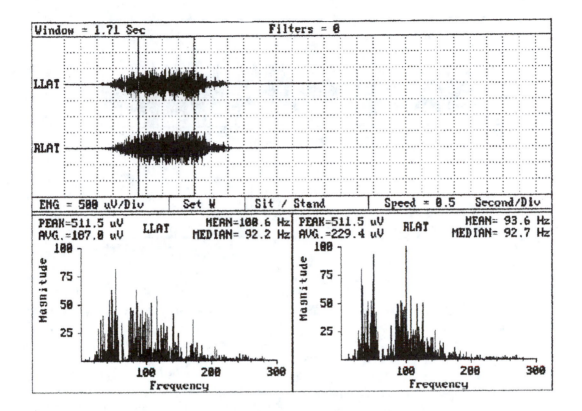

Figure 3–15 Power spectral analysis of an sEMG tracing from a normal contraction of latissimus dorsi. The upper panel shows the raw sEMG recording with the lines in the center representing the portion of the recording submitted for spectral analysis. The lower panel shows the spectral analysis of the sEMG signal. *Source:* Copyright © Clinical Resources, Inc.

analysis), the findings would have yielded a normal sEMG tracing.

Thus, it is important to know the filter characteristics of the sEMG instrument. This will help clinicians interpret the signals correctly. If the sEMG instrument has selective filters, it is important to choose the correct filter for the task at hand. We recommend using a narrow 100-to-200–Hz band pass filter when noise or artifact is problematic for interpretation and cannot otherwise be eliminated. A wider 20-to-300–Hz filter is generally preferred to display the sEMG signal most accurately. This level of band pass is sensitive to muscle fatigue, while the high pass (100-to-200–Hz) filter is not.

TYPES OF SURFACE ELECTROMYOGRAPHY VISUAL DISPLAYS

Once the sEMG signal has been amplified and filtered, it is prepared for visual display and quantitative presentation. There are four primary types of sEMG visual displays: raw sEMG, processed sEMG, spectral analysis, and probability amplitude histogram. Each style of presentation has its benefits and disadvantages.

The Raw Surface Electromyography Display

The raw sEMG display is the oldest form of sEMG presentation. It presents an unprocessed,

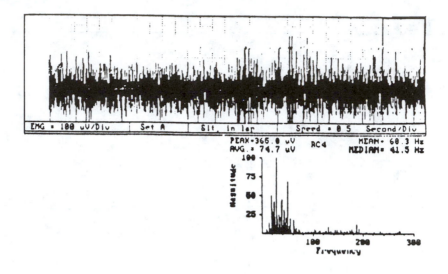

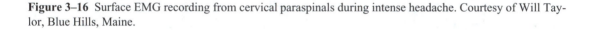

Figure 3–16 Surface EMG recording from cervical paraspinals during intense headache. Courtesy of Will Taylor, Blue Hills, Maine.

peak-to-peak oscilloscopic display of the sEMG signal. As the motor unit action potentials (MUAPs) summate and reach the skin, the small sEMG potentials are amplified and their sinusoidal nature is presented, as they oscillate between the positive and negative poles.

As Figure 3–17 illustrates, the sEMG signal oscillates in both the positive and negative directions, and also varies in its thickness and height. The thickness of the tracing represents the amplitude or strength of the contraction. The thicker the tracing, the stronger the sEMG signal and the stronger the contraction. In this example, the muscle goes from approximately 2 microvolts (μv) (peak to peak) at rest to approximately 200 μv (peak to peak) during the contraction. The unit of measurement for raw tracings is microvolts peak to peak (commonly referred to as pp). This represents the thickness of the tracing.

The advantage of the raw sEMG tracing is that it contains all of the information from the sEMG signal. None of it is processed out. One can readily see the various forms of artifact in the signal. These are explored in greater depth

later in this chapter and include 60-cycle noise, ECG artifact, and movement artifact. In addition, raw sEMG tracings allow clinicians to see postmovement irritability in a muscle that harbors a trigger point. Figure 3–17 demonstrates this phenomenon in a recording taken from the upper trapezius muscle following abduction. Before the movement, the muscle is quiet. During the movement, the sEMG activity rises appropriately and becomes thicker. However, following the cessation of the movement, the sEMG activity level does not return to the resting baseline level. Not only does it remain thicker, but it contains hairlike elements in the left upper trapezius (LUT) (top tracing) portion that extend above the majority of the tracing on a somewhat irregular basis. The right upper trapezius (RUT) (second tracing) also does not return to the baseline levels, but it lacks the hairlike elements. The LUT site contains an active trigger point, and the RUT site does not. The lack of return to premovement baseline levels and the hairlike elements seen in the postrecruitment pattern may represent a disturbance in the muscle spindle

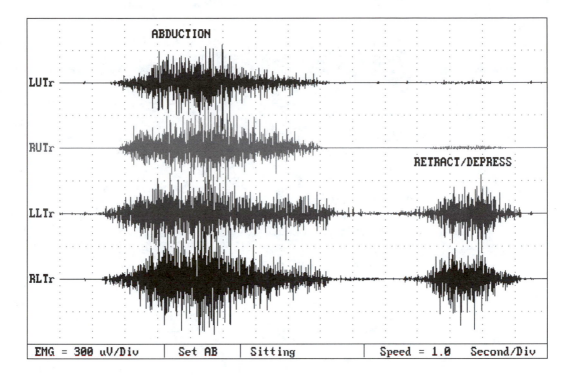

Figure 3–17 Raw sEMG tracing from the trapezius site during abduction and retraction. The signal goes from thin (low activity) to thick (high activity). *Source:* Copyright © Clinical Resources, Inc.

secondary to the presence of a trigger point. The assessment of trigger points is reviewed in Chapter 8.

The primary drawback of the raw sEMG display is that the additional information may make it more difficult for the patient to interpret the signal. This is relevant during biofeedback training sessions, in which the sEMG signal is presented to the patient as a means to guide the use of muscle. Teaching symmetry of movement, for example, may be easier if the two channels of sEMG are overlaid on top of each other so that the patient can see which muscle is higher or lower. In addition, when using a template to teach the patient a particular recruitment pattern, the processed signal is easier to use. An sEMG system that allows both processed and raw displays would be ideal.

The Processed Signal

The manufacturers of sEMG instruments have created ways to process the sEMG signal. This processing may be done either electronically by the resistors, capacitors, and integrated circuits (ICs) that follow the amplifier or digitally by computer software. Researchers have developed ways to process the sEMG signal as a means to make the signal easier to understand, read, and interpret. Because the very nature of muscle is a random, staccotic firing of groups of muscle fibers, finding ways to reduce the variability of muscle activity makes it a little easier to understand. As noted above, this may be especially important when the sEMG instrument is used to train patients in how to control their muscle function. The simpler and easier the

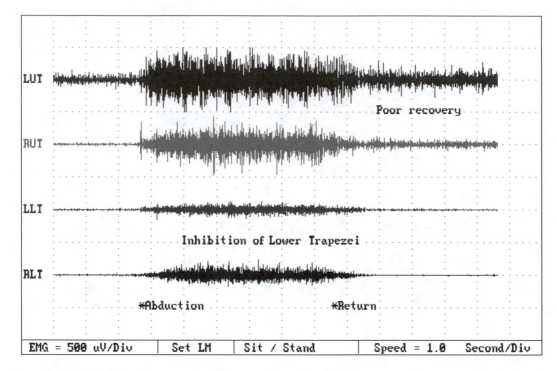

Figure 3–18 Activation and poor recovery for recordings taken from the upper and lower trapezius during abduction and recovery. The left upper trapezius (LUT) (upper tracing) contains an active trigger point. This is noted not only by the lack of recovery of amplitude during the recovery phase, but also by the presence of hairlike elements on the tracing. *Source*: Copyright © Clinical Resources, Inc.

sEMG display is to understand, the better the training effects.

Although the processing of the signal may result in a variety of quantities (ie, RMS, integral average), initially they all begin with a common series of steps. The first step in the process entails rectifying the signal. That is, the portion of the signal that resides below the 0 point (the negative electrical potential) is made positive and artificially placed above the 0 crossing line. This is illustrated in Figure 3–19.

The next step entails smoothing out the signal in some way. This is frequently done mathematically, and is commonly referred to as *digital filtering*. For example, rather than displaying every point of the rectified signal, an average of every six data points of sEMG data is plotted. This is referred to as *integral averaging*. By plotting the average of every six data points, the variability of the sEMG is reduced by a factor of

six. By increasing the number of samples in the average (eg, going from 6 samples to 20 samples), the amount of spontaneous variability in the sEMG signal is reduced. The "odd" sEMG value would get diluted by the 19 other values surrounding it.

Visually, the smoothing process is represented by taking the bumps out of the signal—by reducing its variability. It can be compared to putting shock absorbers on a car so that passengers do not feel every bump in the road. Figures 3–19 and 3–20 visually represent three levels of smoothing the data. Figure 3–19 shows the rectified tracing with very little in the way of smoothing (every six points are averaged and then plotted). Figure 3–20 shows higher degrees of averaging, with (A) representing an averaging of every 12 data points and (B) representing an averaging of every 24 points. The sEMG tracing gets progressively less jagged as the level of pro-

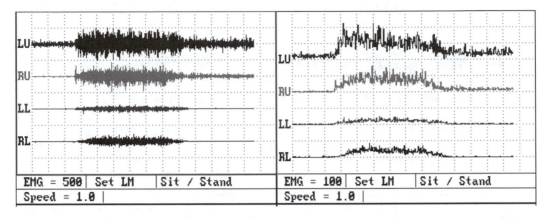

Figure 3–19 The raw sEMG signal of Figure 3–18 is placed side by side with its rectified and averaged display. The raw data points are averaged across every six data points and then drawn to the screen. The amount of upward deflection represents sEMG activity. The moment-to-moment amplitude of the sEMG varies considerably. *Source*: Copyright © Clinical Resources, Inc.

cessing increases. Instrument manufacturers refer to this phenomenon using different terms. Some call it *filtering*, since it is a form of digital filtering. Some call it a *time constant*, a term that comes out of the age of resistors and capacitors and refers to the amount of time it takes for an RC circuit to discharge its stored charge. Some refer to the process as *smoothing*.

QUANTIFICATION OF THE SURFACE ELECTROMYOGRAPHIC SIGNAL

Along with the visual presentation of information related to sEMG amplitude, sEMG information is also processed quantitatively. This process yields numbers that describe the amount of muscular energy expended. Because the sEMG signal oscillates between a positive and negative value or voltage, it is not possible simply to sum up all of the voltages to determine a quantity. This is because all of the positive values would cancel out all of the negative values, and the resulting sum would be zero. For this reason, there are three ways in which sEMG values are commonly derived: peak to peak, integral averaging, and RMS.

Peak to peak is used in raw sEMG recordings. It represents the amount of muscle energy measured from the top to the bottom of the tracing, or its width. Usually the peak-to-peak measure-

ment is summed and averaged over a period of time. Peak-to-peak values in a normal resting muscle might reside between 2 and 10 microvolts, depending upon the spacing of the electrodes, the degree of body fat below the sensors, the muscle that is being monitored, the posture in which it is being recorded, and the particular amplifier characteristics of the sEMG instrument.

Integral average (μv/sec) is used with the processed sEMG signals. It represents the simple arithmetic mean of the rectified sEMG over a given unit of time. The plus and minus signs of the raw sEMG data are ignored (the absolute value). These values are summed over the period of time defined and then divided by the number of values observed. This average would represent 0.637 of one half of the peak-to-peak value. The mean of the sEMG data is represented by the mathematical equation below:

$$\mu v/sec = I\{|m(t)|\} = 1/T \int_t^{t+T} |m(t)|\ dt$$

where T is the period time of integration.

RMS approaches the quantification of the sEMG signal by squaring the data, summing the squares, dividing this sum by the number of observations, and finally taking the square root. For technical reasons having to do with cancellation effects, this method of quantifying sEMG

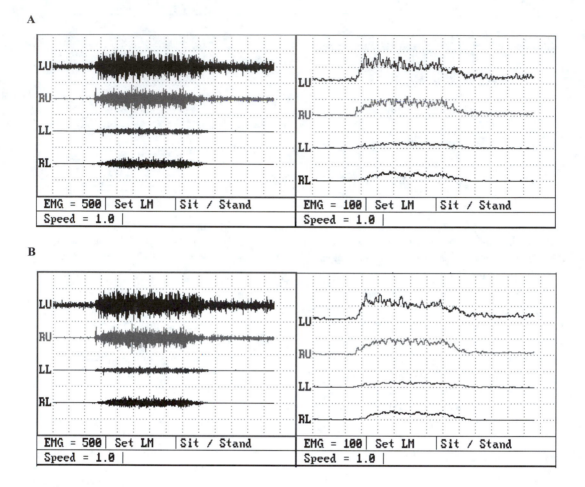

Figure 3–20 The effects of digital filtering or smoothing on the sEMG signal. (**A**) represents an averaging of every 12 data points; (**B**) represents an averaging of every 24 data points. *Source:* Copyright © Clinical Resources, Inc.

information is used more commonly than the integral averaging technique. It is thought to provide less distortion, because it converts an analog signal to a digital form. RMS represent 0.707 of one half of the peak-to-peak value. The RMS conversion is represented by the mathematical equation below:

$$RMS = \{|m(t)|\} = 1/T \, [\textstyle\int_{t}^{t+T} m^2 \, (t) \, dt]^{1/2}$$

where T is the period time of integration.

COMPARISON OF QUANTIFIED SURFACE ELECTROMYOGRAPHY VALUES ACROSS INSTRUMENTS

Each sEMG instrument handles the amplification, filtering, and quantification of the sEMG signal differently. For this reason, it is impossible to compare directly the values obtained on one sEMG instrument with the values obtained on an instrument from another manufacturer. Table 3–1 helps clinicians with this comparison

Table 3–1 Conversion Table for Benchmark

Instrument	Ratio
Benchmark	**1.00**
Davicon (30–300 Hz)	1.67
DMS 4000 (25–450 Hz)	1.17
Flexiplus (100–1000 Hz)	1.07
J&J M-53 (100–200 Hz)	1.00
J&J M-501 (100–200 Hz)	1.00
J&J M-501 (25–1000 Hz)	1.41
J&J I-410 Myoamp (Software Controlled)	1.31
Norodyne 8000 (25–450 Hz)	1.67
Physiotech 4000 (25–450 Hz)	1.17
SRS: Orion (100–1000 Hz)	1.07
SRS: Gemini (100–1000 Hz)	1.65
SRS: Gemini (25–1000 Hz)	2.31
SRS: Gemini (100–200 Hz)	1.08
SRS: Aries (100–200 Hz)	0.90
SRS: Aries (25–1000 Hz)	1.53
Thought Technology: Myotrac (100–200 Hz)	1.27
Thought Technology: Myotrac (20–500 Hz)	1.75
Thought Technology: Myotrac2 (100–200 Hz)	1.21
Thought Technology: Myotrac2 (20–500 Hz)	1.74
Thought Technology: Flexcomp (100–200 Hz)	1.21
Thought Technology: Flexcomp (20+ hi pass)	1.76
Thought Technology: Procomp (100–200 Hz)	1.13
Thought Technology: Procomp (20–500 Hz)	1.60
Verimed Myo2 Dual Channel (20–1000 Hz)	1.22
Verimed VStim 2 (20-1000 Hz)	1.26
Verimed Myo3 Dual (20–1000 Hz)	1.23
Verimed Myo2 (20–1000 Hz)	1.09

process by providing a benchmark basis for comparison. When colleagues want to share findings from different sEMG instruments, they can establish some rough equivalences of the findings from their various instruments. The major weakness of such a comparison is that it is not exact. In fact, it is difficult to make comparisons for sEMG signals in general. One should not directly compare, for example, isometric contractions to concentric contractions or an activity from one muscle to another. Clinicians should always exercise caution when making comparisons. Note that this table does not list all of the sEMG instruments that are commercially available, and that new sEMG instruments are

added over time. This list is not meant to provide an endorsement by the authors for any of the products listed.

The ratios presented in Table 3–1 were derived using the following procedure. Each instrument was provided with a standard input device (a signal generator), whose output provided a pink noise generator with frequencies within the typical range of muscle function and whose amplitudes averaged around 5 microvolts (J&J M-501 benchmark). The signal generator has been described as a "synthetic muscle." This output was sent to the amplifiers of the particular sEMG instruments. Five RMS values displayed by the instrument were recorded and averaged to determine the value for the particular sEMG instrument. A mathematical ratio was then calculated that compares all of the sEMG instruments to the J&J M-501 sEMG amplifier. The formula was:

Ratio = Test Instrument / J&J M-501

This ratio allows the provider to convert the RMS values listed for a particular instrument to a value that is comparable to other instruments. To make this comparison, the practitioner finds the conversion factor for his or her particular instrument, and multiplies the sEMG values by that ratio to obtain a standardized RMS value. The same procedure is used on the second instrument. The resulting values are then roughly equivalent.

COMPARISON OF QUANTIFIED SURFACE ELECTROMYOGRAPHY VALUES ACROSS MUSCLES AND INDIVIDUALS

Comparison of sEMG values both within and between individuals is potentially fraught with problems. Anthropomorphic differences between different recording sites and between individuals suggest cautious use of such comparisons. Some of the factors that might affect these comparisons include: thickness of subcutaneous adipose tissue, muscle resting length, velocity of contraction, muscle mass/cross-sectional area, fiber type, age, sex, subtle changes in posture, interelectrode distance, and impedance of the skin. The effects of the various anthropomorphic moderating variables on comparison between individuals are reviewed in some depth in Chapter 5. The bottom line is that it is possible to compare RMS values across muscle sites for the resting baseline conditions only. Population statistics for the sites of comparison are extremely valuable. However, during dynamic movements, comparison of amplitude measurements alone (ie, peak RMS) across muscle groups can be very misleading without first normalizing the sEMG data.

Researchers and practitioners have attempted to deal with these issues. One technique used to

control for these variables is called *normalization*.[9] There are several forms of normalization, each of which uses some sort of an anchor related to sEMG amplitudes. Each method calculates all other activity as a percentage of that anchor. The most common method is the *maximum voluntary isometric contraction (MVIC)*.[10] Here the patient is asked to make approximately three MVICs for the muscle group of interest. The middle 2 seconds of a 6-second contraction are recorded and then averaged over three trials of the MVIC. Then all subsequent recordings are referenced back to the strongest effort observed as %MVIC. All sEMG data points are then divided by the MVIC value, representing a percentage between 0 and 100%. There are no absolute microvolt values, only relative comparisons to a maximal effort. Thus, all muscle function can be reduced to this common feature of percentage of MVIC, and comparisons between muscles and individuals are made possible. For example, to compare the level of sEMG activity of upper trapezius to that of lower trapezius, one might ask the patient to make a resisted maximum contraction of upper trapezius during shoulder elevation, along with maximum contraction of lower trapezius during shoulder retraction and depression using a manual muscle-testing procedure. These values can then be used to calculate a percentage of MVIC for each muscle to compare the work done by lower trapezius to that of upper trapezius. Because of the differences in cross-sectional area for the two muscles, it would not be accurate to compare the peak RMS contraction of the lower trapezius directly to that of the upper trapezius during a task such as abduction versus flexion.

Unfortunately, this solution is not without its flaws. The primary problem with the technique is that it relies upon a voluntary component. How do we know whether the person has given his or her maximal effort? Is this maximal effort replicable for this individual across time? The illusion of objectivity of the technique should be placed into the context of a subjective, voluntary effort. Working with pain patients complicates this even further because they may choose not to give a maximal effort because it will hurt or because they want to protect themselves from hurting in the future. Restrictions in the range of motion of the patient may also create problems. The motivation of the patient may be suspect. A malingering patient may not put forth his or her best effort because it may hurt a claim or litigation.

Some of these objections may be overcome by requesting that the individual conduct a submaximal voluntary contraction. Here, the practitioner might ask the patient to exert a quantifiable force using a dynamometer, at 50% of what would commonly be seen for that muscle and that movement. Or the practitioner might ask the patient simply to conduct an abduction of the arm to 90 degrees as the standardized reference contraction for the upper and lower trapezius muscles. In either case, the practitioner might ask the patient to hold the position for 15 seconds, taking the middle 5 seconds as reference data. Averaging the middle 5 seconds over four repetitions provides a stable reference value. The reference anchor is used to calculate the %RVC (percentage of reference voluntary contraction). This type of normalization method has a higher reliability across testers compared to the maximum voluntary isometric contraction method.[10]

The next most common method is to record contractions as a function of a dynamic movement cycle, such as walking. Yang and Winter[9] and Knutson et al[10] have studied the submaximal contraction values for the *peak* of the contraction. This method provides a reliable anchor point when at least four repetitions of a movement have been conducted.[11] As a variation to using peak values for a single muscle, one could use the average of several muscles that are being monitored during the same movement as the anchoring point. Like %MVIC, the %RVC is now anchored to the peak or mean value observed during the dynamic movement, and percent values are derived from this. In the case of peak values, the %RVC is usually less than 100%. In the case of the mean value, the %RVC could exceed 100%. An example of this type of normalization might entail monitoring of the soleus, gastrocne-

mius, tibialis anterior, hamstrings, rectus femoris, gluteus maximus, gluteus medius, and tensor fasciae latae muscles during walking. The peak values of each muscle are obtained during at least four gait cycles. The average of the four peaks for each muscle are then used to determine the specific %RVC for each muscle during the gait cycle. In this way, one can compare the activation pattern of one muscle to another during the gait cycle. It is possible to compare not only the peak values, but also the minimum values (rest) as well as the slopes for recruitment and derecruitment of each muscle.

Although the two above techniques are not perfect reflections of a muscular effort, researchers have studied them extensively and know a great deal about them.[10–13] Both the maximal and relative contraction anchors appear to have reasonable test-retest reliability in the upper trapezius (11% to 15% coefficient of variation). The %MVIC appears to be more sensitive to contractions that require more effort and loses its sensitivity at low levels of effort. The %RVC is most appropriate when lower levels of activation are to be studied or assessed. When the above measures are studied on the gastrocnemius muscle for their reliability and relevance to knee-related problems, the %MVIC measure provides more reliable and reproducible data compared to the %RVC measures.[10] Thus, it not possible to select one normalization technique for all occasions. One must choose the best normalization method for the muscle and task to be studied.

Another strategy that can be used to avoid anthropomorphic issues is to study the percentage of asymmetry of a submaximal contraction between homologous muscle groups during a dynamic movement such as forward flexion of the head. The formula for this reflects the difference between the peak of contraction for the right and left aspect of homologous muscles as a ratio of the highest peak:

$$\%\text{asymmetry} = (\text{high peak} - \text{low peak})/\text{high peak}$$

Donaldson[14] has reported that this normalization procedure can differentiate between normal patients and pain patients during forward flexion of the head and torso. In addition, he has presented data that indicate whether a trapezius or sterno-cleidomastoid (SCM) muscle has a trigger point. He has proposed that a 20% cutoff point during the peak of concentric contraction separates out both groups. In reviewing Donaldson's data, it appears that the 40% to 50% range shows greater specificity. The main criticism of this technique is that the percentage of asymmetry may be due to mechanical problems, differences in range of motion, or posture, rather than muscle function. For example, a person may deviate the head slightly to the right during forward flexion because of a facet restriction, thus bringing about a recruitment asymmetry due to mechanical limitations rather than problems in muscle function per se. Careful observation, if not actual measurement of range of motion, should be factored into this type of measurement system. This would more clearly identify possible mechanical reasons for asymmetries. In addition, because this type of assessment requires movement, the asymmetries or levels of activation could possibly change with repetitions. Donaldson has reported that the correlation between the first movement and all other movements is exceptionally poor (personal communication). However, the correlation between the second repetition and subsequent repetitions is much higher. Thus, the practitioner might discard the first % asymmetry score (deeming it a practice movement), and rely more heavily on the third to fifth repetitions. The first and second trials are always discarded.

AMPLITUDE PROBABILITY DISTRIBUTION FUNCTION

The amplitude probability distribution function is a relatively new graphing technique for the sEMG signal, introduced by Jonsson in 1978.[15] Although this style of visual presentation is fairly new, the conceptual framework behind it is not. The curves presented in Figure 3–21 illustrate a way of plotting the variance of the signal. The range of amplitudes is plotted across the

bottom of the graph, instead of along the side. The percentage of time spent at a given amplitude is plotted along the side. When the histogram shows a high value, a large amount of time was spent at that given amplitude. In Figure 3–21, a person has engaged in a very light activity (eg, writing with a pencil) for 10 minutes. The amount of time spent at the continuum of RMS amplitudes is plotted. The high levels at the left-hand side of this curve indicate that a fairly large amount of time was spent at rest (defined as being below 5 microvolts RMS). But in the middle of the graph, another broader elevation indicates the amount of time that work was done. These plots show the probability of a given RMS amplitude—thus the term *amplitude probability distribution function*.

During rest or relaxation-oriented therapies, one would expect the distribution to take on the shape of the curve to the left of Figure 3–21. The curve would have a very narrow distribution located only at the low end of the amplitude spectrum, with perhaps a right-tailed kurtosis (flat tail) as the physiology of the muscle activity runs into the "cellar" of its ability to become more quiet. Cram[16] noted that perhaps it was the reduction of variability that was the "active ingredient" in relaxation-based biofeedback therapies, rather than the reduction in the actual amplitude of the signal. In Cram's study, headache sufferers were offered a relaxation-based biofeedback program or one that taught them to discriminate +/– 10% of the baseline values observed during their baseline condition. At the end of treatment, only the subjects in the relaxation group had learned to lower their general levels of sEMG amplitude for the frontal muscles, but both groups showed reductions in the variability of the sEMG signal. At the end of treatment, both groups showed a significant decrease in headache activity, and at 6-month follow-up the discrimination training group had not only maintained their gains but improved on them. The probability amplitude modulation curves allow the practitioner an opportunity to examine the variability of the sEMG signal.

Clinically, amplitude probability distribution function curves also allow one to examine the

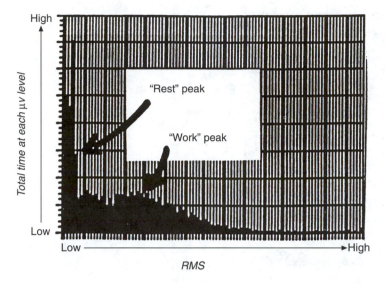

Figure 3–21 Amplitude probability distribution function during light work (writing with a pencil for 10 minutes). The range of sEMG amplitudes is along the *X* axis, while the probability of any given amplitude is plotted along the *Y* axis. Courtesy of Will Taylor, Blue Hills, Maine.

distribution of the sEMG signals for the occurrence of interspersed rest during a work period. Researchers[17,18] have observed that the distribution of the RMS amplitudes during work should be bimodal, as opposed to being unimodal or normally distributed. There should be one peak associated with the effort, and a second peak associated with micromomentary or interspersed rest. Again, an example of this type of configuration is noted in the work distribution of Figure 3–21. In several studies, workers who do not show the rest peak tend to develop muscle pain or tension myalgias in those muscles.[15,17] Usually, rest is defined as sEMG activity below the 5th percentile of either the %MVIC or the %RVC during a work cycle (see above). Using the J&J M-501 benchmark framework, this is approximately around the 5-microvolt RMS level. One can actually calculate the percentage of time spent below such an anchor point. Figure 3–22 illustrates a work pattern of the right and left upper trapezius during a light typing task that occurred over a 10-minute period of time for a patient with a tension myalgia on the right aspect of the shoulder/neck. The tracing for the left

upper trapezius (LUTr) shows a fairly typical distribution. The work amplitudes are relatively low, and there is a clearly defined rest peak present. The percentage of time below the 5-microvolt RMS level is 12.2%. Compared to LUTr, the right upper trapezius (RUTr) graph has a smaller distribution range for the *Y* axis (160 compared to 250). In addition, the RUTr graph shows a significantly greater dispersion of RMS amplitudes, with the highest peak being farther to the right on the graph. The rest peak is greatly diminished compared to the LUTr graph; only 3.8% of the time is spent below 5 microvolts RMS. Some clinicians believe that the percentage of time for rest below the 5-microvolt range should be greater than 5%. When the percentage of time below 5 microvolts RMS is less than 5%, pain is commonly experienced with prolonged exertion. This was the case for the patient example shown in Figure 3–22.

AUDITORY DISPLAYS

The discussion to this point has focused on visually oriented displays. Many sEMG instru-

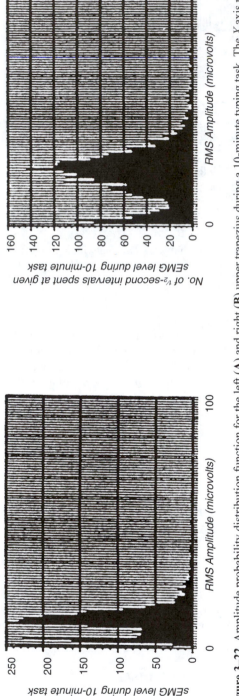

Figure 3–22 Amplitude probability distribution function for the left (**A**) and right (**B**) upper trapezius during a 10-minute typing task. The *X* axis represents 0–100 microvolts RMS. The *Y* axis represents the number of half-second periods of time spent at a given RMS amplitude. Note that the scale for these counts differs for the graphs (**A**) and (**B**). The peak rest and work values for (**A**), the normal side of the patient, are around 2 and 10, respectively. The rest and work peaks for (**B**), the painful side of the patient, are around 2 and 23, respectively. Courtesy of Will Taylor, Blue Hills, Maine.

ments also have auditory capabilities. Some of the finer instruments allow the observer to listen to the raw sEMG signal. This feature is always incorporated in needle EMG systems and provides some of the clues that guide diagnosis. In sEMG, the raw signal sounds like white noise or the ocean. When it is contaminated with 60-cycle interference, one can hear a distinct hum. Many biofeedback instruments convert the sEMG signal into a variety of tones or "musical instruments." For example, the pitch may go higher as the sEMG amplitude goes higher.

Audio tones are commonly linked to thresholds. Here, the practitioner sets an amplitude level, and whenever the sEMG goes above that amplitude, a special tone is played. These thresholds may be used to "shape" the patient's sEMG signals to higher or lower levels. Shaping is a process in which the practitioner gradually increases (or decreases) the threshold as the patient shows improvement in obtaining the threshold goal.

ISSUES REGARDING NOISE AND ARTIFACT

Noise and artifact are functionally defined as anything contained in the sEMG signal that the practitioner does not want. One attribute of an sEMG amplifier is its signal-to-noise ratio. An ideal amplifier has a very high signal-to-noise ratio—all signal and no noise. Below are some of the primary examples of noise and artifact that pertain to the internal noise of the electronic circuitry of the instrument. Noise from outside the instrument may also be a problem.

A common source of noise for the electromyographer is the *ECG artifact*. The ECG is very coherent and much larger than that of the muscles. It is clearly picked up on nearly all of the sites located on the torso. It is primarily seen on the left side of the body, and therefore may lead to asymmetrical RMS values during rest. This artifact is clearly shown in both raw and processed sEMG tracings from the left serratus anterior (LSer) in Figure 3–23. It is also commonly seen in the left lumbar area. ECG artifact is not commonly seen in the extremities, except when wrist-to-wrist or ankle-to-ankle leads are used. ECG artifact can be minimized by placing the electrodes close together and using a 100-to-200–Hz band pass filter. Many practitioners, however, readily accept the ECG artifact as a fact of life and merely educate the patient about this phenomenon. As a side benefit, one could use the ECG as an index of arousal by observing changes in the patient's pulse rate.

Movement artifact is seen as direct current (DC) shifts and/or massive deflections in the sEMG potentials of the raw sEMG recording. This occurs because the electrode slips around on the surface of the skin, generating an electrical potential of its own. The upper panel of Figure 3–23A shows this slippage in the raw sEMG for the left serratus anterior site as a distortion in the DC levels around which the sEMG signal oscillates. In this particular instance, there is a momentary slippage of the electrode as a function of skin distortion (stretch) as the patient moves his or her arms out of abduction and into shoulder elevation. When this tracing is then converted to the processed mode (Figure 3–23B), however, the movement artifact simply appears as an upward deflection. With the process mode, it is difficult to differentiate the movement artifact from the real sEMG signal. Only in the raw mode can the practitioner discriminate movement artifact from the real sEMG recruitment. Movement artifact can be reduced by using floating electrodes rather than direct-contact electrodes. The cushion of paste between the skin and the electrode can absorb the electrode slippage and greatly reduce this type of artifact. An additional strategy involves taping the electrodes to the body of the patient so they do not sway or pull on the electrodes.

Another major source of noise is *60-cycle energy*, which we use to power lights, offices, and the computers used to monitor the sEMG. This is such a significant source of noise that nearly all sEMG instruments have a special notch filter to

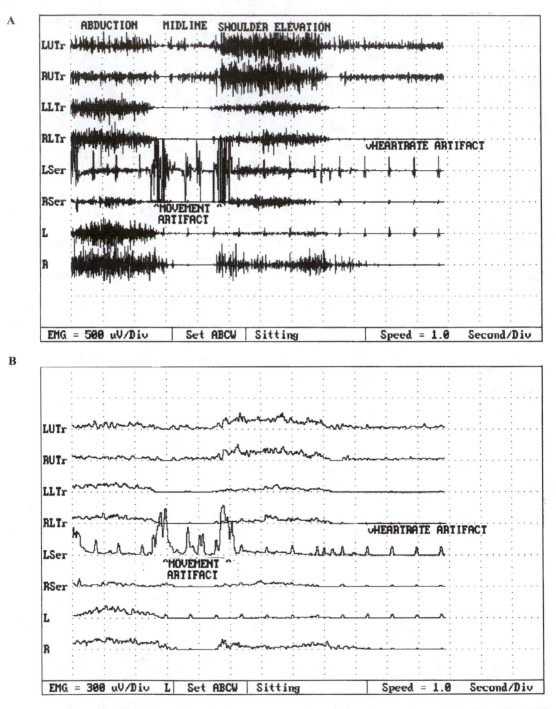

Figure 3–23 (**A**) Raw and (**B**) processed sEMG tracings with clear ECG and movement artifact. The ECG artifact is clearly seen as rhythmic deflections in the serratus anterior (LSer) for both the raw and processed tracings. The movement artifact is seen in the DC shifts in the LSer for the raw tracing. Note how it is difficult to discern the movement artifact in the LSer track of the processed EMG recording. *Source:* Copyright © Clinical Resources, Inc.

try and eradicate it. However, poor electrode connections can easily provide the medium by which the 60-cycle noise exceeds the capacity of the notch filter to eliminate it, and it thus spills over into the visual and quantitative displays. A 60-cycle artifact may be seen in the oscillating pattern in Figure 3–9. It is represented in a more subtle way in the left upper trapezius of Figure 3–24A. This type of artifact is typically easier to see with a raw sEMG display than with a processed one. Figure 3–24B shows the spectral analysis of a 1-second epoch of the tracing in Figure 3–24A. Here, one can see that the 60-Hz portion of the signal has successfully been eliminated. Unfortunately, the harmonics of 60-cycle energy have not been filtered out and contribute heavily to the signal. This is seen as "telephone poles" in the spectral analysis at 120 Hz, 180 Hz, and 240 Hz.

If clinicians observe a 60-cycle artifact, they should begin troubleshooting by replacing the electrodes along with a vigorous abrade. They should reduce the possibility that the electrode leads are acting like an antenna that picks up the noise. Single-stranded leads should be twisted tightly together, and the length of the leads should be shortened if possible. Shielded leads can be tried instead. Clinicians may also want to eliminate any possible sources of 60-cycle noise in the recording environment. One common source of this noise is the computer monitor. The patient should be as far away from the computer as possible (a minimum of 3 feet).

Respiration is another biological artifact commonly seen in sEMG recordings. This artifact is most commonly seen in the upper torso and neck. Specifically, placements on the upper trapezius, scalene, and sternocleidomastoid muscles may show sEMG potentials associated with breathing. This is shown for the scalene muscles in Figure 3–25. Both sets of these muscles are considered ancillary muscles of respiration, and they are invoked when the patient needs to raise the ribs in order to facilitate breathing into the upper lobes of the lungs. This is very common in high-demand situations such as running. During quiet sitting, however, it is highly unusual to see large recruitment patterns associated with respiration in these muscles. The major exceptions to

this rule are patients with chronic obstructive pulmonary disease or patients who breathe in a paradoxical fashion. When this artifact is noted, biofeedback training for the correct respiratory pattern is indicated.

Another possible artifact is caused by radio frequency (RF). Here, the signals from a local radio station are picked up by the antenna effect of the electrode leads and fed into the amplifiers. This phenomenon is fairly rare but does happen. It can be observed most dramatically on sEMG instruments with a raw sEMG audio option, when the radio can be heard on the speaker. Using only the visual display in a processed or raw mode, the practitioner would note large, spontaneous changes in the sEMG signal that have nothing to do with the patient's movements. If RF noise is suspected, it is necessary to move the sEMG instrument into another room or to the other side of the building. Moving the recording environment is the only solution to RF noise.

One other biological artifact is known as cross-talk. This occurs when the energy from a distant muscle reaches the electrodes placed over another muscle site. Although it is the bane of dynamic sEMG, it really does not matter for relaxation-oriented protocols. A very clear example of cross-talk is seen in frontal sEMG recordings when the patient clenches the teeth. This may be seen in Figure 3–26, which illustrates the specificity of the frontal recording site during an eyebrow flash. Cross-talk occurs when the energy of the masseter and temporalis muscles that are recruited during a clench are picked up by the frontal leads.

Careful placement of closely spaced electrodes is the only hope for limiting the cross-talk artifact. It is important to recognize its presence and to monitor from those potentially offending distant muscles.

HOW TO CHECK SPECIFICATIONS OF SURFACE ELECTROMYOGRAPHIC INSTRUMENTS

Not all sEMG instruments are made alike. In a review of 11 sEMG instruments, Rugh and Schwitzgebel[19] noted tremendous variability in

A

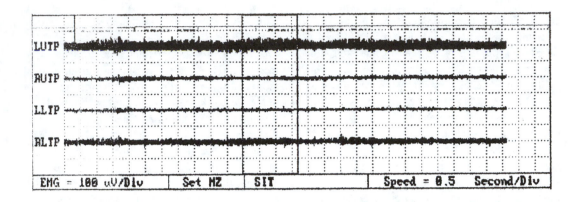

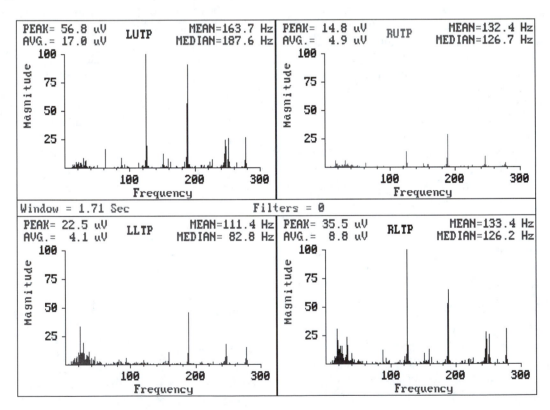

Figure 3–24 (A) Raw sEMG tracing contaminated with 60-Hz noise. **(B)** Spectral analysis of the signal showing the harmonics of 60-Hz noise. *Source:* Copyright © Clinical Resources, Inc.

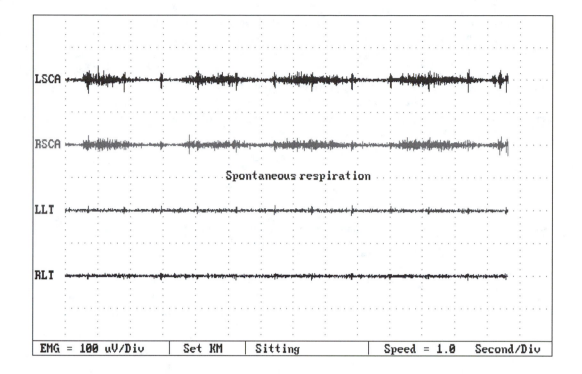

| EMG = 100 uV/Div | Set KM | Sitting | Speed = 1.0   Second/Div |

Figure 3–25 Surface EMG recordings from scalene (LSCA and RSCA) and lower trapezius (LLT and RLT) muscles. The scalene muscles show a clear respiration artifact. *Source:* Copyright © Clinical Resources, Inc.

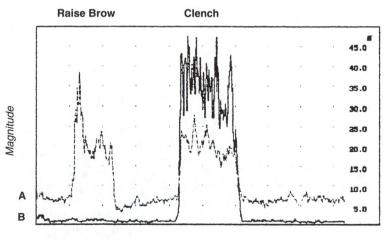

Figure 3–26 Cross-talk from the masseter muscle (**A**) may clearly be seen in the frontal leads (**B**) during a jaw clench.

several key features. It is important for practitioners to know what to look for in the sEMG instruments they are currently using or planning to acquire. The purpose of this section is not to compare one sEMG system directly with another, but rather to recap the instrumentation issues presented in this chapter so that practitioners can note their own instruments' strengths and weaknesses or make an informed choice in an equipment purchase. Table 3–2 reviews the different attributes of sEMG instruments.

As an aid to the practitioner, a checklist is provided that lists all of the attributes of an sEMG instrument (Exhibit 3–1). This form can be used to organize all of the information available on an instrument.

Table 3–2 The Specifications of Surface Electromyographic Instruments

Concept	Desirable Range	Comments
Input impedance	100 kilohm 1 gigaohm	Most commercial machines have 1 megohm input impedance or better. This is more than adequate for medical uses.
Common mode rejection (CMR or CMMR)	70–180 decibels	This determines the ability of the sEMG amplifier to eliminate external noise from the environment, such as noise from energy used to power lights and computers. In general, the higher this value the better.
Instrument noise level	0.1–1.0 microvolt	This represents the lowest level of sEMG an instrument can pick up. It is, in essence, the noise level of the sEMG amplifier. The lower the better. Most commercially available instruments allow detection of 0.5 microvolt or higher.
Band pass filter width General case Relaxation training Musculoskeletal assessment and rehabilitation Facial muscle recordings	20–1000 Hz 100–200 Hz 20–300 Hz 20–600 Hz	Most of the sEMG energy resides between 20 and 300 Hz. The facial muscles are exceptions; because they are closer to the surface, are smaller, and have a high innervation ratio, they can be monitored up to 600 Hz. The band pass width also determines the nature of the noise that is let in. ECG artifact can be all but eliminated by using a 100–200 Hz filter. If the sEMG instrument allows the user to set the band pass filter width, it provides more degrees of freedom. The filter width should be selected to fit the type of work. When working with musculoskeletal dysfunction or soft tissue injury, where the muscle may have a fatigue component, the practitioner should make sure that the lower end of the band pass is around 20 Hz. On the other hand, the 100–200 Hz filter width should work fine with relaxation-based work.

continues

Table 3–2 continued

Concept	Desirable Range	Comments
Range/gain		Range represents the amplitude that can be moni-
General case	0–1000 RMS µv	tored using a particular sEMG instrument. For
	0–1000 RMS µv	dynamic sEMG recordings, the general case of
Dynamic	0–100 RMS µv	amplitude should be possible. If the sEMG
movement		instrument has a range of 0–500 µv and the
Relaxation		practitioner is studying events that exceed that
		amount, the amplifiers would simply saturate at the
		top end of the scale and potentially valuable
		information would be lost. For relaxation-oriented
		work, one would not expect to see amplitudes over
		100 µv. It is best if the instrument allows the
		practitioner to select from several ranges so that
		the recording can be sensitive to what is being
		studied or treated.
Smoothing options	0.1–10 second time constant	The smoothing option on an sEMG instrument may or may not be specified as a time constant. Usually it is necessary to turn a dial or increment a number on a computerized system. Sometimes this feature is referred to as a filter, which refers to digital filtering or smoothing.[20] It is highly desirable for instruments to allow the practitioner to choose how much smoothing or processing of the signal is done.
Visual displays		The visual display is the practitioner's link to the sEMG information. It should be easy to read.
Meter	Linear versus logarithmic	Meters commonly come in two varieties: linear and logarithmic. With linear meters, there is an equal spacing between each number. This is the most common type of meter. Logarithmic meters give more space to the low end than the high end of the scale. We have more precision in how we use our muscles at the low microvolt level than at the high microvolt level. The logarithmic meter makes more sense for relaxation work.
Digital		Digital displays are highly desirable so that the practitioner can see the quantified sEMG as it changes from moment to moment. It is always nice to be able to control how frequently the digital value updates.
Computer	Raw and processed	Computer displays allow the practitioner to see time series scrolls of the sEMG information. Instruments that allow the practitioner to choose between the raw and processed signals offer the greatest versatility. In general, raw sEMG provides greater diagnostic information, while processed visual displays are easier for the patient to understand.

continues

Table 3–2 continued

Concept	Desirable Range	Comments

Audio displays
  Raw sEMG
    audio
  Thresholds
  Binary versus
    analog
	Raw
	Feedback
		The audio portion of the sEMG should be considered. A raw sEMG channel yields valuable diagnostic information to the trained ear. The audio feedback features of an sEMG instrument are essential for retraining purposes. This feedback may be in the form of an analog tone—one that simply varies in pitch. Or it may come in the form of a binary tone that comes on only when the patient is above or below a preset threshold. With today's multimedia computer capabilities, it is possible to play music or complex tones or even have the computer talk to the patient.

Exhibit 3–1 Surface EMG Unit Worksheet for Physical Medicine Practitioners

Check User Priorities *Criteria*	*Unit Name/Model*			
Stand-alone (SA), personal computer (PC), both (B)	SA/PC/B	SA/PC/B	SA/PC/B	SA/PC/B
___ Special computer requirements				
Power source/safety				
___ 3-prong plug, optical isolation	yes/no/NA	yes/no/NA	yes/no/NA	yes/no/NA
___ battery type/life	NA	NA	NA	NA
Electrode compatibility				
___ Any (A), manufacturer's electrode only (M)	A/M	A/M	A/M	A/M
___ Electrode system	active/passive	active/passive	active/passive	active/passive
___ Electrode distance	fixed/modifiable	fixed/modifiable	fixed/modifiable	fixed/modifiable
Lead wires				
___ Electrode connectors	snap/alligator	snap/alligator	snap/alligator	snap/alligator
___ Shielding, general quality	sturdy/okay/flimsy	sturdy/okay/flimsy	sturdy/okay/flimsy	sturdy/okay/flimsy
___ Quality of amplifier connectors	sturdy/okay/flimsy	sturdy/okay/flimsy	sturdy/okay/flimsy	sturdy/okay/flimsy
___ Ground lead	integral/separate	integral/separate	integral/separate	integral/separate
___ Lead length				
Amplifier				
___ Input impedance				
___ **CMRR (common mode rejection ratio)**				
___ Total gain				
Frequency filter				
___ Band width limits/roll–off	/	/	/	/
___ 60-Hz notch filter/roll–off	yes/no	yes/no	yes/no	yes/no
Sampling rate				
Time constant/smoothing range				
Microvolt quantification				
___ RMS, integral avg., other				

continues

Exhibit 3–1 continued

Check User Priorities

Criteria	Unit Name/Model			
Adequate noise suppression	always/not always	always/not always	always/not always	always/not always
Visual display output				
Display type	video/crystal/LED	video/crystal/LED	video/crystal/LED	video/crystal/LED
Display type	linear/log/both	linear/log/both	linear/log/both	linear/log/both
Optional raw display	yes/no	yes/no	yes/no	yes/no
Digital	yes/no	yes/no	yes/no	yes/no
Moving line, oscilloscope-like	yes/no	yes/no	yes/no	yes/no
Variable sweep speed	yes/no	yes/no	yes/no	yes/no
Bar graph	yes/no	yes/no	yes/no	yes/no
Motor templates	yes/no	yes/no	yes/no	yes/no
Games, others	yes/no	yes/no	yes/no	yes/no
Audio output				
Modulating	pitch/click/other	pitch/click/other	pitch/click/other	pitch/click/other
Optional raw audio	yes/no	yes/no	yes/no	yes/no
Audio yoking to signal				
Above goal	yes/no	yes/no	yes/no	yes/no
Below goal	yes/no	yes/no	yes/no	yes/no
Between dual goals	yes/no	yes/no	yes/no	yes/no
Sensitivity	manual/auto only/ manual & auto	manual/auto only/ manual & auto	manual/auto only/ manual & auto	manual/auto only/ manual & auto
Adjustment	yes/no	yes/no	yes/no	yes/no
Adequate low-end response range	yes/no	yes/no	yes/no	yes/no
Adequate high-end response range	yes/no	yes/no	yes/no	yes/no
Choice of sensitivity ranges	okay/limited	okay/limited	okay/limited	okay/limited
Ease of adjustment	easy/okay/difficult	easy/okay/difficult	easy/okay/difficult	easy/okay/difficult
Scale offset available	yes/no	yes/no	yes/no	yes/no
Thresholds/goals				
Easy to see	easy/okay/difficult	easy/okay/difficult	easy/okay/difficult	easy/okay/difficult
Ease of adjustment	easy/okay/difficult	easy/okay/difficult	easy/okay/difficult	easy/okay/difficult
EMG channels				
Number				
Modular additions possible	yes/no	yes/no	yes/no	yes/no
Graphic print capability	yes/no	yes/no	yes/no	yes/no

	Column 1	Column 2	Column 3	Column 4
	max/min/avg/rng ratio/% diff	max/min/avg/rng ratio/% diff	max/min/avg/rng ratio/% diff	max/min/avg/rng ratio/% diff
Comments regarding print functions/ report generation				
EMG data storage capacity				
Statistical management				
Event counter	yes/no	yes/no	yes/no	yes/no
Frequency spectral analysis	yes/no	yes/no	yes/no	yes/no
Download to statistics package	yes/no	yes/no	yes/no	yes/no
Software: general				
Overall ease of operation	easy/okay/difficult	easy/okay/difficult	easy/okay/difficult	easy/okay/difficult
Labeled/dedicated keys	yes/no	yes/no	yes/no	yes/no
Menu driven	yes/no	yes/no	yes/no	yes/no
Mouse drag and click	yes/no	yes/no	yes/no	yes/no
Ability to store patient files	yes/no	yes/no	yes/no	yes/no
Playback ability	yes/no	yes/no	yes/no	yes/no
Other special software features				
Software upgradable	yes/no	yes/no	yes/no	yes/no
External relay for neuromuscular electrical stimulation	yes/no	yes/no	yes/no	yes/no
Ease of EMG-NMES software	easy/okay/difficult	easy/okay/difficult	easy/okay/difficult	easy/okay/difficult
Cost				
Finance/lease arrangements				
Warranty period				
After-purchase services				
Area representative	yes/no	yes/no	yes/no	yes/no
Educational support	yes/no	yes/no	yes/no	yes/no
Trade-ins for upgrades	yes/no	yes/no	yes/no	yes/no
Other				
Other comments				

Courtesy of Movement Systems, Inc., Seattle, Washington.

REFERENCES

1. Peek CJ. A primer of biofeedback instrumentation. In Schwartz M, ed. *Biofeedback: A Practitioner's Guide*. New York: Guilford Press; 1987:45–95.

2. Basmajian JV, DeLuca C. *Muscles Alive*. 5th ed. Baltimore: Williams & Wilkins; 1985.

3. Soderberg GL, ed. *Selected Topics in Surface Electromyography for Use in the Occupational Setting: Expert Perspective*. Washington, DC: US Dept of Health and Human Services; 1992. US Dept of Health and Human Services publication NIOSH 91-100.

4. Cacioppo JT, Tassinary G, Fridlund AJ. The skeletalmotor system. In: Cacioppo JT, Tassinary G, eds. *Principles of Psychophysiology*. New York: Cambridge University Press; 1990:325–384.

5. Kessler M, Cram JR, Traue H. EMG muscle scanning in pain patients and controls: a replication and extension. *Am J Pain Manage*. 1993;3:20–28.

6. DeLuca C. Myoelectric manifestations of localized muscular fatigue in humans. *CRC Crit Rev Biomed Eng*. 1984;11:251.

7. Roy SH, DeLuca CJ, Casavant DA. Lumbar muscle fatigue and chronic back pain. *Spine*. 1989;14:992–1001.

8. Roy SH, DeLuca CJ, Snyder-Mackler L, et al. Fatigue, recovery and low back pain in elite rowers. *Med Sci Sports Exerc*. 1990;22:463–469.

9. Yang JF, Winter DA. Electromyographic amplitude normalization methods: improving their sensitivity as a diagnostic tool in gait analysis. *Arch Phys Med*. 1984;65:517–521.

10. Knutson LM, Soderberg GL, Ballantyne BT, Clarke WR. A study of various normalization procedures for within day electromyographic data. *J Electromyogr Kinesiol*. 1994;1:47–59.

11. Mathiassen SE, Winkel J, Hagg GM. Normalization of surface EMG amplitude from the upper trapezius muscle in ergonomic studies: A review. *J Electromyogr Kinesiol*. 1995;5:197–226.

12. Attebrant M, Mathiassen SE, Winkel J. Normalizing upper trapezius EMG amplitude: comparison of ramp and constant force procedures. *J Electromyogr Kinesiol*. 1995;5:245–250.

13. Bao S, Mathiassen SE, Winkel J. Normalizing upper trapezius EMG amplitude: comparison of different procedures. *J Electromyogr Kinesiol*. 1995;5:251–257.

14. Donaldson S, Donaldson M. Multi-channel EMG assessment and treatment techniques. In: Cram JR, ed. *Clinical EMG for Surface Recordings, II*. Nevada City, CA: Clinical Resources; 1990:143–174.

15. Jonsson B. Kinesiology. With special reference to electromyographic kinesiology. *Cont Clin Neurophysiol EEG Suppl*. 1978;34:417–428.

16. Cram JR. EMG biofeedback and the treatment of tension headaches: a systematic analysis of treatment components. *Behav Ther*. 1980;11:699–710.

17. Veiersted KB, Westgaard RH, Andersen P. Electromyographic evaluation of muscular work pattern as a predictor of trapezius myalgia. *Scan J Work Environ Health*. 1993;19:284–290.

18. Veiersted KB, Westgaard RH. Work related risk factors for trapezius myalgia. *Int Arch Occup Environ Health*. 1990;62:31–41.

19. Rugh J, Schwitzgebel R. Variability in commercial electromyographic biofeedback devices. *Behav Res Methods Instrum*. 1977;9:281–285.

20. J & J Engineering. *USE Language and PC Interface*. Poulsbo, WA: J&J Enterprises; 1988.

Chapter Questions

1. The tissue of the human body acts like:
   a. a high-pass filter
   b. a low-pass filter
   c. a notch filter
   d. an amplifier

2. A differential amplifier
   a. amplifies the difference of two separate muscle sites
   b. finds the difference between two muscles
   c. amplifies everything that is common to the recording electrodes
   d. amplifies everything that is unique to the recording electrodes

3. Which of the following would represent a band reject filter?
   a. 100-to-200–Hz band pass filter
   b. 60-Hz notch filter
   c. 35-Hz low-pass filter
   d. 20-Hz high-pass filter

4. Which of the following amplifiers is considered to have the best common mode rejection?
   a. 70 dB
   b. 50 µv
   c. 140 dB
   d. 10 megohm

5. How much larger should the impedance of the electrode to skin interface be than the input impedance of the amplifier?
   a. 2 times greater
   b. 5 times greater
   c. 10 to 100 times greater
   d. equal to the input impedance of the amplifier

6. How would the sEMG recordings of an obese individual compare to the sEMG levels of a very thin individual?
   a. They would be the same.
   b. They would be higher.
   c. They would be lower.
   d. It doesn't matter.

7. When monitoring the gluteus maximus and rectus femoris muscles during hip flexion and extension, how should the practitioner compare these two muscles?
   a. Compare RMS microvolts only.
   b. Compare only integral averages.
   c. Compare only normalized recordings.
   d. One cannot compare these two muscles.

8. Which filter typically eliminates or dramatically reduces any ECG artifact from sEMG recordings?
   a. 25-Hz high-pass filter
   b. 60-Hz notch filter
   c. 100-to-200–Hz band pass filter
   d. 35-Hz low-pass filter

9. During muscle fatigue, what typically happens to the median frequency of the sEMG power density?
   a. It stays constant.
   b. Its value falls.
   c. Its value rises.
   d. Its value rises in an inverse relation to sEMG amplitude.

10. Raw sEMG tracings are commonly quantified using which of the following methods?
    a. Peak to peak
    b. RMS
    c. Integral average
    d. Raw

11. When examining the sEMG signal for interspersed rest, what is the criterion level at which rest is defined (J&J M501 Benchmark)?
    a. Below 2 microvolts
    b. Below 5 microvolts
    c. Below 20 microvolts
    d. Below 50 microvolts

12. The power spectral density curves used to examine the distribution of muscle energy across the various frequencies of the sEMG recording uses which of the following methods of analysis?
    a. FFT
    b. sEMG
    c. ABC
    d. Mean extrapolation

13. The energy spectrum of sEMG during work commonly resides within which of the following frequency bands?
    a. 20–300 Hz
    b. 100–200 Hz
    c. 20–1000 Hz
    d. 20–40 Hz

14. In sEMG, RMS refers to:
    a. Random motor stimulation
    b. Root mean square
    c. Rotary motion study
    d. Random motion stabilization

15. The ECG artifact is most commonly found where?
    a. on the extremities
    b. on the torso
    c. on the left aspect of the torso
    d. on the cephalic muscles

16. *Smoothing* is a term that refers to
    a. digital filtering
    b. how to abrade the skin for electrode placement
    c. the quality of a movement pattern during training
    d. relaxation training protocols

17. What can be said about sEMG amplitudes and force?
    a. There is a one-to-one relationship.
    b. There is a curvilinear relationship.
    c. There is no relationship.
    d. It actually doesn't make sense to focus on this relationship because the issues are far too complex.

18. The impedance at each recording electrode should be:
    a. low
    b. high
    c. low and balanced
    d. high and balanced

CHAPTER 4

Electrodes and Site Selection Strategies

ELECTRODE SELECTION

Electrodes are like tiny microphones that are used to listen to the muscles. Because there are several types of electrodes available on the market, practitioners should know the intended use of each and select the electrode that provides the highest quality of surface electromyography (sEMG) recording. Figure 4–1 shows a variety of electrodes available for the practitioner.

In making the selection, practitioners should consider the size of the electrode. Electrodes with smaller detection areas (and housings) allow closer interelectrode spacings and thus a higher level of selectivity.[1] Small electrodes are important in recordings from the facial muscles and from some of the muscles of the upper extremities. These electrodes might be 0.5 cm in diameter and placed at an interelectrode distance of 1 cm. For larger, broad muscles, electrodes with larger surface areas are desirable and may be placed farther apart. For example, a very common electrode on the market provides a 1-cm diameter pellet, placed an interelectrode distance of 2 cm. This size and spacing works for many sites. As the interelectrode spacing increases to 3 cm, larger, broader muscles may be monitored. As the interelectrode distance increases, the specificity of the recording decreases and recordings become more "regional." A 2-cm spacing on upper trapezius provides a very specific recording for that muscle. The wide trapezius placement provides a regional re-

cording of the upper back. Here, the recording electrodes are placed quite far apart, with one electrode on the right and one electrode on the left aspect of trapezius.

Some electrodes are placed in direct contact with the skin, while others float on a cushion of paste above the skin. *Direct contact electrodes* are small disks that are placed directly on the skin and held in place by tape. These are the type of electrodes originally used for sEMG. In the past, these electrodes were usually made of silver or gold, and a small amount of saline paste was placed between the electrode and the skin. Some practitioners soldered a lead to a silver quarter or nickel and then taped it over the muscle of interest. Today, direct contact electrodes are commonly 0.5 to 1 cm in diameter and are made of a disposable silver-impregnated plastic that is coated with a thin layer of silver chloride to help stabilize the electrical potentials of the skin. They are held in place with a small adhesive or foam collar that is slightly larger than the pellet. The adhesive quality of collars varies greatly. Some are diaphoretic (allowing perspiration through). One should consider the adhesion properties of the collar or electrode when choosing the appropriate electrode for the site of interest. For example, electrodes placed on the low back need to adhere very well to the skin because the area is subject to extreme skin distortions and stretching during dynamic movements. However, when recording from the facial muscles, some patients cannot tolerate an ex-

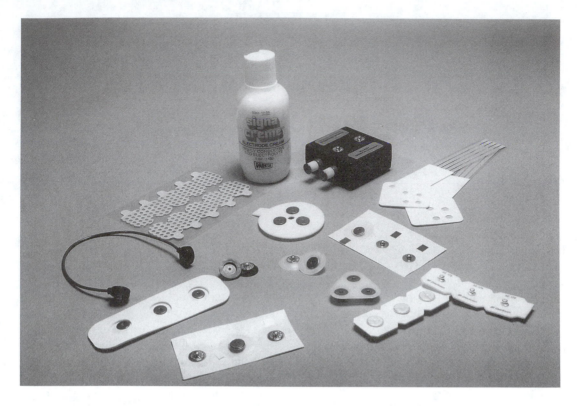

Figure 4–1 Types of sEMG electrodes.

tremely adhesive pad. Hydrogel electrodes (see below) provide a very gentle adhesive to be used on patients with sensitive skin.

Direct contact electrodes are ideal for quiet sEMG recordings (ie, relaxation-based therapies). Because they reside directly on the skin, they are more subject to movement artifact (see Chapter 3) and, therefore, are not recommended for recording of dynamic movements. Activity of the body may create movement of the electrode itself upon the skin's surface, thus creating a direct current (DC) offset potential or movement artifact. Such artifacts commonly occur during vigorous movement, but may even be present during soft, quiet movements.

Floating electrodes are recommended for recording of dynamic movements. They are created in such a way that the electrode is housed inside a cup, elevated above the skin by a millimeter or so. The cup is then filled with an elec-

trolytic medium. An electrode paste or gel provides the bridge between the electrode and the skin. This potentiates the biological signal from the skin to the electrode and provides a cushion that absorbs the movement of the electrode (housing) on the skin's surface.

Floating electrodes may take more time to prepare and are usually a little more expensive than direct contact electrodes. While the electrolytic cushion reduces the movement artifact, it may not totally eliminate it. In addition, the use of pastes and gels may lead to a bridging of electrode paste between two active electrodes. This may be true when electrodes are placed only 2 cm apart. One can reduce the probability of bridging by applying only a light pressure to the cup electrodes when they are applied to the skin. Firm pressure may accidentally force the paste in one cell over to the adjoining cell. When such bridging occurs, the impedance at the electrode site is radically reduced or short-circuited. The biological energy seen by the sEMG amplifiers is significantly reduced, yielding a digital reading that is atypically low for the site and that does not change in a predictable way as a function of vigorous muscle contraction. If the practitioner is monitoring multiple sites, the sEMG readings for the site with bridging appear quite low in comparison to the other sites. It is necessary to remove the bridged electrode, abrade the skin again, and replace the electrode before a high-quality recording may be obtained. Some patients may be allergic or sensitive to the electrode paste or gel. Patients with such sensitivities should be offered hydrogel electrodes.

Hydrogel electrodes were initially developed for providing electrical stimulation to the skin (ie, transcutaneous electrical nerve stimulation, or TENS) and have since been used to record biological potentials. They commonly consist of a silver chloride disk electrode covered with a dry, sticky layer of gel as large as the usual adhesive collar. Sometimes the electrode consists of a foil with a tab. Hydrogel has a water and acidity content that is similar to the skin and, thus, does not adversely affect the skin. Although hydrogel allows the electrical potentials from the muscles to flow into the amplifiers, it has a higher impedance than the direct contact electrode or floating electrode and, thus, may be a bit noisier. In addition, the adhesion to the skin is lighter, thus allowing easy removal of the electrode. Hydrogel electrodes may be moved from one electrode site to another, although this practice is not recommended. In a sense, these electrodes are replaceable. The lightness of the adhesion also means that the electrode may come loose when perspiration occurs or during movements that place a strain on the lead attached to the electrode. To ensure good adhesion, hydrogel electrodes are typically large in surface area. They are probably best used for relaxation or other forms of quiet training and are the solution for patients with sensitive skin.

Electrodes for recording from the perineum (pelvic floor) have been developed. These so-called *vaginal and rectal electrodes* may take on the dumbbell shape seen in Figure 4–2. Two or three electrodes are located on the middle part of the electrode. They are inserted into the rectum or vaginal barrel and allow recording from the perianal muscles or the muscles of the pelvic floor. They are somewhat intrusive and, therefore, may not be appropriate for children. In addition, sterilization of the electrode may be an issue. Therefore, it is wise to use a single-user type of electrode. This means that the patient can clean and keep the sensor for repeated uses, but the same sensor is not used on multiple patients.

Ribbon electrodes are relatively new and consist of a silver ink electrode array and lead wires printed onto a thin sheet of Mylar and then covered by a thin foam pad with "cells" that define the electrode size and allow for electrode paste

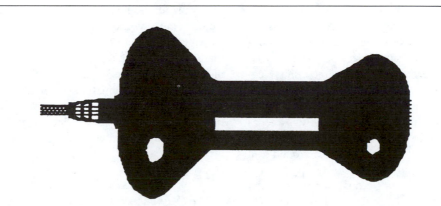

Figure 4–2 Vaginal recording electrode. Courtesy of Self Regulations Systems, Redmond, Washington.

or gel. Such an electrode is shown in Figure 4–3. These electrodes are ideal for recording from predetermined sets of muscles, such as those on the face. They are currently being used to monitor the facial displays of emotion from the muscle activity of frontalis and corrugator, or zygomaticus and orbicularis oculi during surgical procedures.[2] In addition, the flat pad allows for recordings when the patient is face down. This would be impossible with pellet types of electrodes. Ribbon electrodes will certainly be extended to other applications in the future.

ELECTRODE LEADS AND CABLES

The lead wires transmit the sEMG signals to the sEMG amplifiers. Leads should be kept as short as possible and be shielded. This is because electrode leads may act as antennas and pick up 60-Hz noise from the walls, fluorescent lighting, computers and monitors, or radio signals from a nearby transmitting tower. The longer the leads, the greater the probability of this phenomenon. Short leads (18 inches or so) not only minimize the antenna effect, but also reduce the sway of wire, which can introduce movement artifact. When a wire is moved through a magnetic field (in this case, the earth's magnetic field) a current is induced into the wire. This small current is then amplified and displayed as if it is coming from the muscles. Therefore, elimination of any unnecessary wire sway is highly desirable.

Movement of the electrode leads may be reduced by taping them to the skin or the clothing. This also provides strain relief, so that the wires do not pull on the electrodes and cause a secondary movement artifact. If electrode leads are not shielded, the leads from the two recording electrodes should be in a tightly twisted pair. Usually, the two tightly twisted wires are placed within the same plastic sheath. If there is a separate lead wire for each electrode, they should be twisted or braided together with the ground lead such that they approximate the tightly twisted pair concept. This is because when two lead wires run in parallel, any external noise tends to affect both wires equally and simultaneously;

the external noise would be eliminated by the common mode rejection of the amplifiers.

Lead wire noise problems have also been addressed by the *active electrode*. Using surface mount technology, sEMG manufacturers have developed small plastic housings that place the preamplifier directly at the electrode site. The snaps on the electrodes plug directly into the preamplifier, and this eliminates lead wire noise. The big benefit of the active electrode is noise reduction from wire sway and 60-cycle energy. In applications where this type of noise is an issue, an active electrode should be considered. The disadvantage of these electrodes is that they have a fixed interelectrode distance. This may be altered, however, by the use of short stem leads to allow for different interelectrode distances. If the electrodes are snapped directly into the plastic housing of the active electrode, one should remember that the plastic housing is a flat surface that works best when placed on another flat surface. Unfortunately, there are not many flat surfaces on the human body. This mismatch may lead to poor electrode contact and faulty recordings. Practitioners should always verify their signals and electrode connections carefully when using this type of arrangement. Finally, the active electrodes are slightly heavier than typical electrode housings and, thus, may require a stronger adhesive to maintain adequate contact with the skin.

Researchers hope that, in the future, sophisticated telemetry systems will virtually eliminate the need for lead wires. Here, a tiny transmitting device would be located within the active electrode, which would use a radio frequency to transmit the muscle's energy to a receiving unit that would store the data, process the signal, and display it on a video screen for analysis. Unfortunately, today's telemetry systems are quite expensive and tend to introduce some unwanted noise into the signal transmission. They are primarily used in recording athletic events.

SITE PREPARATION

The electrode-skin interface is a delicate matter. It is important to keep the impedance of the

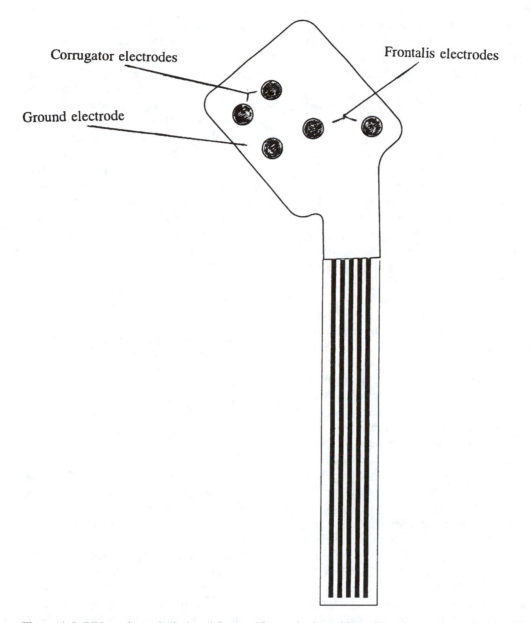

Corrugator electrodes

Frontalis electrodes

Ground electrode

Figure 4–3 Ribbon electrode designed for specific monitoring of frontalis and corrugator muscles of the face. Courtesy of Patient Comfort, Inc., Nevada City, California.

skin as low and balanced as possible. Although some equipment manufacturers claim that electrode site preparation requires little attention because of the high input impedance or special characteristics of their sEMG amplifiers, these claims have not been justified. This is because no matter how high the input impedance of the amplifier, the impedance at the electrode site could be higher. For example, with a dry, scaly skin; skin with oil-based makeup; or skin with a deep layer of hair, the impedance of the electrode at the skin could be infinite (ie, it could produce a faulty connection). Site preparation is strongly recommended as part of all clinical protocols.

To prepare the skin, use an alcohol-soaked pad and rub the electrode site with approximately six vigorous strokes. The pad should contain some rag content so that it is a little rough. Some electrode preparation pads actually contain a small amount of pumice to facilitate abrasion. Avoid cotton balls and tissues for this purpose. They simply do not do the intended job of removing the oils and top layer of dead or hornified skin so that the biological potentials can easily reach the recording electrodes. When the task is done well, a slight rubor is commonly seen.

Site preparation sometimes includes the application of a small amount of electrode paste or gel directly onto the recording site. A way to accomplish this is to take a cotton swab, dip it into the electrode paste to the skin, and then spin it lightly at the location where the electrode will be placed. Whether the practitioner preapplies electrode paste to the skin, applies it directly to the electrode, or uses pregelled electrodes, the electrolytic medium penetrates the sweat glands and provides a link to the potentials residing below the skin. This greatly facilitates the transfer of the motor unit action potentials.

In situations where the instrument manufacturer provides dry electrodes for the active electrodes, these electrodes eventually become moistened by perspiration of the skin. When the dry electrodes are applied to the skin, the skin eventually opens up its pores and exudes sweat in the body's natural attempt to shed the foreign object. Thus, the body supplies its own electrolytic medium. However, this may be somewhat unpredictable and take several minutes. Cram and Rommen[3] have compared the impedance characteristics of several types of site preparation. As can be seen in Figure 4–4, the impedance improves rapidly for site preparations that include electrolytic mediums. Only in the case of the dry electrode does impedance take a long

time. During this accommodation period, the impedance of the electrode site falls along with the sEMG amplitude reported by the instrument. Changes in impedance affect the sEMG amplitudes as well. The amplitudes drift downward over time, along with improved impedance.

Skin temperature is another factor that may noticeably affect the impedance of the site and thus the sEMG recordings. Skin temperature may fluctuate as a function of room temperature, but it is more likely affected by vigorous exercise. As skin temperature increases, the impedance reduces; such fluctuations can also alter the sEMG recordings. This is particularly true if the initial impedance was poor.

STRATEGIES FOR ELECTRODE PLACEMENT

Because the electrodes are the listening devices for picking up sEMG activity, knowing where to place the electrodes is a very important part of the process. Although only a small amount of information is available on this topic, Fridlund and Cacioppo[4] have highlighted six elements that can improve the fidelity of sEMG recordings:

1. Select the appropriate proximity of a proposed site to the underlying muscle mass, keeping the minimum amount of tissue between the electrodes and the muscle fibers themselves.

2. Select the appropriate position of the electrodes relative to the muscle fibers. Whenever possible, the electrodes should be placed parallel to the fibers to maximize sensitivity and selectivity (see Figure 4–5). Perpendicular placements tend to lead to greater common mode rejection and less selectivity.

3. Avoid straddling the motor end plate region. If this is done, the amplitudes observed are typically lower due to differential amplification. Placing electrodes a little off the center of the muscle will accomplish this goal.

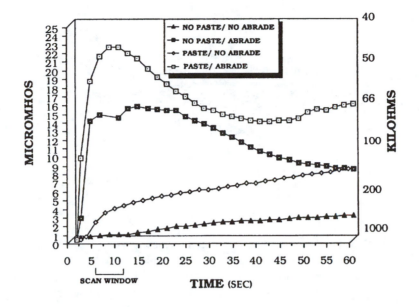

Figure 4–4 Impedance as a function of the type of electrode site preparation. *Source:* Reprinted with permission from JR Cram and D Rommen, Skin Preparation and Validity of EMG Scanning Procedure, *Biofeedback and Self Regulation*, Vol 14, No 4, pp 75–82, © 1989, Plenum Publishing.

4. Choose sites that are easy to locate (sites that have good anatomical landmarks to facilitate reliable placement of electrodes during subsequent recording sessions).
5. Choose sites that do not unduly obstruct vision or movement. Avoid areas that present problems from skin folds, bony obstruction, etc.
6. Minimize cross-talk from proximal deep or superficial muscles by selecting the best electrode size and interelectrode spacing.

The practitioner must also decide which muscles are of clinical interest. One strategy for doing this is the educated guess. Here the practitioner considers which muscle or muscles might be associated with the clinical phenomenon being studied or treated. The practitioner then places the electrodes over those muscle sites to test his or her clinical assumptions. This is a good model, because it encourages the practitioner to learn about muscle synergy patterns and to begin to see the movement and postural and emotional patterns as part of a larger whole.

A common but naive strategy is the placement of electrodes only over the area that hurts or is dysfunctional. For example, the practitioner might study only the upper trapezius muscle in someone with neck or shoulder pain. Although this may be a reasonable place to start, such a narrow focus on sEMG recordings for solitary muscles places artificial limits on the information that is obtained. This becomes clear when one considers the possibility that pain may be referred from a more distal site. An alternate strategy is to use validated clinical protocols for sEMG recordings for specific disorders. For the patient with upper quarter pain, protocols have been developed that explore asymmetries and synergies of not only the upper trapezius but also the lower trapezius, and perhaps the serratus anterior.[5] Such protocols are designed to provide the practitioner with a limited, but very practical approach to understanding the roles that muscles play in a given dysfunction. Protocols often

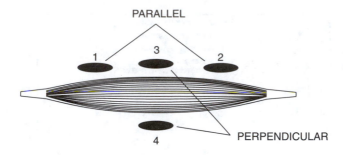

Figure 4–5 Relationship of muscle fibers to electrode placement. *Source:* Copyright © JR Cram, *Clinical EMG for Surface Recordings: Volume 2*, Clinical Resources, Inc.

work well; but when they fail, the practitioner must give further thought. An extension of the protocol strategy is to develop variations based upon clinical reasoning, knowledge of anatomy, and pathokinesiology. For the shoulder pain patient, the practitioner may want to consider also monitoring the deltoids, the infraspinatus, or the pectoralis. And finally, the practitioner should be open to the possibilities that the disorder may be due to postural or emotional components or have its source in fascia, bone, or vessel. Given the complexity of the problem, the practitioner should have a strategy of going from one level of assessment to another, until all of the possible contributors have been examined.

In considering the strategy for assessing the postural component of dysfunction, it helpful to incorporate the sampling technique called *muscle scanning*.[6] Instead of studying just one or two sites while the patient is sitting and standing, muscle scanning allows the right and left aspects of multiple muscle groups to be studied in both the sitting and standing positions quickly using a handheld scanner. The handheld scanner provides a chassis for two (or three) direct contact electrodes. These recording electrodes are held in place over a muscle by hand with a light pressure. For more information, see Chapter 6. The values that are obtained are then compared to either a normative reference group or are normalized and compared within the individual to determine which muscles are relatively hyperactive versus hypoactive. Right and left asym-

metries may be considered within the context of various vertebral segments. Weight shifting or antalgic postures are commonly observed. Imbalances in the upper back can better be understood when imbalances in the lower back are also included. Once these relationships have been determined, attach electrodes to gain a better understanding of how these relationships affect movement.

Strategies for studying or identifying the emotional aspect of the neuromuscular system also should be considered. It is common for practitioners to place widely spaced electrodes on the frontal muscle, expose the patient to stressful events, and record the patient's reactions. Although such a recording procedure allows the practitioner to measure some of the major negative emotional states seen on the human face (eg, anger, fear, and sadness), it does not provide information concerning specific emotional activation at the injured site or its homologous counterpart. One may broaden the search for an emotional component by placing a set of electrodes on the right and left aspects of the area of reported pain. Flor and associates, for example, have demonstrated exquisite specificity of emotional reactions in the erector spinae muscles of low back pain patients, with little or no involvement of the facial muscles.[7]

Strategies associated with general relaxation are commonly used to treat the emotional component of dysfunction. Electrode placement for general relaxation typically involves widely spaced electrodes that cross the midline. Rather than monitoring and treating one muscle group, it is better for the practitioner to monitor and treat muscular regions. Placement of widely spaced electrodes on the frontal region increases the probability that the practitioner will see any emotional events of the patient's face. Widely spaced electrodes on the trapezius group allow the practitioner to see any activations of the neck and upper back. Wrist-to-wrist electrode placements allow the practitioner to see clearly any holding patterns or activations in the upper extremities, upper back, and chest. The ankle-to-ankle leads do the same for the lower extremities, buttocks, low back, and abdomen. In dynamic relaxation protocols, such as the ones developed by Ettare,[8] the right and left aspects of general regions are considered. For example, the right and left trapezius placement strategy would allow the practitioner to monitor the right and left aspects for the region of the upper back. Treatment would be directed at teaching the patient how to quiet the muscles quickly following their activation.

Strategies of electrode placement associated with specific muscle monitoring typically involve closely spaced electrodes that are placed parallel to muscle fibers or in areas with the least cross-talk. They are most commonly placed directly over or slightly lateral to the belly of the muscle. The electrode placement strategy for specifically monitoring the upper fibers of trapezius, for example, is to place the recording electrode on the ridge of the shoulder, slightly lateral to the center of the muscle belly, and with the electrodes running in the direction of the fibers. In considering placement of electrodes for muscles that are partially covered by another muscle or a muscle that has very close proximity to neighboring muscles, it is sometimes possible to place recording electrodes on a distal portion of the muscle to avoid or minimize cross-talk. Recordings from flexor digitorum in the forearm is a good example of this. Although this placement is not directly over the belly of the flexor digitorum muscle, it does detect enough of the action potentials from the distal portion of its muscle fibers to reflect finger (as opposed to wrist) movement. Specific placements of electrodes may be used to assess patterns of muscle recruitment associated with movement. They are commonly used to treat the patient by teaching the patient to activate ("uptrain") a specific muscle to improve the muscular effort. They may also be used to "downtrain" a specific muscle—to teach the patient specifically to turn off the recruitment of a muscle following its use.

Chapters 5 and 6 explore in great detail where to place the electrodes for both static and dynamic procedures. These chapters contain specific recommendations about placement sites, along with examples of what one would expect to see given a particular electrode placement.

REFERENCES

1. Loeb GE, Gans C. *Electromyography for Experimentalists.* Chicago: University of Chicago Press; 1986.

2. Bennett H, Kornhauser S. Assessment of general anesthesia by facial muscle electromyography (FACE). *Am J Electromed.* 1995;6:94–97.

3. Cram JR, Rommen DR. Skin preparation and validity of EMG scanning procedure. *Biofeedback Self Regul.* 1989;14(4):75–82.

4. Fridlund AJ, Cacioppo JT. Guidelines for human electromyographic research. *Psychophysiol.* 1986;23:567–598.

5. Taylor W. Dynamic EMG biofeedback in assessment and treatment using a neuromuscular reeducation model. In: Cram JR, ed. *Clinical EMG for Surface Recordings, II.* Nevada City, CA: Clinical Resources; 1990:175–196.

6. Cram JR. EMG muscle scanning and diagnostic manual for surface recordings. In: Cram JR, ed. *Clinical EMG for Surface Recordings, II.* Nevada City, CA: Clinical Resources; 1990:1–142.

7. Flor H, Turk D, Birbaumer N. Assessment of stress-related psychophysiological reactions in chronic back pain patients. *J Consult Clin Psychol.* 1985;53(3):354–364.

8. Ettare D, Ettare R. Muscle learning therapy: a treatment protocol. In: Cram JR, ed. *Clinical EMG for Surface Recordings, II.* Nevada City, CA: Clinical Resources; 1990:197–234.

Chapter Questions

1. Which type of electrode is ideal for dynamic movement studies?
   a. direct contact electrode
   b. cup or floating electrode
   c. dry electrode
   d. tri-electrode

2. When bridging of electrode paste between two electrodes occurs, what impact does it have on the resulting sEMG amplitudes?
   a. It quickens the response time of the sEMG signal.
   b. It artificially increases the sEMG levels.
   c. It artificially decreases the sEMG levels.
   d. It sends the amplitude to 0.

3. Which electrode is ideal for the patients who are allergic to either the paste or the adhesive collar?
   a. direct contact electrode
   b. cup/floating electrode
   c. hydrogel electrode
   d. percutaneous fine-wire electrode

4. Which of the following represent problems or artifact that may be introduced into the sEMG signal by the electrode leads?
   a. 60-Hz noise (the antenna effect)
   b. movement artifact
   c. radio frequency interference
   d. all of the above

5. Strain relief refers to:
   a. removing the weight of the electrode leads from the electrodes themselves
   b. the effect of placing the muscle on stretch
   c. the effect on the electrode when the patient moves through the range of motion
   d. the effect of taking the muscle off of stretch

6. Site preparation for electrode placement:
   a. is always recommended
   b. is needed only with low-input impedance amplifiers
   c. is needed only with high-input impedance amplifiers
   d. is not needed

7. Poor electrode contact usually has what effect on the sEMG recording?
   a. It artificially decreases the sEMG amplitudes.
   b. It artificially increases the sEMG amplitudes.
   c. It reduces the response time of the sEMG to changes in muscle function.
   d. It only changes values in instruments with high input impedances.

8. When placing the sEMG electrodes for dynamic sEMG procedures, the practitioner should consider:

a. symmetry of recording electrode placement
b. agonists and antagonists (myotatic units)
c. the anterior compartment
d. the posterior compartment
e. all of the above

9. When conducting assessments for the postural component of muscle dysfunction, which of the following procedures yields the most complete picture?
   a. muscle scanning
   b. dynamic sEMG protocols
   c. frontal sEMG recordings
   d. palpation examination

10. When assessing for the emotional component of dysfunction, the practitioner should:
    a. place the electrodes on the facial muscles (wide spaced frontal)
    b. place the electrodes on the site of injury or pain
    c. place the electrodes over the zygomaticus
    d. both a and b

11. When conducting a general relaxation training session, it is extremely useful to:
    a. use widely spaced electrodes
    b. place the recording electrodes across the midline
    c. use closely spaced electrodes
    d. place the electrodes so that they run parallel to the muscle fibers
    e. both a and b

12. When placing sEMG electrodes for dynamic protocols, the practitioner should:
    a. place the electrodes over the belly of the muscle fibers of interest
    b. place the electrodes over the compartment of the muscle of interest
    c. place the electrodes such that they avoid cross-talk from other muscles
    d. all of the above

CHAPTER 5

General Assessment Considerations

In the healing arts it is commonly believed that treatment should naturally flow from the practitioner's diagnostic impressions. For surface electromyography (sEMG), this diagnosis is not the same type of *medical* diagnosis that is seen with intramuscular EMG studies; these intramuscular, needle studies have to do with structure and tissue damage. With sEMG, the practitioner makes a *functional* or clinical diagnosis; instead of diagnosing tissue damage, the practitioner considers the use or misuse of muscular energy by the central nervous system. George Whatmore, one of the pioneers of sEMG, referred to this misuse of muscular energy as *dysponesis*, or the bad use of energy.[1]

As in formal diagnosis, a strong functional diagnosis requires the practitioner to "correctly" interpret the information collected during assessment, basing the sEMG treatment protocol upon this interpretation. To that end, this chapter focuses on the interpretation of sEMG information and strategies for using sEMG to correct the observed anomaly.

FACTORS THAT AFFECT INTERPRETATION

The process of forming a clinical diagnosis begins with understanding some of the possible moderating variables that could affect the sEMG recording. This is particularly true if the practitioner is using a "standardized" assessment protocol (ie, a protocol with a clear set of rules to

allow replication). Although standardized protocols provide the practitioner with a basis to compare one patient with another and a means of communicating findings to colleagues, they fail to honor the uniqueness of the individual patient. Moderating variables provide some guidelines upon which the practitioner begins to build in this individuality, adding depth and meaning to the interpretation. There are many moderating variables for the practitioner to consider, several of which are explored below.

Anatomical and Physiological Considerations

Whenever practitioners apply surface electrodes over muscle, it is very important to palpate the site and possibly have the patient do a resisted isometric contraction of the muscle ("manual muscle test") to verify that the electrode is over the muscle of interest. Only then can the practitioner ascertain that the map or atlas corresponds to the particular patient. Two practitioners have argued that morphological characteristics of the human body (muscle mass, muscle length, source of sEMG, adipose tissue) vary so widely among individuals so as to preclude the use of standardized electrode sites, let alone any associated normative values.[2,3] All practitioners, of course, recognize that people come in a variety of shapes and sizes, as do their muscles. So, rather than summarily dismissing the notion of any standardized electrode placement sites, recording procedures, and associated reference data, the practitioner must adjust the electrode placement, the clinical procedures, and the interpretation of the normative values based upon the unique presentation of the patient's anatomy. It is the establishment of standardized electrode placement sites and clinical protocols that helps practitioners to communicate with colleagues concerning assessment findings and treatments.

In the assessment and treatment of tension myalgias for the upper quarter, for example, placement of electrodes on the upper trapezius muscle is quite common. In a recent review of the literature on this topic, Mathiassen et al[4] argue strongly for standardization of research and clinical procedures so as to facilitate the understanding of findings across labs and clinics. One of the standardization issues concerns electrode placement over the trapezius. For many years, clinicians and researchers have used a placement described by Zipp,[5] in which the electrodes are placed at 50% of the distance between the seventh cervical vertebra (C-7) and the acromion. However, more recent research by Veiersted clearly demonstrated that a slight lateral shift from the middle position is preferable.[6] This placement provides a stronger and more reliable signal. Clinicians are strongly encouraged to learn from the experience of others and to use this new standardized placement for trapezius (it is clearly delineated in the electrode atlas in Part II).

Consider sEMG recordings obtained during a static versus dynamic assessment procedure. The recordings obtained during the static phase of assessment are generally less problematic than recordings obtained during dynamic assessment procedures. This is because, during dynamic studies, the muscles change their resting length and move differentially in relationship to the skin. The sEMG electrodes do not stay over the "belly" of the muscle during the entire course of the movement. Consider the placement of the electrodes 2 cm apart, parallel to the spine over the belly of the erector spinae at the L-3 (third lumbar vertebra) level with the patient in

the neutral standing posture. As the patient engages in forward flexion, the distance between the recording electrodes widens as the skin stretches to accommodate the lengthening of the back. In fact, practitioners always have to use strategies to stop the recording electrodes from "popping" or coming loose during this movement. During extension, back to midline, these electrodes return to their original interelectrode distance. Then, if the patient is asked to extend backwards, the electrodes come closer together as the muscle shortens. So, movement systematically alters the interelectrode distance, and thus the recording field.

Consider another example—the placement of the electrodes over the belly of the sternocleidomastoid (SCM) during axial rotation of the head. During rotation of the head, the SCM radically changes its resting length by 50%, and the recording electrodes drift either ahead of or behind the belly of the muscle, depending upon the direction of the head turn. As the electrodes move from their intended location directly above the SCM, from which muscle(s) is the electrode recording (digastric? scalene?)? The electrodes probably continue to record primarily from the SCM due to volume conduction, unless one of the surrounding muscle groups (such as scalene) is also dysfunctional and fires briskly as a function of axial rotation. Donaldson has also made this observation, using multisite recordings around the circumference of the neck (personal communication). DeLuca suggests one possible solution to this dilemma.[7,8] In all of his studies of sEMG, DeLuca uses a sustained isometric contraction (activation without a change in muscle length). DeLuca goes so far as to state that, because of this electrode movement phenomenon, sEMG recordings observed during dynamic movement are meaningless. This is, of course, an extreme position to take. What is important to note here is that there are some dynamically related changes in length-tension relationships that make the sEMG:force relationships variable or even unknown. Such considerations do not enter into sEMG activity during the static phase of the assessment.

Considering all of the possible contributing and contaminating factors associated with dynamic sEMG recordings, it is remarkable that we see any consistency in the sEMG recordings at all. But the truth is that both dynamic and static sEMG recordings provide reliable,[9,10] predictive,[11–13] and descriptive[14,15] information that is valuable for researchers and practitioners.

Adipose Tissue

Adipose tissue is well known for its insulating and attenuating effects on the sEMG signal. Because of this, it is important for the practitioner to remember that the dispersion of adipose tissue differs across individuals, within individuals, and between the two sexes. For example, females tend to carry more of this tissue in their upper chest and thighs, while males tend to carry more in the abdominal region. Because of the problems with adipose tissue dispersion, ideally the practitioner should measure and record the thickness of the adipose tissue directly at the electrode site, rather than relying upon some global measure of percentage of body fat from impedance measurements. In a small, unpublished pilot study of 16 subjects, Cram conducted skin-fold measurements on six sites prior to sEMG recordings; he observed the correlation between adipose tissue thickness and sEMG levels in the quiet resting state to be around 0.5, and 0.25 during moderate levels of contraction. Adipose tissue, then, seems to bear more directly on resting or static sEMG measurements than measurements that involve recruitment or activation of the muscle. This is because resting tone is commonly associated with low sEMG activity, which is more readily absorbed by the insulating effects of the fat. In the active muscle, higher amplitudes of sEMG activity prevail. The high amplitude allows more of the energy to pass through the fatty tissue.

Thus, information about adipose tissue helps clinicians and researchers interpret and report the sEMG data, particularly in the resting state. Until further research is conducted, however, it is difficult to provide the electromyographer with a precise correction factor for the effects of adipose tissue on the integrated levels of sEMG. Unfortunately, one rarely sees any information concerning adipose tissue in the scientific literature or clinical reports on sEMG. Nonetheless, the practitioner would be well advised to observe and record such information. This practice would allow the sEMG interpretations to be globally scaled upward or downward. Because of the current state of this knowledge, when clinicians conduct sEMG assessments on the torso and upper extremities, it is recommended that they use Donoghue's[16] four-site method of skin caliper measurement—in which the thickness of the upper arm (above biceps and triceps), upper back (just below the scapula), and lower back (just above the iliac crest) is sampled and then compared to normative data for percentage of body fat. The percentage of body fat would then provide the basis for the scaling of the interpretation. Finally, clinicians should note that the uses of a single-subject or within-patient design for sEMG assessment does not eradicate the problems associated with adipose tissue. As we have all noticed in the mirror, there is an uneven distribution of adipose tissue, even within the single subject.

Therefore, when interpreting the amplitudes associated with sEMG information, it is wise to consider the patient's adipose tissue. Obese individuals tend to have much lower amplitudes than thin individuals. Within the individual, assessment of symmetry would not necessarily be affected by adipose tissue levels. Comparisons of amplitudes at various body parts (ie, upper back versus lower back) may be affected. Practitioners should remember that static values seem to be affected more by the presence of adipose tissue than recordings of dynamic procedures.

Position, Posture, and Dynamic Movement

Position, posture, and dynamic movement constitute another set of related variables that moderate the level of muscle energy reaching the electrode. During the static evaluation, the patient is typically studied in a neutral posture of standing or sitting unsupported. Here, the muscles are working against gravity, and any disturbance in the muscular activation patterns is considered to be associated with a disturbance in postural homeostasis.[17] Such a postural disturbance may be due to one or several factors: pain (antalgic postures); postural habits (slouching); anatomical features (eg, leg length discrepancy, scoliosis, etc); neurological impairment (eg, due to cardiovascular accident, spinal cord injury, herniated disk); or emotional arousal (eg, bracing, acting "uptight"). It is not enough for the practitioner to note a disturbed activation pattern during a static assessment and let it go at that. Slight postural adjustments of the upper extremity or torso, for example, affect the resting tone in the erector spinae muscle group.[18] The practitioner must incorporate information gained from the clinical interview, physical examination, and visual observation of posture/movement in order to place the sEMG reading into perspective.

For the static evaluation, practitioners should use caution in the verbal instructions given to the subject regarding posture. Matheson et al,[19] for example, observed a significant sex difference in the midback region when his subjects were instructed to "sit up straight." The power of this language caused the female subjects to vest significantly more energy in the midthoracic spine, thus bringing them into a more upright posture similar to what their mothers had presumably taught them to do. It is strongly recommended that the practitioner/scientist use neutral words, such as "sit comfortably." In addition, it is recommended that the practitioner/scientist have the person sit on an adjustable chair or backless stool, with the chair height set so that the patient's knees are flexed at 90 degrees. When the patient is standing, the arms should be allowed to hang comfortably at the sides.

In addition, it is important to recognize that different muscle groups have different resting tones (sEMG levels), and that the resting tone may vary as a function of posture. Some practitioners, such as Headley,[2] have advocated the use of a general criterion value for all sites. For example, the practitioner might use the "rule of 5," which holds that any sEMG value that is greater than 5 microvolts root mean square (RMS) is considered abnormal. Unfortunately, this approach is somewhat simplistic and can lead a practitioner to erroneous conclusions. A better solution to this problem is to use normative data collected for the various muscle sites while the patient is in various positions. Such a normative database for static recordings may be found in Chapter 6. Using such a reference group for comparison purposes, the resting tone of a patient with low back pain was recorded using the muscle scanning procedure for two neutral postures (see Table 5–1). The patient appears to put on a "muscular corset" as he moves from sitting to standing; this is seen in the dramatic increase in activation in the low back area during standing. In addition, note the suprasegmental organization of the paraspinal muscles with the neck muscle activating along with low back muscle during standing. Normative comparisons for the various sites can assist practitioners in their initial understanding of relationships between muscle groups and neutral postures.

Some practitioners have proposed conducting the static scanning procedure while at the end range of motion (ROM). Chiropractors usually do this to complement an end ROM study conducted as part of the clinical exam.[20,21] To date, one study by Leach et al has provided information concerning a static assessment at full forward flexion of the low back, in an attempt to assess the flexion relaxation response.[22] These authors found that end ROM values of several low back sites during forward flexion differed between normal subjects and low back pain patients. There are three major problems, however, in using the static procedure for end ROM studies: (1) electrode movement artifact due to the handheld sensors, (2) potential accommodation of the sEMG amplitudes due to stretch receptor adaptation associated with the time necessary to conduct multiple samples, and (3) disturbances in low back patients' neuromuscular activation patterns associated with pain when left in a flexed posture for short periods of time. It would

Table 5–1 Scan Summary Demonstrating a Strong Postural Component for a Patient with Low Back Pain

Muscle Site	Sitting		Standing	
	Left	Right	Left	Right
C-2 Paraspinal	5.6*	3.6	9.2**	7.6*
C-4 Paraspinal	5.2*	3.5	7.2*	6.1*
C-6 Paraspinal	4.9*	4.5	5.5*	6.2*
Trapezius	4.9	4.2	4.7	5.0
T-2 Paraspinal	2.1	2.5	4.3	5.7
T-4 Paraspinal	3.4	2.5	4.9	5.0
T-6 Paraspinal	3.6	3.0	4.8	5.7
T-8 Paraspinal	3.3	3.0	9.1	9.2
T-10 Paraspinal	3.2	3.2	7.2	8.8
L-1 Paraspinal	3.4	3.4	9.9	15.6
L-3 Paraspinal	7.5*	9.3*	15.8***	26.6***
L-5 Paraspinal	5.6	5.3	9.1*	10.2**

*1 SD above the mean

**2 SD above the mean

***3 SD above the mean

Note: A J&J M-501 with a 25 to 1000 Hz filter was used.

seem more natural and more appropriate to use a dynamic recording procedure to study sEMG during a ROM. These dynamic procedures allow the practitioner to examine the pattern and timing of recruitment of sEMG, along with recovery from the perturbation of the movement.

Position and posture are also important issues for dynamic sEMG protocols. Practitioners who are trained in manual muscle testing procedures are familiar with the issues pertaining to assessment of recruitment patterns in muscles. The essence of these principles is that, by correctly positioning the limbs or torso, the practitioner may inhibit or potentiate attempts to isolate a given muscle group. For more information on manual muscle testing procedures, see Kendall, Kendall, and McCreary.[23]

Middaugh et al describe a common example of how posture and position may affect dynamic evaluation and treatment.[24] These authors approach the assessment of upper quarter pain primarily through the monitoring of the cervical paraspinal and upper trapezius muscle groups. They pay careful attention to the position of the head and the arms, noting forward head and arm position for augmentation of the resting tone of these sites. They study simple movements such as shoulder elevation, abduction, and forward flexion for pattern of recruitment and cessation of recruitment following request to terminate the movement. They note that recruitment patterns are inefficient when the posture is poor, becoming more efficient once the "correct" posture has been obtained. The corrected posture entails placing the elbows closer to the side of the torso and moving the head into a more neutral position. When working with a patient, the therapist may need to stretch and strengthen certain muscles to allow the patient to retract the head back over the shoulders.

Dynamic recruitment patterns may change as a function of slight alterations of limb position. Several examples of this are presented in the electrode atlas in Part II. For example, recruitment of biceps during elbow flexion changes when the hand is pronated rather than supinated (see Figure 14–33D). Recruitment of the infraspinatus during abduction differs when the arm is medially or laterally rotated (see Figure 14–24B).

In summary, both static and dynamic sEMG recordings may be affected significantly by posture, position, and movement. The astute practitioner must understand these relationships and use them in assessment and treatment protocols. It is important to note these issues in the documentation.

Volume Conduction

Another factor that affects the sEMG is volume conduction. *Volume conduction* (or far-field potentials) refers to the source of the sEMG signal residing at some distance from the surface EMG sensors. Years ago, Basmajian[25] discussed cautions regarding volume conduction. He cautioned that the frontal (wide) electrode placement is nonspecific and may record from muscle as far away as the first rib. Although far-field potentials from the ancillary muscles of respiration (ie, scalene) have been noted in widely spaced electrodes at frontal site, it is much more common to see volume conduction at this site from the corrugator, temporalis, or masseter muscles. The point is that recordings from a single set of electrodes placed over a particular muscle group may lead the practitioner to an erroneous conclusion about that muscle. It is helpful for the practitioner to know which sites are more easily contaminated by volume conduction or cross-talk, and which sites lend themselves to cleaner specific recordings. Volume conduction and cross-talk are typically more problematic for dynamic recordings than static sEMG recordings. However, static recordings are not immune to this phenomenon.

The purpose of a muscle scanning technique is to encourage the practitioner to consider the muscular system as a whole rather than drawing conclusions based on one set of electrodes. Muscle scanning technique emphasizes sampling from a variety of muscle sets, looking to identify active or inhibited sites. It is helpful in searching for the problems areas, particularly if one is not sure where to begin. For example, consider a patient who is clenching his or her jaw (activation of masseter and temporalis). If the practitioner conducts a single-site recording at frontalis, he or she might conclude that the patient had elevated resting tone at that site. Such a conclusion would be misleading. In conducting multisite recording from the facial musculature, the practitioner would be able to observe that the sEMG activation from masseter and temporalis is volume conducted, elevating the amplitudes observed at the frontalis sites as well (see Table 5–2). From the multisite recording, the practitioner would observe that the highest level of microvolt activity is seen at the masseter site. Such a "within-patient" pattern analysis of the multiple site suggests that the practitioner consider volume-conducted activity from the masseteric activation. As Iacona[3] notes, such a single-subject or within-patient analysis is an essential part of correctly interpreting a static evaluation. Sole reliance upon a normative database comparison in this case would lead one to conclude that the masseter, temporalis, frontalis, and SCM sites were all significantly elevated. The practitioner must sort out these volume-conduction issues.

It is also important for evaluation of dynamic procedures to contemplate volume-conducted

Table 5–2 Scan Summary on Person Who Is Clenching Teeth Intentionally

Muscle Site	Sitting	
	Left	*Right*
Frontalis	22.0*	24.2*
Temporalis	35.2*	41.1*
Masseter	57.2*	65.2*
SCM	12.1*	14.6*
Trapezius	2.6	2.0
T-2 paraspinal	2.3	2.1

*Severe elevations

Note: A J&J M-501 with a 25 to 1000 Hz filter was used.

activity and place electrodes accordingly. The same type of examination of the facial muscles can be done with multiple-site dynamic sEMG recordings. Figure 14–1B demonstrates volume conduction to the frontal leads during a clench. Some sites are more vulnerable to volume conduction than others. For example, Perry and colleagues have reported that only 36% of the sEMG activity recorded at the soleus site is due to the soleus muscle. The rest is volume conducted from gastrocnemius and related muscles.[26] Considerable cross-talk can also happen in the muscles of the forearm. The electrode atlas (Part II) orients practitioners about the possibility of cross-talk and which muscles may contribute to this phenomenon.

Problems with volume conduction are also paramount when attempting to record from a "deep" muscle—that is, a muscle that resides underneath another muscle. With surface electrodes, how does one know whether the recording comes from the more superficial muscle or the deeper muscle group? This question is even more difficult to answer when both the superficial and deep muscles are synergists, performing slightly different functions yet being activated by the same movement. The supraspinatus versus middle trapezius muscles, and the quadratus lumborum versus latissimus dorsi (or abdominal oblique) are two such examples. For this reason, the electrode atlas focuses on monitoring these deeper muscles by their location or site rather than by the muscle itself. For example, these two electrode placements would be called suprascapular/supraspinatus and lateral low back/quadratus, respectively.

While it would be nice to think that sEMG recordings at multiple sites are totally independent, they are not. Just as some of the Minnesota Multiphasic Personality Inventory (MMPI) scales share some of the same stimulus items, source EMG may find its way to sensors at some distance. With sEMG (unlike intramuscular needle or fine-wire recordings), practitioners must learn to think in terms of populations of motor units, muscle synergies, and muscle dyssynergies. The system is tied together, into myo-

tatic units.[27] Muscle scanning and multisite dynamic sEMG recording allow one to see the "bigger picture." Normative data or benchmark values for each site provide the background for beginning the interpretation, with a single-subject/within 1-1 patient analysis of the pattern of activation and inhibition as a complementary step. Focusing upon both types of comparisons helps the practitioner to reach sound conclusions.

Age and Gender

Age and sex variables may play a substantial role in physiological functioning and should be considered in sEMG recordings. Indeed, Wolf et al[28] and Brown[29] have noted that for dynamic procedures, the level of sEMG recruitment decreases with age. This is probably the result of a loss of muscle bulk due to inactivity that comes with age. However, for sEMG recordings of static procedures, these differences disappear. Three studies have examined sEMG activity in the static, neutral posture across ages and between sexes.[11,23,28] All three studies note a lack of correlation between age and sEMG levels at rest. Sex differences, likewise, show too much random variation under static conditions to provide a meaningful distinction between sexes for resting tone.

SURFACE ELECTROMYOGRAPHY AND CLINICAL SYNDROMES

From a clinical perspective, the aberrant sEMG patterns that relate to myogenic etiologies for pain may arise from different types of psychophysiological and musculoskeletal dysfunctions. Below is a partial list of clinical syndromes for which a dynamic sEMG assessment may be used:

- simple postural dysfunction
- emotional dysfunction
- learned guarding or bracing
- peripheral weakness or deconditioning
- acute, reflexive spasm or inhibition
- learned inhibition

- direct compensation for joint hypermobility or hypomobility
- chronic faulty motor program

An introduction to a scheme for syndrome recognition and treatment planning, developed in large part by Kasman,[30] is presented below. Note that the presentation is simplified, and that a more detailed exploration of these principles can be found in *Clinical Applications in Surface Electromyography* by Kasman et al.[31] Also note that clinical syndromes presented in this framework are not mutually exclusive. Patients may exhibit qualities of one or more syndromes. Procedures that are alluded to in this framework are intended as a starting point in the practitioner's evaluation. These guidelines should be modified and tailored to the individual patient. In some cases, a team approach to patient care is required to complete the assessment.

To determine which syndromes are relevant for a given patient, the practitioner should begin by asking some of the following questions:

1. What are the significant findings from the history, intake, and clinical examination? Although the issues to consider are as varied as the patients themselves, it is helpful to consider some of following elements: trauma, vocation, medical history, type of pain description, pain-related movements, temporal aspects of pain, respiratory distress, cognitive dysfunction, visual/balance dysfunctions, headache, incontinence, paresthesia, weakness, medications, substance abuse, major life stressors, affect, coping mechanisms, impaired activities of daily living, etc.
2. What specific aberrant sEMG patterns are observed? Consider amplitude, timing, and muscle groups involved.
3. Under what conditions are the aberrant patterns displayed? Consider activity/work-related aspects, posturally related aspects, and emotional overtones.
4. Under what conditions are the aberrant patterns not displayed? When are they normal? Consider environmental, emotional, postural, and movement aspects.
5. How do questions 1 through 4 come together? What is the bigger picture?

Below are some simplified descriptions for the clinical syndromes listed above. One case example is briefly described to provide an illustration of each of the concepts presented. Treatment considerations for these different syndromes is presented in Chapter 9.

Simple Postural Dysfunction

Aberrant motor activity can be a direct function of posture. Take a case example of a patient with headache and tension myalgia of the upper quarter and neck associated with work as a keyboard entry person. Postural examination shows that the patient sits with the head forward and with the arms extended slightly while typing. Surface EMG recordings show hyperactivity primarily in the cervical paraspinal and upper trapezius. These sEMG levels greatly improve when the patient achieves "correct" postural alignment.

Emotional Dysfunction

Heightened muscle activity may be due to maladaptive coping with stressful situations or may be a conditioned response to a traumatic event (posttraumatic stress disorder). Consider the patient who comes to the practitioner four weeks after a motor vehicle accident in which she sustained a flexion extension injury to her neck and shoulder region. Traditional medical and physical therapies do not produce long-term gains. A stress-profiling procedure is done, in which the offending muscle (wide trapezius) site and a muscle that indicates general emotions (wide frontal) are monitored as the patient recounts the details associated with the accident. Large emotional recruitment patterns are noted during the patient's discussion of the accident scene. Appropriate treatment of the posttraumatic stress disorder should precede or be done concurrently with the physical therapy.

Learned Guarding or Bracing

Heightened muscle activity is a learned (emotional) response to pain that occurs upon movement or postural loading. Responses are performed in an attempt to avoid pain and the possibility of further injury. In some cases, the syndrome may involve complex behavioral dysfunction that may include responses performed to declare pain and disability. Consider an example of a patient with litigation pending, following a trauma to the left shoulder area associated with a fall two years ago. This patient commonly clutches at the neck and shoulder region, and periodically attends a session with her own cold pack on the area. There is diffuse activation of the upper quarter and neck observed on the muscle scan during quiet sitting and standing, and electrodes attached to the right and left upper and lower trapezius bear this out. Simple abduction indicates that the upper trapezius on both the right and left sides have peak amplitudes that are four to seven times greater than those of the lower trapezius muscles. The right upper trapezius has a peak amplitude that is twice that of the injured left side. Anticipated and small movements of the left arm or shoulder tend to fire the right upper trapezius. With attention and sEMG feedback training, this muscle activation improves during the session, but the patient is slow to transfer gains from session to session and from the office to home. The patient responds well to relaxation-based therapies. Pain management is a key feature.

Peripheral Weakness or Deconditioning

This syndrome refers to patients who have become impaired due to simple muscle disuse. This may be caused by immobilization after injury or surgery, or as the cumulative effect of poor motor habits and decreased activity. The condition may include atrophic loss of muscle cross-sectional area, inefficient vascularization, and compromised biochemical and physiological function. Symptoms may include a gradual decrease in peak torque, power deficits (ie, inability to sustain force through ROM arcs), and impaired fatigue resistance.

Consider the case of a patient who has had his knee immobilized and weight bearing restricted for 6 weeks after sustaining a leg fracture. The quadriceps has undergone disuse atrophy during the period of immobilization. Range of motion, strength, endurance, and functional mobility are impaired during the rehabilitation period. If the knee patient is cleared for active strengthening and is examined with sEMG, the recorded activity will likely differ between the involved and uninvolved lower extremities. Maximal effort sEMG activity will probably be decreased on the involved side, although submaximal contractions may show increased activity, presumably reflecting decreased neuromuscular efficiency. The asymmetrical sEMG activity will be associated with obvious findings of weakness and deconditioning on physical examination.

Acute, Reflexive Spasm/Inhibition

Elevated or inhibited (depressed) muscle tension presumably occurs via reflex mechanism induced by pain and/or effusion. Take an example of a patient with a bulging or herniated disk with pain in the left aspect of the low back, radiating down into the left hip and leg. The patient has decreased range of motion of the torso and poor sitting tolerance. The patient might present with a flexed and laterally shifted trunk posture, and visibly and palpably elevated lumbar paraspinal tone. Pain is on the same side as the bulging disk. The patient may show discrete activations of the erector spinae muscle on the ipsilateral side of reported pain. Occasionally, this activation pattern is more diffuse to both sides of the low back, and extends clearly into the midback region as well. Pain is increased with sitting (supported or not), and the sEMG activation level also increases. Any movements, active or passive, of the lower extremity lead to an activation of the left erector spinae muscles.

An example of acute, reflexive inhibition might be seen in a patient with a recent history of trauma and physical examination findings of swelling, tenderness, and inability to tolerate vigorous manual muscle testing of the lower extremity. Surface EMG monitoring would show a discrete focal drop in sEMG amplitude recorded from the quadriceps during a painful portion of the knee range-of-motion arc. The focal drop in sEMG activity in this case would be as a consequence of neurophysiologic inhibition. Similar scenarios regarding spasm and inhibition could result from the cumulative effects of subtle, recurrent trauma to a joint.

Learned Inhibition/Weakness

This is a rare syndrome, but one worth considering. Here the patient unconsciously learns to inhibit motor activity so as to avoid pain. This is similar to the protective guarding syndrome discussed above, but with inhibition rather than spasm. Take, for example, an otherwise healthy patient who sustains recurrent strains of the hip adductor muscles while playing racquetball. The pain becomes severe and exacerbated whenever the adductor muscles vigorously contract during functional activities. To evade the contraction-induced pain, the patient learns to reduce firing of the adductors while performing stressful physical activities. Over a period of time, the altered patterns become unconsciously incorporated into the patient's selection of motor programs.

The adductor sEMG amplitude of the patient described above appears symmetrical on the uninvolved side during walking and low-level activities. However, activity appears to be markedly decreased and impaired during higher-velocity and loading conditions such as sustained unilateral stance, lunging, or formal manual muscle testing. When the patient is subjected to an unanticipated postural perturbation, the adductors recruit to a level that exceeds their voluntary activation. Thus, the muscles are recruited with postural reactions to help prevent a fall. Inconsistent activation patterns might also be observed with novel tasks for which motor programming schema have not been learned, especially if there are simultaneous cognitive distractions.

Direct Compensation for Joint Hypermobility or Hypomobility

Aberrant sEMG activity may occur as a consequence of chronic joint hypermobility or hypomobility. The neuromuscular system compensates by attempting to stabilize lax joint structures, by affecting movement against joint stiffness, or by subserving linked compensatory movements over kinetic chains. Although sEMG activity is aberrant, the primary problem is a biomechanical articular fault (joint dysfunction). The articular fault causes a compensatory motor control pattern, which may spontaneously resolve upon improvement in joint mechanics. Chronic joint dysfunction may lead to motor control problems that themselves contribute to deterioration of the kinetic segment and persist even after joint mobility improves. The distinction is made because if aberrant motor activity is believed to be directly compensatory to articular dysfunction, then biofeedback is not a first choice of treatment. The joint dysfunction should be addressed and then sEMG activity should be reassessed.

As an example, a patient with jaw pain is found on physical examination to display hypomobility at the left temporomandibular joint (TMJ). There is a deviation of the midline of the jaw during opening and closing, and a palpable difference between the motions of the left and right mandibular condyles. As opening is initiated (or closing completed), the condyles are felt to spin in place. The condyles are then felt to translate forward as opening continues. This rolling/gliding relationship is necessary for normal jaw range of motion and is expected to be symmetrical at the left and right TMJs. In this case example, sEMG activity shows greater recruitment at the right masseter during jaw opening/closing range of motion. In this case, the right mandibular condyle translates a greater distance along the articular surface of the zygomatic process. The right masseter is activated to a greater degree to subserve the greater range of movement than the right TMJ. The fundamental problem, however, is not that the right masseter sEMG activity is greater than the left, but that the left joint has less mobility than the right. Surface EMG spontaneously becomes symmetrical once the left TMJ is mobilized with manual techniques or exercises.

Chronic Faulty Motor Programs

With chronic faulty motor control, it is assumed that the central nervous system learns to cope with pain, muscle weakness, joint instabilities, trigger points, myofascial extensibility issues, etc. As a result of this, there is a learned disruption of the normal agonist-antagonist-synergist relationships. The assessment (and treatment) of this broad syndrome requires sEMG monitoring along with assessment of coincident joint segment dysfunction, soft tissue dysfunction, and behavioral analysis.

Consider a patient with chronic cervical paraspinal and suprascapular pain following lifting activities at work. Motion takes place throughout the shoulder girdle to elevate the arm forward. This includes upward rotation of the scapula, achieved by the coordinated actions of the upper trapezius, the lower trapezius, the lower fibers of the serratus anterior, and numerous other muscles with direct and indirect stabilizing roles. A motor program is a planned set of commands from the central nervous system that serves to coordinate the actions of muscles so that a specific goal is achieved—in this case, shoulder flexion. If an inefficient motor program is selected, then one muscle might contract with excessive or reduced tension relative to its synergist, resulting in abnormal loading patterns of both myofascial and articular tissue. With this patient, the sEMG activity of the upper trapezius is increased on the involved side, whereas the activity of the lower trapezius or lower serratus anterior is decreased, each relative to the uninvolved side. It is also the case that the latter two muscles are slower to increase their activity on the involved side through an equivalent left/right range-of-motion arc. These findings are associated with passive tightness of the upper trapezius and maximal manual muscle test weakness of the lower trapezius or serratus anterior. With close visual inspection, there are visual differences in the pattern of the scapular displacement between the two sides. Physical and emotional stress tend to increase the aberrant patterns. The patient has a poor ability to recognize tension and to manipulate the sEMG signals on the involved side.

ASSESSMENT/TREATMENT LINK: AN UPPER QUARTER EXAMPLE

The clinical diagnosis should lead practitioners to a treatment plan of some sort. And, as practitioners treat their patients, it is not uncommon to continue to assess all along the way, and to move from one treatment strategy to the next, based upon the successful acquisition of neuromuscular skills. Taylor has developed a good protocol-driven approach for the upper quarter, in which assessment and treatment are intimately linked.[32] For a more in-depth examination of this protocol, please refer to Taylor's chapter in *Clinical EMG for Surface Recordings: Volume 2*.[32] While the upper quarter is much more complicated than is depicted in this protocol, Taylor takes the approach advocated by Janda,[33] in which upper quarter dysfunctions are best described as an imbalance between the postural and phasic muscles. He then provides a good model for assessing and treating this type of disorder. Further exploration of Taylor's approach to treatment is presented in Chapter 9.

Phase 1: Postural Muscle Relaxation

Relaxation of the postural tone is the first step in treatment (see Figure 5–1). Because posture is the foundation upon which movement rests, paying attention to the resting tone is essential to successful treatment outcomes. The bilateral placement refers to independently monitoring the right and left aspects of upper trapezius using a narrow placement (see electrode atlas). Resting tone is tested in two postures—hands in the lap and arms hanging at the sides. If elevated levels are noted, the practitioner should begin by

Phase 1: Postural Muscle Relaxation

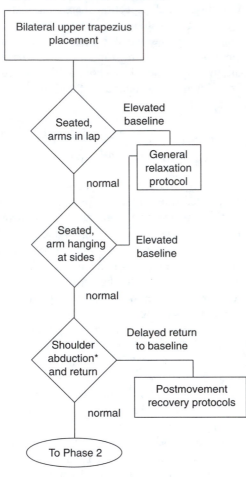

*and/or flexion or shrug

Figure 5–1 Phase 1: Postural muscle relaxation assessment and treatment linkage. *Source:* Copyright © 1990, JR Cram, *Clinical EMG for Surface Recordings*, Clinical Resources, Inc.

making general postural adjustments. For example, by simply asking the patient to lower the shoulders, the activation pattern might disappear. If not, a relaxation-based treatment protocol is indicated. Second, the resting tone is checked out following movement. This is described in more detail in Chapter 8. If the muscle does not return to a good resting baseline following movement, the practitioner should begin by teaching the patient how to rest the muscle com-

pletely following a given movement. These movements might include abduction to 90 degrees, flexion of the arms, or a shoulder shrug. Once a good resting tone is present, the practitioner can proceed to Phase 2.

Phase 2: Postural Muscle Stretching

The site for assessment may stay with the trapezius or it may focus on the scalene muscles. Muscle shortness may be a substantial contributor to problems in this region. In addition, the problem may be linked to respiration. The practitioner should examine the recording for large activation patterns that follow the breath, or ask the patient to take a deep inspiration and look for symmetrical recruitment patterns here. For initial treatment, Taylor suggests a stretching protocol similar to that suggested by Travell and Simons[27] for this site. He recommends lateral bending of the head, a passive stretch, and a protocol in which the patient is asked to breathe into the stretch and then relax into the stretch (relax-in-stretch). If the patient shows increased sEMG activity with the stretch, the goal is to teach the patient to reduce this activity while on stretch (see Figure 5–2). Once the patient's muscle is at a better resting length, the practitioner can continue to Phase 3.

Phase 3: Isolation of Phasic Muscles

The practitioner typically begins this phase as a result of the observation that when the patient abducts the arms, the upper trapezius clearly dominates over the lower trapezius (with normal functioning, there is a better balance between the two muscles). This imbalance is thought to reflect inhibited lower trapezius activity, rather than overactive upper trapezius activity. This is discussed in greater detail in Chapter 8. The electrodes are placed on both the right and left aspects of the upper and lower trapezius. The patient is asked to engage in an activity that would recruit the lower trapezius. If poor recruitment patterns are noted, then isolation training is initiated (see Figure 5–3). The goal here is

Phase 2: Postural Muscle Stretching

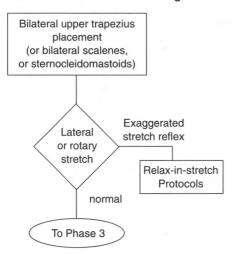

Phase 3: Isolation of Phasic Muscles*

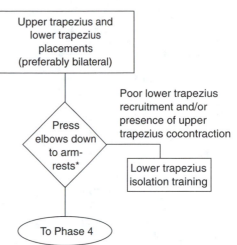

*See Lewit[34] for other isolation exercises.

Figure 5–2 Phase 2: Postural muscle stretching assessment and treatment linkage. *Source:* Copyright © 1990, JR Cram, *Clinical EMG for Surface Recordings*, Clinical Resources, Inc.

Figure 5–3 Phase 3: Isolation of phasic muscles assessment and treatment linkage. *Source:* Copyright © 1990, JR Cram, *Clinical EMG for Surface Recordings*, Clinical Resources, Inc.

to be able to activate the lower trapezius, without cocontractions from the upper trapezius or contralateral lower trapezius. Such training is described in Chapter 9. Once the patient can isolate and contract the lower trapezius, the practitioner can move to Phase 4.

Phase 4: Postural/Phasic Muscle Balance

The purpose of this phase is to bring other muscles into play and to seek proper synergy patterns among them (see Figure 5–4). Again, the upper and lower trapezius are monitored. The patient does a simple abduction to 90 degrees. Two levels of assessment are considered: (1) the relationship between upper and lower trapezius and (2) the relationship between contralateral muscle groups. If the upper trapezius continues to dominate, the practitioner should have the patient use the skill developed in Phase 3 to learn how to turn on the lower trapezius as part of the movement. Templates of the desired recruitment pattern are very useful and assist the patient in acquiring the proper timing of the new response pattern. This is termed "motor copy,"

and Wolf et al[35] have demonstrated that it accelerates learning of motor skills. Once the upper and lower trapezius can work in proper synergy, the practitioner should work on any right and left asymmetrical recruitment patterns. Once the patient has attained proper synergy patterns, it is time to move to Phase 5.

Phase 5: Stereotyped Movement Patterns

In this phase, electrodes are usually placed on the upper and lower trapezius. However, the serratus anterior may be substituted for the lower trapezius if the task at hand suggests this new placement. The goal of this phase is to transfer the skills learned in one posture to other postures and to more complex movement patterns. A very strong focus on activities of daily living is encouraged. If excessive upper trapezius activity returns, more work is needed to promote generalization. In fact, it is better not to assume that the generalization of motor skills will occur. The training of the neuromuscular system is typically very specific, and generalization should be built into treatment procedures (see Figure 5–5).

Phase 4: Postural/Phasic Muscle Balance

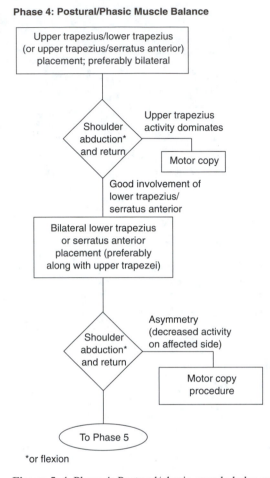

*or flexion

Figure 5–4 Phase 4: Postural/phasic muscle balance assessment and treatment linkage. *Source:* Copyright © 1990, JR Cram, *Clinical EMG for Surface Recordings*, Clinical Resources, Inc.

Phase 5: Stereotyped Movement Patterns

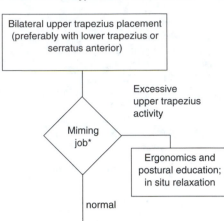

*and other tasks, eg, driving, typing, shaving, hair care

Figure 5–5 Phase 5: Stereotyped movement patterns assessment and treatment linkage. *Source:* Copyright © 1990, JR Cram, *Clinical EMG for Surface Recordings*, Clinical Resources, Inc.

CONCLUSION

Muscle dysfunction cannot be divided into disciplinary boundaries. The well-rounded practitioner must be alert to the many roles that muscles play and how muscles are affected by their external and internal environments. To be unaware of the postural aspects of muscle is to ignore the effects of gravity. To be unaware of the psychophysiological aspects of muscle is to deny the reality of emotions. To be unaware of the movement aspects of muscle is to ignore life. The rich and varied life experiences of patients must be considered and incorporated into practitioners' assessments. Along with activity or activation of the muscles, practitioners should consider the role of rest on a macro level as well as a micro level. To ignore the muscle as an organ system tied to bones is to forget the physical reality of what we are working with. Practitioners should determine when function gives way to structure and should attend to the repair of the structure before working on restoring function.

Each practitioner needs to recognize fully the limits of his or her own knowledge. It is probably impossible to be knowledgeable about *all* aspects of muscle energy and function, although the practitioner should attempt to do so. However, sometimes the best that can be hoped for is an awareness of one's own limits, along with knowledge that someone outside the practitioner's immediate discipline might have something additional to offer to the patient. In the best of all worlds, the patient is treated within a truly interdisciplinary setting where all of the various aspects of muscle function can be integrated into a comprehensive and complete treatment plan. Sometimes psychological or behavioral issues need to be resolved before physical issues can be addressed. A patient with a high level of stress or with major behavioral issues relating to pain will probably need to have these issues resolved before the physical treatments will be effective. Likewise, patients with a major contribution to dysfunction from a physical source (eg, joint mobility issues) will probably need to have this issue resolved before sEMG feedback for functional gains will be effective. A practitioner who knows his or her own discipline but is also aware of the other areas of concern, can more effectively treat the patient through cross-referral when appropriate.

REFERENCES

1. Whatmore G, Kohli D. *The Physiopathology and Treatment of Functional Disorders.* New York: Grune & Stratton; 1974.

2. Headley B. *Muscle Scanning.* Boulder, CO: IPR; 1990.

3. Iacona C. Muscle scanning: caveat emptor. *Biofeedback Selfregul.* 1991;16:227–241.

4. Mathiassen SE, Winkel J, Hagg GM. Normalization of surface EMG amplitude from the upper trapezius muscle in ergonomic studies: a review. *J Electromyogr Kinesiol.* 1995;5:197–226.

5. Zipp P. Recommendations for the standardization of lead positions in surface electromyography. *Eur J Appl Physiol.* 1982;50:41–54.

6. Veiersted KB. The reproducability of test contractions for calibration of electromyographic measurements. *Eur J Appl Physiol.* 1991;62:91–98.

7. DeLuca C. Myoelectric manifestations of localized muscular fatigue in humans. *CRC Crit Rev Biomed Eng.* 1984;11:251.

8. DeLuca C. Keynote presentation. Presented at the Applied Psychophysiology and Biofeedback Conference; March, 1992; Colorado Springs, CO.

9. Ahern DK, Follick MJ, Council JR, Laser-Wolston N. Reliability of lumbar paravertebral EMG assessment in chronic low back pain. *Arch Phys Med Rehab.* 1986; 76:762–765.

10. Cram JR, Lloyd J, Cahn T. The reliability of EMG muscle scanning. *Int J Psychosom.* 1990;37:68–72.

11. Cram JR, Steger JC. Muscle scanning and the diagnosis of chronic pain. *Biofeedback Selfregul.* 1983; 8:229–241.

12. Klein AB, Snyder Mackler L, Roy S, DeLuca C. Comparison of spinal mobility and isometric trunk extensors forces with electromyographic spectral analysis in identifying low back pain. *Phys Ther.* 1991;71:445–453.

13. Triano J, Schultz AB. Correlation of objective measurement of trunk motion and muscle function with low back disability ratings. *Spine.* 1987;12:561–565.

14. Dolce JJ, Raczynski JM. Neuromuscular activity and electromyography in painful backs: psychological and biomechanical models in assessment and treatment. *Psychol Bull.* 1985;97:502–520.

15. Robinson ME, Cassisi JE, O'Connor PD, MacMillan M. Lumbar iEMG during isotonic exercise: chronic low back pain patients vs controls. *J Spinal Disord.* 1992;5:1.

16. Donoghue W. *How To Measure Your Percent Bodyfat.* Plymouth, MN: Creative Health Products; 1990.

17. Cram JR. EMG muscle scanning and diagnostic manual for surface recordings. In: Cram JR, ed. *Clinical EMG for Surface Recordings, II.* Nevada City, CA: Clinical Resources; 1990:1–142.

18. Wolf L, Segal R, Wolf S, Nieberg R. Quantitative analysis of surface and percutaneous electromyographic activity and lumbar erector spinae of normal young women. *Spine.* 1991;16:155–161.

19. Matheson D, Toben TP, De Lacruz DE. EMG scanning: normative data. *J Psychopathology Behav Assess.* 1988;10:9–20.

20. Berman FS, Marcarian D. The Berman technique: a proposed standard protocol for chiropractic EMG scanning. *Am Chiropractor.* November 1990:34–40.

21. Kent C, Hyde R. Potential applications for EMG in chiropractic practice. *Digest Chiropractic Econ.* 1987; 9:20–25.

22. Leach RA, Owens EF, Giesen JM. Correlates of myoelectric asymmetry detected in low back pain patients using hand held post style surface electromyography. *J Manip and Phys Ther.* 1993;16:140–149.

23. Kendall FP, Kendall E, McCreary BA. *Muscles, Testing and Function.* 3rd ed. Baltimore: Williams & Wilkins; 1983.

24. Middaugh SJ, Kee WG, Nicholson JA. Muscle overuse and posture as factors in the development and maintenance of chronic musculoskeletal pain. In: Grzesiak RC, Ciccone DS, eds. *Psychological Vulnerability to Chronic Pain.* New York: Springer Publishing Co; 1994:55–89.

25. Basmajian JV. Fact versus myth in EMG biofeedback. *Biofeedback Selfregul.* 1976;4:369–371.

26. Perry J, Easterday CS, Antonelli DJ. Surface versus in-tramuscular electrodes for electromyography of superficial and deep muscles. *Phys Ther.* 1981;61:7–15.

27. Travell J, Simons D. *Myofascial Pain and Dysfunction: A Trigger Point Manual, I and II.* Baltimore: Williams & Wilkins; 1983.

28. Wolf S, Basmajian J, Russe C, Kutner M. Normative data on low back mobility and activity levels. *Am J Phys Med.* 1979;58:217–229.

29. Brown WF. *The Physiological and Technical Basis of Electromyography.* Boston: Butterworth; 1984.

30. Kasman GS. *Surface EMG in Physical Therapy: Applications in Chronic Musculoskeletal Pain.* Seattle, WA: Movements Systems; 1995.

31. Kasman G, Cram JR, Wolf S. *Clinical Applications in Surface Electromyography.* Gaithersburg, MD: Aspen Publishers: 1997.

32. Taylor W. Dynamic EMG biofeedback in assessment and treatment using a neuromuscular reeducation model. In: Cram JR, ed. *Clinical EMG for Surface Recordings, II.* Nevada City, CA: Clinical Resources; 1990:175–196.

33. Janda J. Postural and phasic muscle in the pathogenesis of low back pain. Presented at the Tenth Congress of International Society Rehabilitation; 1969; Dublin, Ireland.

34. Lewit K. *Manipulative Therapy in Rehabilitation of the Locomotor System.* Boston: Butterworth Heinemann; 1991.

35. Wolf S, LeCraw D, Barton L. Comparison of motor copy and targeted biofeedback training techniques for restitution of upper extremity function among patients with neurologic disorders. *Phys Ther.* 1988;69:719–735.

Chapter Questions

1. Surface EMG can be used:
   a. to diagnose nerve damage
   b. to diagnose herniated disk
   c. as a "clinical" diagnosis only
   d. all of the above

2. How does adipose tissue (the fat layer) affect sEMG recordings?
   a. It makes them invalid.
   b. It reduces the sEMG amplitude.
   c. It increases the sEMG amplitude.
   d. It has a stronger impact on dynamic than static recordings.

3. During the static evaluation, what approach should one take toward controlling the posture of the patient?
   a. Standardize the posture by asking the patient to "sit or stand up straight."
   b. Retain as much of the patient's natural posture by asking him or her to sit or stand comfortably.
   c. Ask the patient to go to the end range of motion.
   d. None of the above.

4. Surface EMG recordings appear to change as a function of age. In general, what statement can be made concerning this finding?
   a. Dynamic sEMG amplitudes diminish over the years (decades).
   b. Dynamic sEMG amplitudes become higher over the decades.
   c. Static sEMG amplitudes become higher over the decades.
   d. Both a and c.

5. Issues regarding volume-conducted sEMG are best addressed using the following:
   a. single-site sEMG recordings
   b. multiple-site sEMG recordings
   c. an ohm meter
   d. a volume conductor

6. Some muscle sites are more affected by volume conduction than others. Identify the muscle site below with the lowest probability of being affected by volume conduction:
   a. frontalis
   b. upper trapezius
   c. quadratus lumborum
   d. supraspinatus

7. Which of the following is not one of the clinical syndromes described in the chapter?
   a. simple postural dysfunction
   b. weakness or deconditioning
   c. acute reflex spasm or inhibition
   d. bruxism

CHAPTER 6

Static Assessment and Clinical Protocol

STATIC ASSESSMENT

The static evaluation is used to assess the "tonic" or resting state of the muscle. It provides an objective assessment of this resting tone, which correlates exceptionally well with any hypertrophied muscle mass noted during a palpation exam. To this extent, the static evaluation provides an objective measurement of chronically hyperactive muscles. In the more acute phase, these hyperactive muscles could be described as *muscle spasms*. Muscle spasms are similar to chronically hyperactive muscles, in that both are involuntary increases in alpha motor activity; however, unlike chronically hyperactive muscles, muscle spasms cannot be voluntarily released, they prevent lengthening of the muscle involved, and they are due to a painful stimulus impinging on the lower motor neuron.[1] Chronic hyperactive muscle activity may have lost its nociceptive origin and is functionally defined as excessive muscle effort that is outside the patient's conscious awareness. Resting tone is an attribute that normally resides outside the general awareness of the patient. When we execute our conscious volition, we use primarily our alpha motor system (our large extrafusal fibers), with a secondary emphasis upon gamma motor activity (the posture in which we do the movement). The resting tone is the foundation upon which volitional movement rests. It is the basis for posture. Thus, when the resting tone of

a muscle is observed to be above normal and expected levels, chronic hyperactive muscle activity or muscle spasm is identified. Usually, this is a low-grade activity, and not the obvious level of spasm noted in a "cramp."

Reliance on palpation alone can lead the practitioner to erroneous conclusions about muscle activity. Perhaps this is why some practitioners find that the term *spasm* has limited clinical use. When the practitioner palpates the muscle, it may feel hard to the touch. If the muscle is also electrically active, it is called a hyperactive muscle. However, in the case where the muscle feels hard and is electrically silent, the muscle is in a physiologically shortened resting length. Usually this is brought about because of the lack of use or complete range of motion for the muscle. It adaptively shortens its resting length to fit its range of use. Thus, a hard, silent muscle will be treated differently than a hard, active one. With the former condition, the practitioner might begin with heat and gentle stretches to begin the process of lengthening the muscle, and then proceed with retraining it. With the latter condition, the practitioner would examine the agonist/antagonist/synergist relationships in the context of pain to try to determine what drives the muscle into chronic hyperactivity.

In painful conditions, it is not unusual for the patient to adopt an *antalgic posture*—a postural shift to avoid pain. This reflects the patient's unconscious or a suprasegmental reflexive movement away from a painful sensation. When placed into an avoidant learning paradigm, the negative reinforcement (pain) leads the patient to learn the antalgic posture. This postural shift may become one of the signs of a painful condition and a perpetuating factor associated with the painful condition. Therefore, the muscle scanning procedure for assessing the static component of muscle is a tool for assessing hyperactive muscle and antalgic postures.

In addition, when evaluating antalgic postures, it is advantageous to assess the right and left aspects of axial muscles in both the sitting and standing postures. It is difficult to fully describe a postural shift if the practitioner monitors only one muscle site such as the trapezius or the erector spinae muscles at the third lumbar vertebra (L-3). The practitioner could obtain a stronger description by monitoring both sites or, better yet, by looking at the activation patterns for the right and left aspects of multiple sites along the spine.

NORMATIVE DATA

In understanding muscle function, it is useful to have a sense of what the "normal" surface electromyography (sEMG) amplitudes are for a given muscle. The atlas in Part II provides a "benchmark" approach for certain muscles, but only under static load conditions. These represent an approximate level associated with a given resting posture and are listed as a guide for interpretation. No norms are provided for dynamic procedures because of the complexity of the issues. The use of *normalized values* is recommended for dynamic procedures.

With any normative group comparisons, one should always be knowledgeable of the intended use of the testing instrument, how the test was constructed, on what populations it has been normed, how the standardized procedures were administered and scored, and the guidelines for the interpretation of the test results. The guidelines for the clinical administration of the muscle scanning procedure along with specific interpretive information for specific sites may be found at the end of this chapter.

Chapter 5 discussed factors that can confound the normative data. The practitioner should weigh these factors and moderate the interpretation of the sEMG data accordingly. For example, with some obese or exceptionally lean individuals, these factors may negate the validity of the normative data. Consider the use of normative data in psychometric/personality testing. Reading level may play a significant role in the validity of psychometric testing of personality using a paper-and-pencil instrument like the Minnesota Multiphasic Personality Inventory (MMPI). If the patient's reading ability is below that of the test construction or if the patient is significantly impaired due to the effects of a therapeutic drug, the results of the personality assessment would be invalid. Hopefully, clinical examination in conjunction with pattern recognition of the test scores would help the provider to determine the validity of the test. Although such moderating factors can invalidate the use of test norms on an individual basis, such factors do not negate the potential clinical utility of standardized testing in general.

The population upon which the norms for a given test are based is very important. Standards may be developed for a variety of populations: "normal" subjects, different patient populations, vocational groups, etc. In addition, normative databases may vary in size, thus affecting our ability to generalize from them. The larger the sample population, the greater our ability to generalize. In the normative database presented for the muscle scanning procedure, the comparison group was the "normals." What is meant by *normal?* Does this mean "really healthy," or is it just the average for the population? Attempts to describe *normal* are difficult, so knowing the description of the reference population is very important. The normative data presented in Tables 6–1 and 6–2 are based on a study by Cram and Engstrom,[2] in which *normal* was defined as not having a pain-related problem requiring a physician's visit for at least two years. So, *normal* in this case was defined as "the absence of the symptoms." To comprise this sample, 104 subjects were drawn from a subset of the stu-

Table 6–1 Normative Data Based on the J&J M-501 (100 to 200 Hz Filter)

Muscle Site	Sitting				Standing			
	Left		Right		Left		Right	
	Mean	SD	Mean	SD	Mean	SD	Mean	SD
Frontal	2.0	2.1	1.8	1.9	2.0	2.0	2.1	2.0
Anterior temporalis	2.4	2.0	2.4	2.2	2.5	2.1	2.1	2.0
Sternocleidomastoid	1.3	1.2	1.3	1.9	1.3	1.7	1.6	1.6
C-2 paraspinal	1.9	1.9	1.9	1.9	1.8	1.8	1.8	1.8
C-4 paraspinal	1.9	1.2	1.9	1.1	1.8	2.0	1.8	1.9
C-6 paraspinal	2.0	2.0	2.0	2.0	2.5	2.5	2.5	2.5
Trapezius	2.2	2.5	2.3	2.8	3.1	2.7	3.3	2.9
T-2 paraspinal	2.4	2.1	2.2	1.7	2.7	2.7	3.1	3.0
T-4 paraspinal	2.3	2.3	2.3	2.3	2.3	2.3	2.3	2.3
T-6 paraspinal	2.6	2.9	2.5	2.6	2.2	2.9	2.3	3.0
T-8 paraspinal	2.4	2.4	2.4	2.4	2.7	2.7	2.7	2.7
T-10 paraspinal	2.4	2.9	2.1	2.8	2.9	3.1	3.2	3.1
L-1 paraspinal	2.0	2.0	2.0	2.0	3.1	3.1	3.1	3.1
L-3 paraspinal	2.1	2.7	1.8	2.6	3.3	3.6	3.3	3.4
L-5 paraspinal	2.0	2.0	2.0	2.0	3.1	3.1	3.1	3.1

Note: Mild = Mean + 1 SD; Moderate = Mean + 2 SD; Severe = Mean + 3 SD.

Table 6–2 Normative Data Based on the J&J M-501 (25 to 1000 Hz Filter)

Muscle Site	Sitting				Standing			
	Left		Right		Left		Right	
	Mean	SD	Mean	SD	Mean	SD	Mean	SD
Frontal	2.8	2.9	2.5	2.7	2.8	2.8	2.9	2.8
Anterior temporalis	3.6	2.8	3.4	3.0	3.5	2.9	2.9	2.8
Sternocleidomastoid	1.8	1.7	1.8	2.7	1.8	2.4	2.2	2.2
C-2 paraspinal	2.7	2.7	2.7	2.7	2.5	2.5	2.5	2.5
C-4 paraspinal	2.7	1.7	2.7	1.5	2.5	2.8	2.5	2.7
C-6 paraspinal	2.8	2.8	2.8	2.8	3.5	3.5	3.5	3.5
Trapezius	3.0	3.5	3.2	3.9	4.3	3.8	4.6	4.0
T-2 paraspinal	3.4	2.9	3.0	2.4	3.8	3.7	4.3	4.2
T-4 paraspinal	3.2	3.2	3.2	3.2	3.2	3.2	3.2	3.2
T-6 paraspinal	3.6	4.0	3.5	3.6	3.0	4.0	3.2	4.2
T-8 paraspinal	3.4	3.4	3.4	3.4	3.8	3.8	3.8	3.8
T-10 paraspinal	3.4	4.0	2.9	3.6	4.0	4.3	4.8	4.3
L-1 paraspinal	2.8	2.8	2.8	2.8	4.3	4.3	4.3	4.3
L-3 paraspinal	2.9	3.8	2.5	3.6	4.6	5.0	4.6	4.4
L-5 paraspinal	2.8	2.8	2.8	2.8	4.3	4.3	4.3	4.3

Note: Mild = Mean + 1 SD; Moderate = Mean + 2 SD; Severe = Mean + 3 SD.

dents attending adult education classes at the University of California at Irvine. One could argue that this normative population is limited in size and diversity.[3] One might ask, for example, are the muscles of students the same as muscles of truck drivers, car mechanics, or carpenters? To answer such a question, one would need to study a sample of "normal" individuals from each of these vocations and compare that database to the database for students. More research is obviously needed. One might predict that a particular vocational population would differ from students to the extent that the group systematically developed or used some muscle more than other populations as a function of the work. Finally, the larger the sample and the wider the base of the sampling technique, the more confidence there is in generalizing the database to the population as a whole. For the normative database described below, the number of people studied is more than adequate to establish population statistics. However, the practitioner who uses this database should be aware of the limitations noted above.

Table 6–1 presents the mean sEMG value and standard deviation (SD) for a variety of cephalic and paraspinal muscle sites. Table 6–2 represents a mathematical extension of the narrow filter data to a wider filter. Here, a factor of 1.41 was used to provide the practitioner an additional set of values to help interpret recordings from wider filters. Using the conversion factors presented in Table 3–1, the practitioner may convert the data in Table 6–1 to equivalents for his or her own particular sEMG instrument.

WITHIN-PATIENT ANALYSIS

An alternative method of analysis for muscle scanning data is the "within-patient" analysis suggested by Iacona.[3] Here, the sEMG values for all of the sampled muscle sites in a given posture are analyzed for their central tendencies (ie, the mean and standard deviation are calculated). Then, each of these sites is placed in relationship to the central tendency for that particular patient and in that particular posture by comparing its value to that of the mean plus the standard deviation. This allows for a statistical description of both hyper- and hypoactive patterns for the particular patient. The hypoactive sites or patterns are only statistically visible when using the within-patient analysis method. This is because using population statistics, the standard deviation at a given site is usually only slightly smaller than the mean. Thus, a standard deviation of 1.0 below the mean normally lies within the noise level of the sEMG instrument and, thus, is meaningless. The within-patient analysis provides a basis for observing both hyper- and hypoactive sites by normalizing each site to the average of all sites for the particular patient. Thus, the highs and the lows become more visible. Tables 6–3 and 6–4 show group norm data and within-patient data on a patient with neck pain and headache. The hyperactive pattern at the C-4 paraspinal site noted by the group norm comparison also has a significant hypoactive pattern on the contralateral side, as shown by the within-patient analysis. Such findings may indicate a disturbance of the gamma motor system for that myotatic unit.

Within-patient analysis is most efficiently done with computer programs that calculate the mean sEMG value and standard deviation for the sitting posture and the standing posture. These programs then mark the data fields, as in the examples below, with some sort of notation. The legend below the data explains the notation. Where the practitioner wants to do a "thumbnail" of a within-patient analysis on a field of data, the practitioner would calculate the mean for the sitting posture. In the example in Table 6–4, the mean is 2.45. The standard deviation is likely to be approximately one half of the mean. We estimate it to be 1.2. Thus, the practitioner would add and subtract 1.2 from 2.45 to find the first standard deviation levels. They would be 1.2 for hypoactive and 3.6 for hyperactive. From the field of data in Table 6–4, only one value fits the hypoactive level—left C-4, with a value of 1.1. The only value to fit the hyperactive level is found at right C-4, with a value of 6.3. To estimate two standard deviations, add an additional

Table 6–3 Scan Summary Using Group Norm Data (J&J M-501, 25 to 1000 Hz Filter)

Muscle Site	Sitting		Standing	
	Left	*Right*	*Left*	*Right*
Frontalis	2.2	2.5	2.5	2.5
Anterior temporalis	2.4	2.6	2.7	2.5
Masseter	2.0	2.1	2.3	2.2
Sternocleidomastoid	1.9	1.8	1.7	1.8
C-4	1.1	6.3*	0.8	8.3**
Trapezius	2.6	2.6	2.7	3.0
T-2	2.1	2.0	2.0	2.3

*Mild activation

**Moderate activation[2]

1.2 to 3.6 (the total is 4.8); to estimate three standard deviations, add yet another 1.2 (the total is 6.0). The right C-4 value of 6.3 is greater than 6.0; therefore, it is at least three standard deviations away from the mean and qualifies as being "severely elevated."

In addition, the within-patient analysis is highly desirable for individuals with "unique" morphologies. This is particularly true for patients who have an extremely thin or thick layer of adipose tissue. Table 6–5 shows muscle scan findings in an individual who is extremely thin. Many of the microvolt readings are moderately high due to the lack of adipose tissue to impede the conduction of the muscle action potentials, and the group norms comparison identifies many elevated or activated sites. When the same data are submitted to a within-patient analysis (Table 6–6), only a few sites show activation. The within-patient activation pattern corresponds to the clinical examination through palpation (ie, the hyperactive sites associated with hypertrophied muscle mass). Table 6–7 shows scan findings for an individual who is obese. All of the microvolt readings are very low and appear to be within the normal range due to the ab-

Table 6–4 Scan Summary Using Within-Patient Analysis (J&J M-501, 25 to 1000 Hz Filter)

Muscle Site	Sitting		Standing	
	Left	*Right*	*Left*	*Right*
Frontalis	2.2	2.5	2.5	2.5
Anterior temporalis	2.4	2.6	2.7	2.5
Masseter	2.0	2.1	2.3	2.2
Sternocleidomastoid	1.9	1.8	1.7	1.8
C-4	1.1†	6.3***	0.8†	8.3***
Trapezius	2.6	2.6	2.7	3.0
T-2	2.1	2.0	2.0	2.3

***Severe activation

†Mild inhibition

Table 6–5 Group Norm Analysis of an Extremely Thin Patient (J&J M-501, 25 to 1000 Hz Filter)

| | Sitting | | Standing | |
Muscle Site	Left	Right	Left	Right
Capitis	3.0	3.5	6.4*	6.2*
C-4	8.2***	5.2*	8.6**	2.1
C-6	9.0**	7.0*	1.1	6.2
Trapezius	52.4***	15.4***	47.8***	19.7***
T-2	5.1	5.7*	12.3**	7.6
T-4	4.8	4.8	3.8	5.4
T-6	5.0	6.5	3.1	4.1
T-8	10.7**	17.2***	4.2	7.8*
T-10	11.2*	18.7***	1.8	16.1**
L-1	2.6	3.8	2.1	9.3*
L-3	1.8	2.6	3.7	6.6
L-5	1.8	2.7	4.2	2.7

*Mild activation[2]

**Moderate activation[2]

***Severe activation[2]

Table 6–6 Within-Patient Analysis of an Extremely Thin Patient (J&J M-501, 25 to 1000 Hz Filter)

| | Sitting | | Standing | |
Muscle Site	Left	Right	Left	Right
Capitis	3.0	3.5	6.4	6.2
C-4	8.2	5.2	8.6	2.1
C-6	9.0	7.0	1.1	6.2
Trapezius	52.4***	15.4	47.8***	19.7*
T-2	5.1	5.7	12.3	7.6
T-4	4.8	4.8	3.8	5.4
T-6	5.0	6.5	3.1	4.1
T-8	10.7	17.2	4.2	7.8
T-10	11.2	18.7	1.8	16.1
L-1	2.6	3.8	2.1	9.3
L-3	1.8	2.6	3.7	6.6
L-5	1.8	2.7	4.2	2.7

*Mild activation

***Severe activation

Table 6–7 Group Norm Analysis of an Obese Individual (J&J M-501, 25 to 1000 Hz Filter)

Muscle Site	Sitting		Standing	
	Left	Right	Left	Right
Capitis	3.1	2.8	4.2	1.9
C-4	1.6	1.7	1.2	1.4
C-6	1.8	1.4	1.6	1.8
Trapezius	1.7	1.7	1.9	1.6
T-2	2.8	2.8	1.9	2.4
T-4	3.0	2.8	1.9	2.4
T-6	3.3	3.7	2.7	3.0
T-8	1.9	1.8	3.0	2.3
T-10	2.2	2.5	3.4	1.7
L-1	1.8	1.7	3.2	1.3
L-3	2.6	2.9	2.1	1.7
L-5	1.6	2.3	1.6	6.7

Note: No sites were determined to be outside the "normal limits."[2]

sorption of the muscle action potentials by the adipose tissue. However, when the same data are submitted for a within-patient analysis (Table 6–8), a more meaningful activation pattern emerges from the data. Clinicians should be aware that all of the information regarding group norms and within-patient analysis presented above would also apply to data recorded during dynamic evaluations. Both static and dynamic sEMG information must conform to the same laws of physiology and statistics. The normalization of sEMG data as discussed in Chapter 3 provides the within-patient analysis perspective for sEMG recordings during dynamic procedures.

It is recommended that practitioners always use within-patient analysis on patients whose morphology is outside of the norm (ie, thin and obese patients). The within-patient analysis also provides a basis for examining the muscles for hypoactive sites, which is impossible using group norms. The group norms are useful in determining when the patient's activation patterns are outside the data set of an external reference group. This is particularly helpful if the analysis is required for litigation.

SENSITIVITY AND SPECIFICITY

The issues of sensitivity and specificity in sEMG research are complicated due to the complex nature of the relationship of sEMG to pain. Some of the classic reviews of the literature of headache[4] and back pain[5] have found that the relationship between the location of pain and sEMG values has a concordance rate of approximately 33%. However, it would be unwarranted, naive, and premature to conclude that sEMG lacks sensitivity in pain assessments. This is because the involvement of the central nervous system in pain is more complex than a simple one-to-one relationship. For example, the response to pain via muscle may bring about a protective guarding pattern in which the painful side is "spared," while the contralateral homologous muscle group becomes activated and is overused. In this case, it is the contralateral side that would be active, not the ipsilateral side, and the one-to-one correspondence of sEMG to pain would appear to break down. A second factor in the complicated relationship between sEMG and pain entails the spatial dislocation of pain associated with trigger points. Here the source of the

Table 6–8 Within-Patient Analysis of an Obese Individual (J&J M-501, 25 to 1000 Hz Filter)

Muscle Site	Sitting		Standing	
	Left	Right	Left	Right
Capitis	3.1*	2.8	4.2*	1.9
C-4	1.6†	1.7	1.2†	1.4
C-6	1.8	1.4†	1.6	1.8
Trapezius	1.7	1.7	1.9	1.6
T-2	2.8	2.8	1.9	2.4
T-4	3.0*	2.8	1.9	2.4
T-6	3.3*	3.7**	2.7	3.0
T-8	1.9	1.8	3.0	2.3
T-10	2.2	2.5	3.4	1.7
L-1	1.8	1.7	3.2	1.3
L-3	2.6	2.9	2.1	1.7
L-5	1.6†	2.3	1.6	6.7***

*Mild activation

**Moderate activation

***Severe activation

†Mild inhibition

painful sensation (the trigger point) may lie at a distance from the perceived location of pain.[6] When a muscle harbors a trigger point, its effect on muscle activity may not be clearly seen until the muscle is recruited during dynamic movement.[7] This is explained in more detail in Chapter 8. Suffice it to say that when the practitioner considers protective guarding and trigger points, the relationship between pain and sEMG comes into a clearer focus.

Cram and Steger[8] originally studied the sensitivity and specificity of the static evaluation technique. They compared the sEMG data on two groups of patients—headache patients and low back pain patients. They collected sEMG data from the right and left aspects of 10 muscle sites, both in the sitting and standing postures. They found that headache patients tended to show activation patterns in the cephalic and related muscles, while patients with low back pain tended to show asymmetries in the paraspinal (low back and neck) muscles. A later study by Cram and Engstrom[2] compared 104 normal subjects to 200 chronic pain patients. This study established that the muscle scanning technique separated pain patients from the normal population. These authors suggested that these differences occurred at a number of muscle sites, and that posture played a significant role in some muscles but not others. Scanning of the low back muscles (L-3 and T-10), for example, more clearly separated normal patients from low back patients during the standing posture. It was primarily the left aspect of the back that afforded this distinction. The trapezius muscles showed a much larger activation pattern upon standing, as well. This study was later replicated by Kessler, Cram, and Traue[9] in a well-controlled study with a well-defined group of low back pain patients matched with controls for age and sex.

RELIABILITY

The reliability of a procedure is a key to its use. Tests for the reliability of the muscle scanning procedure have been conducted on two occasions with two distinct populations in different locations. In an initial and preliminary assessment of the reliability of the scanning technique,[10] a 5-minute test-retest study was conducted on a small sample of 16 patients. Here, the test-retest correlations were found to be 0.92. Later, Cram, Lloyd, and Cahn[11] studied the reliability of the scanning technique; they studied 102 patients at three points during the day. The patients had come into a multidisciplinary clinic and were scanned upon their arrival. Next, they saw either the physician or psychologist, and then were scanned around midday. They were then seen by the second provider and scanned for the final time toward the end of the day. In this study, the test-retest reliability scores had a mean correlation of 0.64, indicating that the various samples of the sEMG data accounted for 64% of the variance. This figure is within the range of acceptable values for psychological tests in general,[12] and the authors believe that it is more than adequate for this type of physiological recording. The difference in correlations between the first to the second and the first to the third evaluation was not significant. This study establishes stability of the nature of the findings from muscle scanning across the course of one day. Further study of the stability of findings from muscle scannings across days, weeks, or months would be desirable. Information regarding longer-term reliability for single-site recordings using attached electrodes suggests that the longer the interval between test and retest, the lower the correlation coefficients[13] (see Chapter 8).

STABILITY OF THE SIGNAL

Because the scanning procedure entails holding the electrode over the patient's muscle site by hand and sampling from the site for relatively short periods of time, information regarding the stability of the sEMG signal during the actual data collection phase of the procedure would be of great use. When one initially places the scanning electrode onto the skin, there is an "electrical explosion" at the skin electrode interface. Soon the impedances begin to settle in, and the electrical noise of this event begins to settle out.

In some instruments (eg, J&J M-57 or M-501), this settling time is approximately 4 to 8 seconds, after which the signal becomes fairly stable. In other instruments that use an "active electrode" (eg, Thought Technology "Smart Sensor"), this settling time is two to three times longer. If one watches the integrated sEMG amplitudes (ie, bar graphs on stand-alone instruments or curves on the computer screen) during the scanning procedure, one can see the initial large drop in the signal amplitude associated with this settling time. After that, the signal has significantly less variability. One study[14] has examined the stability issue and found that the sEMG signal obtained with the handheld scanning tool is more than adequate. Figure 6–1A illustrates the nature of this stability. The researchers suggest that a 10-second integration time yields slightly greater stability than 2 seconds; but the differences are relatively small and any integration between 2 and 10 seconds should adequately represent the signal. Figure 6–1B demonstrates that by 4 to 6 seconds, the signal has significantly less variability.

Because the sEMG signal varies somewhat once the settling has occurred, some practitioners wonder when they should collect the sample of data. In general, if the practitioner takes the sample just a few seconds after the sEMG has settled down, that sample would be the most representative. In the Thompson et al study[14] noted above, data collection was initiated at this point in time, and a 10-second epoch was averaged. However, if practitioners wait too long, looking for an extremely flat and stable signal before taking a sample, they will miss the mark. Some variability in the sEMG signal ($\pm10\%$) should always be expected. In general, practitioners simply strive to minimize that variability. Cram and Kall have introduced an alternative algorithm into the data collection schema for muscle scanning software.[15] Some computerized scanning systems have deemed this "autocollect" feature. It assesses the amount of variance around the sliding average; when this variance becomes small enough, a 2-second sample is allowed to be collected.

A

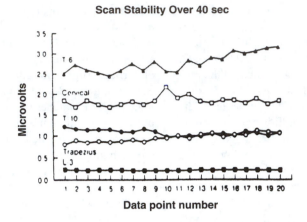

B

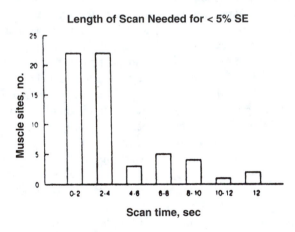

Figure 6–1 (**A**) Stability of sEMG signal at different sites for one subject. (**B**) Muscle sites grouped by length of time to achieve < 5% standard error. *Source:* Reprinted with permission from JM Thompson, EP Rolland, and KP Offord, EMG Muscle Scanning: Stability of Hand Held Surface Electrodes, *Biofeedback and Self-Regulation*, Vol 14, No 1, pp 55–61, © 1989, Plenum Publishing.

INTERPRETATION OF STATIC FINDINGS

The interpretation of scanning information is best guided by comparison of the patient data to the reference database collected by Cram and Engstrom.[2] This recommendation should be replaced with the within-patient analysis when the patient is extremely thin (<15% body fat) or extremely obese (>50% body fat), or when the acti-

vation pattern seen with group norm comparison does not coincide with the palpation exam. As Callet has stated: "Know what is normal, then you can discriminate what is abnormal."[16] The patient's sEMG information is examined for its level of activation or inhibition, its degree of asymmetry, and how much it is altered with postural change (see Exhibit 6–1). Once the sEMG information is collected, it is compared to information from the clinical examination.

Exhibit 6–1 Keys to Clinical Interpretation of Static Surface Electromyography Data

- *Site of activation/inhibition:* Greater than two standard deviations higher (activation) when compared to the population norms or two standard deviation lowers (inhibition) for within-patient normalization
- *Degree of symmetry:* 40% asymmetry between right and left sides[17]
- *Impact of posture:* Greater than two standard deviations difference between two postures
- *Comparison to clinical examination:* Sites of activation should correspond to palpation exam for hypertrophied sites

HEADACHE EXAMPLE

Muscle scanning can play an important role in the examination of the headache patient, because it allows the practitioner to suspend the one-to-one model of pain sensation to causation. Consider the data from two headache patients (Tables 6–9 and 6–10). Both patients present with identical dull, bifrontal headaches that are worse in the afternoon. Examination of the first patient (Table 6–9) suggests a myogenic headache associated with an activation pattern in the frontal region. With such a patient, attached sEMG electrodes might be placed on the frontal region using the wide frontalis placement from the atlas. Further evaluation using stress profil-

ing could be explored at this site. The examination of the second patient (Table 6–10), however, is more complex. It suggests referred headache pain associated with activation patterns in the cervical and trapezius region. This patient also exhibits asymmetry, along with a mild postural disturbance. Together, these findings suggest a potential biomechanical contribution to the patient's headache disorder. The practitioner might conduct further evaluation with at least two sets of attached electrodes, using the wide cervical trapezius placement listed in the atlas. Further recordings might consider the impact of stress, posture (sitting versus standing), and dynamic movement.

The scan data should always be compared with the clinical examination of the patient. The second patient, for example, was found to have a restricted range of motion in the cervical region, along with trigger points in the left trapezius muscle group that projected pain to the temporal region. This is an excellent case of the spatial dislocation of pain, where the pain is experienced at a different site than the site of origin.

Thus, the muscle scanning procedure adds one more dimension of data to the clinical findings. It does not replace a thorough clinical exam. In addition, the muscle scan findings suggest treatment options. With the first patient, the practitioner might consider a relaxation training procedure, aided with biofeedback from the frontal EMG site. The second patient, on the

Table 6–9 Headache of Frontal Origin

Muscle Site	Sitting		Standing	
	Left	Right	Left	Right
Frontalis	7.3*	9.2*	8.2*	9.4*
Temporalis	6.0*	6.4*	6.1*	6.8*
Masseter	1.8	1.6	1.6	1.8
Sternocleidomastoid	1.0	1.1	1.1	1.1
Cervical	1.9	1.6	2.2	2.3
Trapezius	0.8	0.9	0.7	0.9
T-2 paraspinals	1.9	1.8	1.9	1.9

*Outside the normal and expected levels[2]

Table 6–10 Headache of Cervical or Trapezius Origin

Muscle Site	Sitting		Standing	
	Left	Right	Left	Right
Frontalis	3.1	3.0	3.2	3.0
Temporalis	2.8	3.2	3.0	3.3
Masseter	0.9	0.8	0.9	0.9
Sternocleidomastoid	0.6	0.5	0.6	0.6
Cervical	7.7	2.7	5.6	3.3
Trapezius	10.7*	3.0	14.0*	8.0
T-2 paraspinals	4.9	3.8	5.6	4.2
T-6 paraspinals	5.5	4.7	5.2	4.3

*Outside the normal and expected levels[2]

other hand, might initially be approached with a stretch-to-relax protocol[18] or post-isometric relaxation protocols[19] assisted by sEMG feedback. This might be followed by dynamic movement retraining suggested by Donaldson et al.[20] In addition, the practitioner might consider the more traditional treatments for the identified trigger point.

LOW BACK PAIN EXAMPLE

Back pain is another disorder that can be evaluated with the muscle scanning procedure, because the back muscles are orchestrated and work together.[21] The multiple site approach of scanning matches the multijointed, suprasegmental nature of the back muscles. But, which sites should the practitioner monitor? Is the upper back involved in a low back patient? One would not know for sure without assessing multiple sites. The muscle scanning procedure provides a quick and reliable basis for deciding where to place attached electrodes for further study. Below are three scanning studies conducted on patients with low back pain. The first study (Table 6–11) shows an example of protective guarding, the second patient (Tables 6–12 and 6–13) show an instability in the pelvis that is posturally mediated, and the third patient (Table 6–14) provides an example of splinting in response to a neurological event.

The first study (Table 6–11) represents an individual with a primary complaint of low back pain, with no objective findings on traditional tests (physical exam, plain films, magnetic resonance imaging, needle EMG). He was injured 5 months ago, when he strained his back muscles while lifting and turning. Unfortunately, traditional conservative care has not led to a diminution of his pain. The EMG scan data show high levels of EMG activation only in the erector spinae group at L-3 and T-10. This appears to worsen upon standing, as if the patient puts on a neuromuscular corset as he goes from the sitting to the standing posture. This type of postural change commonly reflects *protective guarding*, a learned muscle activation pattern used to avoid pain. In addition, there is a striking asymmetry, with the right side more active than the left. In cases such as this, a hemipelvis or leg length discrepancy may have been discovered during the physical exam. However, if the pain complaint is on the opposite side of the activation pattern, the asymmetry usually represents a protective guarding mechanism. Here, the patient consciously or habitually shifts his or her weight away from the pain. It is far more common for the activation to be on the side opposite the pain rather than the ipsilateral side.

The findings of this scan suggest that further sEMG assessment using attached electrodes should be conducted. Because the upper back

Table 6–11 Low Back Pain Patient Protocol

Muscle Site	Sitting		Standing	
	Left	Right	Left	Right
Frontalis	3.5	3.8	1.2	1.3
Temporalis	3.5	3.5	4.6	3.6
Masseter	1.3	1.5	1.5	1.6
Sternocleidomastoid	1.2	1.5	0.8	0.9
Cervical	1.6	1.7	1.9	1.9
Trapezius	2.2	2.3	3.0	2.5
T-1 paraspinals	1.5	1.5	1.3	1.1
T-6 paraspinals	3.7	3.5	4.7	4.4
T-10 paraspinals	9.6*	19.2*	44.8*	59.2*
L-3 paraspinals	2.2	11.2*	19.2*	30.4*
Abdominals	1.3	1.5	1.6	1.8

*Values are outside the normal and expected limits.[2]

does not appear to be involved, a multiple electrode array in the low back area would be indicated. This is reviewed in greater detail below. It also suggests that biofeedback treatment should be directed toward the low back musculature. Here, the patient might strengthen the abdominal muscles, while using sEMG feedback to teach the patient how to use this musculature in a more biomechanically efficient fashion (ie, anterior pelvic tilt) while standing. The equality of weight distribution, using a weight scale under each foot, would be useful feedback.

The second low back patient represents a 35-year-old male who received a traumatic blow to his midback region while working in the logging industry. The muscle scan shown in Tables 6–12 and 6–13 was conducted using the 25 to 1000 Hz filter. Both the group norms and the within-patient analysis are presented because of the patient's moderate level of obesity. The results of both analyses are similar. The major difference is that the within-patient analysis identifies the cervical musculature and left low back sites while sitting as hypoactive. Otherwise, there is a shift in the symmetry patterns from left to right as the patient changes from the sitting to the standing posture. Note how the activation patterns in the low back shift from right low back to

left low back, while the upper back shows a compensatory shift from the left upper back to the right upper back as the patient changes from the sitting to the standing posture. Such a shift in the activation pattern strongly suggests a hemipelvis. This finding was verified during the clinical examination and was treated through joint mobilization techniques. In addition, external support with cushions or orthoses could be used to normalize the nature of this imbalance.

The third low back pain patient presents during a recurrent flare-up of a long-standing pain problem. The patient reports that the pain is very severe and radiates down into his right buttocks. Radiographic studies indicate a bulging disk at L-3 and L-4. The EMG scan data shown in Table 6–14 indicate activation patterns at the L-3 and T-10 sites, with the sitting posture evoking the higher level of activation. This type of finding—an activation pattern in the T-10 to L-5 region that is stronger when sitting than when standing—has been observed in a series of 12 patients with bulging or herniated disks (Cram and Dike, unpublished). It is thought that the additional pressure on the disk from sitting creates a larger bulge and thus places pressure on the nerve, creating a nociceptive environment that evokes an acute muscular splinting pattern around the in-

Table 6–12 Low Back Pain: Postural Shift Shows Instability in the Pelvis, Group Norms Analysis

Muscle Site	Sitting		Standing	
	Left	Right	Left	Right
Capitis	2.4	2.5	1.9	1.6
C-4 paraspinals	4.8*	4.5*	3.5	3.7
C-6 paraspinals	3.3	4.2	5.3	4.5
Trapezius	5.4	3.2	4.3	8.5
T-2 paraspinals	4.8	4.6	5.5	11.4*
T-4 paraspinals	8.2*	3.9	5.5	10.9**
T-6 paraspinals	5.5	4.8	5.0	4.7
T-8 paraspinals	6.4	5.7	5.7	4.0
T-10 paraspinals	3.7	7.6*	8.6*	8.3
L-1 paraspinals	2.9	10.1**	7.6	9.6*
L-3 paraspinals	2.6	6.7*	10.0*	7.2
L-5 paraspinals	2.3	5.1	12.9**	7.1

*Mild activation[2]

**Moderate activation[2]

Table 6–13 Low Back Pain: Postural Shift Shows Instability in the Pelvis, Within-Patient Analysis

Muscle Site	Sitting		Standing	
	Left	Right	Left	Right
Capitis	2.4†	2.5†	1.9†	1.6†
C-4 paraspinals	4.8	4.5	3.5†	3.7
C-6 paraspinals	3.3	4.2	5.3	4.5
Trapezius	5.4	3.2	4.3	8.5
T-2 paraspinals	4.8	4.6	5.5	11.4*
T-4 paraspinals	8.2*	3.9	5.5	10.9*
T-6 paraspinals	5.5	4.8	5.0	4.7
T-8 paraspinals	6.4	5.7	5.7	4.0
T-10 paraspinals	3.7	7.6*	8.6*	8.3
L-1 paraspinals	2.9	10.1**	7.6	9.6*
L-3 paraspinals	2.6†	6.7	10.0*	7.2
L-5 paraspinals	2.3†	5.1	12.9**	7.1

*Mild activation

**Moderate activation

†Hypoactivation

jured nerve to help minimize further damage. Such reflexively based splinting patterns are suggested when the pain complaint is on the ipsilateral side of the activation. In this particular case, there is a mild asymmetry on the ipsilateral side of the patient's pain. If such an sEMG scan pattern is observed in a patient without radiographic studies, radiographic studies should be considered. One should never diagnose a herniated disk or neuropathy from sEMG data alone. For this patient, EMG biofeedback therapy might best be used within the context of McKenzie-type therapies.

Through the systematic sampling of multiple muscle sites in these two neutral postures, the sEMG scanning procedure provides a framework for identifying potential sites of activation. Scanning of multiple sites may identify potential contributions missed by a more limited study. Its major weakness is that it represents only a "snapshot" of the potential contribution of the muscles in pain-related disorders. The dynamic EMG evaluation is needed to assess the impact of pain on movement.

To summarize, the muscle scanning technique may elucidate the following interpretive elements:

- identification of which muscle groups have been affected
- identification of antalgic (painful) postures
- identification of protective guarding
- identification of splinting
- identification of mechanical postural components

THE CLINICAL PROCEDURE ASSOCIATED WITH THE STATIC ASSESSMENT

Although a static assessment can be done with attached electrodes moved about during rest conditions, it is somewhat slow and involves a fair amount of supplies. A muscle scanning tool has been developed to make this procedure fast and reliable. A new tool to do static assessments first appeared in the 1970s as a picture in *Muscles Alive* (3rd edition) by John Basmajian.[22] In this picture, a specially engineered device with "post-style" direct contact electrodes was shown assessing the zygomaticus muscle; the electrodes were held in place by hand, rather than being attached with adhesives. While Basmajian had seen the wisdom of being able to sample and assess specific muscles quickly using these post-style electrodes, this technology essentially went unnoticed and undeveloped until its reintroduction in a commercialized form simultaneously by J&J Enterprises and Davicon (circa 1980).

The purpose of this section is to review the technical aspects of the static assessment procedure using a muscle scanning tool. It describes

Table 6–14 Low Back Pain Patient with Herniated Disk

Muscle Site	Sitting		Standing	
	Left	Right	Left	Right
Cervical	1.2	1.5	1.5	1.7
Trapezius	2.2	3.3	3.2	3.5
T-1 paraspinals	1.2	1.3	1.2	1.2
T-6 paraspinals	3.7	3.8	5.2	5.4
T-10 paraspinals	10.3*	17.1*	4.4	5.9
L-3 paraspinals	10.4*	15.2*	4.2	5.1
Abdominals	1.3	1.5	1.6	1.8

*Outside the normal and expected limits[2]

the sites for electrode placement, discusses interpretation of findings for each site, and briefly highlights some of the pitfalls associated with the technique.

Although the general principles of muscle scanning are quite simple, one must adhere to the principles outlined below or the sEMG study will be significantly flawed, providing a false view of the neuromuscular system.

1. It is important to keep the impedance (resistance) at the recording site as low as possible. One must abrade the site to be scanned, so that it is free of oils and the dead or horny layer of skin.
2. If the scanning electrodes allow this, the practitioner should coat the scanning electrodes lightly with electrode paste or cream prior to placing them onto the site. This will add ions to the electrode skin interface, thus lowering the impedance while potentiating the biological signal.
3. The practitioner should hold the sensors in place with a light pressure and avoid pressing too firmly. Too much pressure might push the patient off the center of gravity, thus creating an artificial recruitment pattern. Some practitioners have asked whether excess pressure might place the muscle on stretch. Cram has attempted to demonstrate this on many occasions and in many ways, and has not found this to be a source of artifact.
4. Because scanning electrodes are not held in place with adhesive tape, the electrodes must be held motionless by hand for a period of 6 to 20 seconds. It takes the signal 4 to 8 seconds to stabilize from the electrical explosion that occurs when the scanning electrodes initially make contact with the skin. In addition, going much beyond 30 seconds does nothing but add potential movement artifact into the signal. Intentional or accidental movement or sliding of the scanning electrode must be avoided, because it generates an offset potential that artificially elevates the levels of energy seen on the instrument.

A Step-by-Step Description of the Clinical Procedure

The clinical procedure described below has evolved over 10 years of refinement. Many different strategies have been tried over the years, and the following procedure yields reliable results.

- *Step 1.* Identify the muscle group of interest. Think about the origin and insertion of the muscles and the direction of the muscle fibers. Visually or tactually locate the belly of the muscle.
- *Step 2.* Abrade and clean the scan site with a rough alcohol swab. The practitioner might think of the phrase "rub to rubor." Do not use cotton balls. Let the site air dry. Clean all of the sites that will be scanned (see Figure 6–2). The reference electrode simply needs to be on the patient's body.
- *Step 3.* Ask the patient to sit or stand comfortably. Do not otherwise verbally or physically prompt the patient's posture. Make visual observations of the "natural" posture.

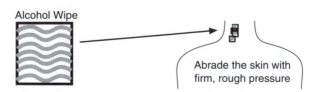

Alcohol Wipe

Abrade the skin with firm, rough pressure

Figure 6–2 Abrade the placement site with a rough alcohol swab. *Source:* Copyright © 1992, JR Cram, *SIS 3000 Manual*, Clinical Resources, Inc.

- *Step 4.* If appropriate, run a bead of electrode paste or cream on a tissue. Dip the scanning electrodes in the bead and lightly coat them with this paste. Avoid ending up with globs of paste on the electrodes (see Figure 6–3).
- *Step 5.* For recording from specific muscle groups, place the scanning electrodes so that they run parallel to the muscle fibers of the muscle of interest. When comparing data to the normative data presented in Tables 6–1 and 6–2, be certain to use the electrode placement guide used in the normative study. Once the electrodes are on the skin, hold them motionless with a light pressure (see Figure 6–4).
- *Step 6.* Observe the EMG recording. Allow it to settle from its initial contact artifact. This usually takes 4 to 20 seconds, depending upon the sEMG instrument. The signal is considered stable (±10% in its fluctuations) and free of artifacts (swallowing, movement) and noise (60 Hz). The level of heart rate artifact, if present, should be noted.
- *Step 7.* When the stability of the sEMG signal seems satisfactory, record that EMG

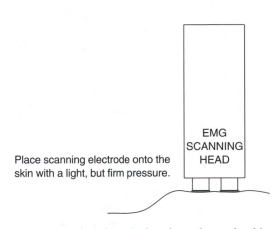

Place scanning electrode onto the skin with a light, but firm pressure.

Figure 6–4 Place the scanning electrodes on the skin and hold in place with a light, but firm pressure. *Source:* Copyright © 1992, JR Cram, *SIS 3000 Manual*, Clinical Resources, Inc.

value as the best representative sample of sEMG activity for that site. The total scanning procedure for a given site commonly takes about 10 to 30 seconds.

- *Step 8.* If a site shows values in the "severe" range (see normative database), verify that this value is the result of sEMG signals rather than noise of some type. If the values are excessively low, consider the possibility of bridging of electrode paste. In either event, clean the site again and rescan it to see if it remains stable in its elevation.
- *Step 9.* Study the right and left aspects of each muscle site. If the sEMG system has dual-channel scanning capacity that allows the practitioner to monitor the right and left sides simultaneously, use it. If postural muscles are monitored, conduct the scan in both the sitting and standing postures.

Potential Problems and Pitfalls of the Procedure

There are five problems that commonly enter into the scanning procedure: exceptionally low value, exceptionally high values, variable EMG values, obesity, and physical appliances.

1. *Exceptionally low sEMG readings* (in the noise range for the sEMG amplifier).

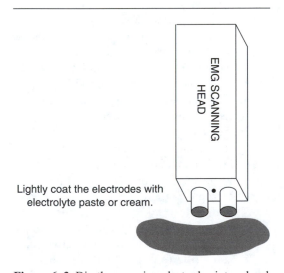

Lightly coat the electrodes with electrolyte paste or cream.

Figure 6–3 Dip the scanning electrodes into a bead of electrode paste. *Source:* Copyright © 1992, JR Cram, *SIS 3000 Manual*, Clinical Resources, Inc.

These readings occur when there is a bridging of paste between the two active electrodes. If the procedure is done while the skin is still moist from the alcohol abrade, the patient's natural salts may join the moisture of the alcohol to form an electron bridge. Exceptionally low values should always be suspect. Clean the site again, let it dry, and scan it a second time.

2. *Exceptionally high sEMG values* (above 25 to 40 microvolts on most sEMG instruments). Surface EMG values seldom go above these amplitudes, except in posturally active muscles or muscles in "spasm." High readings may also be due to 60-cycle noise entering the amplifiers. This is commonly associated with poor contact of the electrode with the skin. If the skin has not been adequately abraded, and natural oils or oils from makeup have not been removed, 60-cycle noise can easily invade the signal. This problem is often associated with scanning at the hairline. Here, the practitioner may adequately abrade the skin in the cervical region, but not into the hairline; or the practitioner may use adequate electrode paste for the skin but not enough to penetrate through the hair. If there is a radical difference in the level of impedance between the two recording electrodes, the differential amplifier is defeated and becomes very vulnerable to 60-cycle noise. Practitioners are discouraged from scanning up into the hairline to reduce the probability of impedance. Listening to the raw sEMG for the muscle action potentials (rather than the hum of the 60-cycle noise) can increase the practitioner's confidence in the validity of a high EMG reading. If the raw sEMG is not available, check the skin preparation and adequacy of electrode paste and rescan the site.

3. *Excessive variability of the sEMG values.* Sometimes the practitioner places the scanning electrodes onto the skin and the sEMG values do not appear to stabilize enough. Because no consistent value is generated, it is difficult to tell which sample is the best representation of the true sEMG value. Most of the time, this problem occurs when a person who is new to scanning stays on the site too long. Typically, the signal drops rapidly and then stabilizes for some 10 to 20 seconds, after which the level of variability increases. This variability likely has to do with the effects of holding the scanner in place by hand. In essence, the patient begins to sway, as he or she subtly presses back against the pressure of the scanning electrode. The practitioner should stay on the site for as little time as possible. As soon as the signal has stabilized, record that value. A second source of variability has to do with respiration artifact. Some individuals (especially smokers and patients with chronic obstructive pulmonary disease) tend to use their ancillary muscles instead of the diaphragm for respiration. Surface EMG readings of the muscles of the upper trapezius and the dorsal region seem to be most affected by this type of artifact. When it is observed, one can easily note the correlation between the variability of the sEMG reading and the patient's respiration cycle. If this is the case, the correct sEMG value to record would be the one associated with the pause between expiration and inspiration.

4. *Obesity.* Because adipose tissue is an effective insulator, it attenuates or reduces the amount of sEMG signal reaching the skin's surface, which causes the sEMG levels on an obese individual to be much lower than normal. One should exercise extreme caution in the interpretation of scan values taken from an obese individual. When comparing an individual patient's data to that of a normative population (see Tables 6–1 and 6–2), there is a high probability of a false negative finding.

5. *Physical appliances* (such as dentures, glasses, shoes, lifts, etc). Although physi-

cal appliances may introduce an alteration in muscle activity, they may also provide powerful diagnostic clues about the etiology of pain and dysfunction. Recordings from the temporalis muscle group provide a good example of this phenomenon. Cram has noticed that patients who wear dentures have a higher probability of bracing with these muscles; where this bracing is clearly seen, the patient is having problems with loose-fitting dentures and is using the temporalis muscles to hold the dentures in place. He has also noted problems with frontalis and cervical muscles in patients who are having difficulties with glasses (usually bifocals); this problem may come from frowning, squinting, or tilting the head excessively to see through the correct area of the lens. Shoes and/or lifts may also introduce another level of variance in the sEMG values. It is up to the practitioner to inquire and make astute observations to allow for these factors in the interpretive framework.

NORMATIVE DATA COMPARISON CONSIDERATIONS

To develop normative data, the initial clinical protocol entailed the scanning of the right and left aspects of 11 muscle groups, first in the sitting and then in the standing postures. This was later extended to additional muscle groups. The normative data collected on 104 normal subjects is presented in Tables 6–1 and 6–2. For practitioners to compare the EMG values collected on an individual patient to the normative data, it is essential to follow the procedure and protocol described below. The filter selection, skin preparation, patient instructions, posture, and electrode placement must be exactly the same as those used in the collection of the normative data. The step-by-step procedure outlined in the previous section should be followed closely. Below is a description of the instructions given to patients regarding their posture.

- *Sitting posture:* The therapist asks the patient to sit on an adjustable, backless stool or to sit sideways on a chair so that there is no support given to the back. The sitting surface should be parallel to the ground and lightly padded. It is even better if the height of the sitting surface can be altered to accommodate the leg length of the patient. If the height is fixed, the therapist will need to use devices such as pillows or boxes to create a 90-degree angle at the knee and to allow the patient's feet to rest comfortably on a surface. The patient is asked to place his or her hands in the lap, and to "sit in a comfortable fashion." Words such as "sit up straight" are avoided. The patient is requested not to help the therapist by altering posture. For example, if the patient leans the head forward to help with scanning the cervical paraspinals, the therapist gently redirects the patient to sit comfortably. No further instruction concerning posture is given. The object is for the patient to take on as natural a sitting posture as possible.
- *Standing posture:* The therapist asks the patient to "stand comfortably" in an unsupported fashion with hands at the sides. Again, the patient is requested not to alter his or her posture to help make the scan easier. If the patient does this, the therapist redirects the patient to stand comfortably. No further instruction about posture is given. The goal is for the patient to take on the natural/habitual posture for standing.

LOCATION OF SCAN SITES AND INTERPRETATION FOR EACH SITE

As the placement for each site is presented below, consider the anatomical markers described to aid in the placement. Examine the graphic depiction for the original 11 scan sites displayed in Figure 6–5, along with the additional extended scan sites displayed in Figure 6–6. An interpretive framework for the recordings of each site is given. The practitioner should remember that the site labels refer most clearly

A

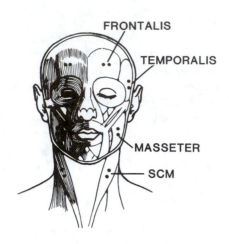

FRONTALIS

TEMPORALIS

MASSETER

SCM

B

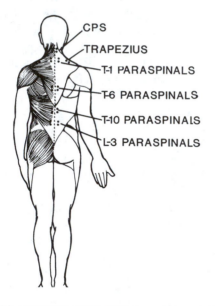

CPS

TRAPEZIUS

T-1 PARASPINALS

T-6 PARASPINALS

T-10 PARASPINALS

L-3 PARASPINALS

Key: CPS, cervical paraspinals; SCM, sternocleidomastoid

Figure 6–5 The original scan sites (**A**) for the face and (**B**) for the back. Abdominal site is not shown. *Source:* Copyright © 1992, JR Cram, *The Cram Scan Manual*, Clinical Resources, Inc.

to the location of the scanning electrodes rather than to the muscles actually recorded from. Further information on the location and interpretation of each of these sites also can be found in the electrode atlas in Part II. The practitioner

should be aware that the muscle scanning procedure is most appropriately used in assessing postural muscles and emotional tone. In the sites described below, phasic muscles are also included. These will be flagged by an asterisk (*). Use of the scanning protocol to assess these muscles should be limited to evaluation of the resting state and exploration of possible emotional contributions. Practitioners should not attempt to use muscle scanning to assess these phasic muscles during dynamic movement. They may use scanning to study isometric contractions but only with extreme caution.

Low Frontalis

Placement

The scan electrodes are placed parallel to the eyebrow, and approximately 1/2 inch above it. The space between the two electrodes is centered over the iris of the eye. This configuration of the recording electrodes runs perpendicular to the muscle fibers of the frontalis muscle. This is a nonspecific recording that records from a small region on the forehead—including frontalis, corrugator, orbicularis oculi, and temporalis.

Interpretation

The primary function of this muscle or region is the nonverbal display of emotions. The emotions of anger, fear, sadness, and surprise activate this region. It may also be associated with intense concentration or squinting of the eyes. Elevations noted here may represent an emotional contribution to the presenting problem. It has been suggested that elevations on the left aspect may be seen in patients who are prone to cardiac problems.

Anterior Temporalis

Placement

The scan electrodes are placed in a vertical direction. The lowest of the recording electrodes is placed across from the notch of the eye socket

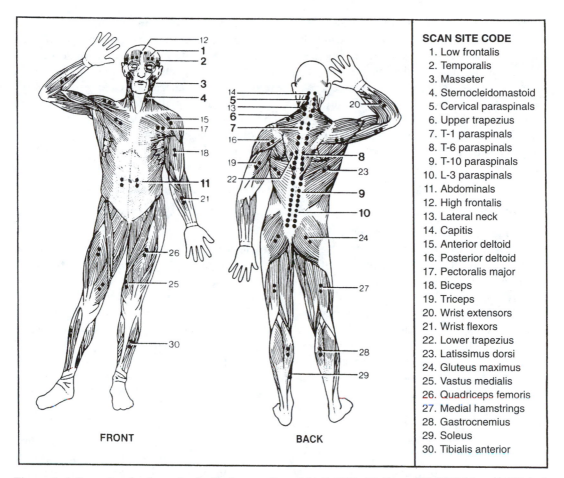

SCAN SITE CODE
1. Low frontalis
2. Temporalis
3. Masseter
4. Sternocleidomastoid
5. Cervical paraspinals
6. Upper trapezius
7. T-1 paraspinals
8. T-6 paraspinals
9. T-10 paraspinals
10. L-3 paraspinals
11. Abdominals
12. High frontalis
13. Lateral neck
14. Capitis
15. Anterior deltoid
16. Posterior deltoid
17. Pectoralis major
18. Biceps
19. Triceps
20. Wrist extensors
21. Wrist flexors
22. Lower trapezius
23. Latissimus dorsi
24. Gluteus maximus
25. Vastus medialis
26. Quadriceps femoris
27. Medial hamstrings
28. Gastrocnemius
29. Soleus
30. Tibialis anterior

FRONT   BACK

Figure 6–6 Scan sites for the entire body. *Source:* Copyright © 1992, JR Cram, *SIS 3000 Manual*, Clinical Resources, Inc.

approximately 1/2 inch laterally. The electrodes run parallel to the muscle fibers of the anterior temporalis.

Interpretation

The temporalis is a major muscle of mastication and stabilization of the mandible. It elevates the jaw bone. Patients who clench their teeth during times of stress may show elevations at this site. Asymmetrical patterns (right versus left) may suggest involvement of the temporomandibular joint, which can contribute to headache conditions. The practitioner might consider inquiring about symptoms of temporomandibular joint dysfunction, which typically include

clenching, grinding, bruxing, splinting, making popping sounds, and feeling the jaw lock up.

Patients who wear dentures may show excessive activation in this muscle group. They appear to use the temporalis muscle to stabilize loose-fitting dentures. Noted elevations in this muscle group should be followed by an inquiry about the use of dentures.

Masseter

Placement

The practitioner can easily palpate the masseter muscle by placing fingers on the patient's jaw and asking the patient to clench his or her teeth. The goal of electrode placement for the masseter muscle is to place the scanning electrodes over the belly of the muscle, with the electrodes running parallel to the muscle fibers. To do this, the practitioner should draw an imaginary line from the corner of the jaw to the cheek bone and place the scanning electrodes along this line over the belly of the muscle. Scanning of this site on men with beards is impossible and should not be attempted.

Interpretation

The masseter muscle is the major muscle of mastication. The vectors of force form concentric pressure on the teeth and allow chewing. When one is not chewing, swallowing, or talking, this muscle should be quiet. Elevations and/or asymmetries in this muscle are commonly associated with dental problems (such as temporomandibular joint dysfunction, myofacial pain dysfunction, bruxing) and may suggest an etiology for headache. In addition, such as examination could be of interest to dentists who want to determine the appropriate splint fabrication for patients with temporomandibular joint dysfunction.

Sternocleidomastoid (SCM)

Placement

This muscle runs from the back corner of the skull (mastoid process) to the collarbone (clavicle). If the practitioner asks the patient to rotate the head to the right and elevate the head slightly, the belly of the SCM on the left may be easily seen. The scanning electrodes are placed parallel to the muscle fibers of the SCM and halfway between the mastoid process and the clavicle. The head is in the midline position during the scanning.

Interpretation

The major function of this muscle is the rotation of the head. The SCM on the side that is opposite the direction of the head turn is active.

The SCM also plays a minor role in respiration. Rhythmic sEMG oscillations that follow the patient's respiration pattern may suggest excessive use of the ancillary muscles of respiration. Asymmetrical patterns are clearly seen in torticollis (an abnormal twisting of the neck) and may be seen in patients with acceleration injuries to the neck. The activity in this muscle is typically quite low.

Cervical Paraspinal Muscles (C-4)

Placement

The scan electrodes are placed parallel to and approximately 1/4 to 1/2 inch from the spine over the belly of the muscle. If the electrodes are placed too far laterally, slightly off the belly of the muscle, the EMG values will be significantly lower. The upper scanning electrode should be below the hairline, approximately in the vertical center of the neck. (This differs from the capitis or C-2 placement, where the upper scanning electrode may reach into the hairline.) In conducting the scan of this site, it is important to notice whether the patient attempts to help the practitioner by leaning the head slightly forward. This error is common, because so many people have been trained by the barber or beautician to help in this way. If the patient does lean forward, the practitioner should simply say that it is not necessary to help in this way and should instruct the patient to return to a comfortable sitting or standing posture, facing forward.

Interpretation

There are many layers of muscles in this region; the scanning electrodes collect from the upper fibers of the trapezius, the splenius capitis, the splenius cervicis, and the semispinalis cervicis. These muscles are primarily involved in the support and rotation of the head. With unilateral activations of these muscles, rotation or lateral flexion of the head may occur; with bilateral activation, extension of the head may occur. In patients with poor posture, where the head is held in front of its center of gravity, these muscles are required to provide chronic muscular support for the 15-pound weight of the head. In such cases, these muscles may become fatigued, and 100 to 200 Hz filter recordings may not adequately represent the nature of muscular dysfunction. In another common variation, the cervical muscles may appear to have very low EMG values, especially in comparison to trapezius T-1 or T-6. When this occurs, the patient's posture may be such that he or she has "unloaded" the cervical muscles, transferring the work to these lower muscles. This pattern of activity is an inappropriate muscle synergy. Even though the cervical muscles show low EMG values, activations in related muscle groups make these values suspect. If evaluating this region, the practitioner should consider pattern analysis of one site to other sites.

The cervical muscles have been indicated in headaches located in the occipital and frontal regions. There may be a concordance in activation between the frontalis muscle and the cervical paraspinal muscles. Such a concordance may indicate an emotional overlay in the patient, suggesting that stress plays a major role in the headache.

Upper Trapezius

Placement

The scanning electrodes are placed so that they run parallel to the muscle fibers of the upper trapezius. Their direction follows the ridge of the shoulder. They are placed approximately 1 inch from this ridge, toward the back. They are located approximately halfway between the spine and the lateral edge of the acromion, just lateral to the belly of the muscle. The belly of the muscle may easily be determined by palpation.

Interpretation

The primary function of the upper trapezius has to do with stabilization or movement of the shoulder. It is also used in lateral bending or rotating the head. In addition, the shoulder region is considered a strong emotional display system.

Patients may elevate their shoulders when they feel threatened or are anxious and uptight. When EMG activation or asymmetries are noted on the trapezius, one or both shoulders are probably elevated.

This muscle is strongly affected by posture. Its static level of discharge may be radically different during standing compared to sitting. The position of the arms in relationship to the torso may be a major factor. In addition, there appears to be a left-sided dominance in this region, with the left aspect generally more active than the right. Some have argued that this is associated with "handedness." Others have suggested that this is associated with heart rate artifact. Because this left-sided dominance is more predictably seen during standing than during sitting, it is difficult to imagine how it might be associated with heart rate artifact.

Using the normative database, the relative activity of the trapezius should always be compared to the activity of other muscles, particularly those of the lower and midback. Compensatory shifts may be seen in some cases, where a left-sided asymmetry at the L-3 level is associated with a right-sided asymmetry at trapezius. In addition, the trapezius may be overly active as a result of too much inhibition of the dorsal (T-8 and T-10) muscle groups. Elevations in trapezius sEMG activity may be associated with temporal headache or neck, upper back, and shoulder pain.

T-1 and T-2 Paraspinal Muscles

Placement

The scanning electrodes are placed so that they run parallel to the spine and approximately 3 cm out from the vertebral ridge. The landmark for this placement is the C-7/T-1 prominence, which clearly stands out in most adults. To find it, the practitioner should follow the spinal processes in the cervical region down into the upper back until reaching the most prominent spinal process in the upper back; the chances are good that this is the C-7/T-1 prominence. The uppermost scanning electrode is placed across from this prominence.

Interpretation

There are multiple muscles at this recording site. Contributions from trapezius (upper/middle fibers), longissimus, semispinalis, splenius capitis, and multifidus muscle groups may contribute to the sEMG recordings. The primary use of these muscles is the stabilization and support of the head and neck. This site appears to be a major stress point for postural support.

Elevations at this site commonly are in concordance with elevations in the trapezius muscle group. High sEMG levels of these muscles when the cervical muscles show very low sEMG values suggest that these muscles may be doing some of the work of the cervical muscles. Elevations and asymmetries at this site may be noted in patients who complain of headache or neck or upper back pain.

T-6 Paraspinal Muscles

Placement

The scanning electrodes are placed so that they run parallel to the spine and are approximately 3 cm out from the vertebral ridge. The vertical level of placement is approximately between the shoulder blades (or scapulae). If the spinal processes can be clearly seen or palpated on the patient, the practitioner can count down six vertebrae from T-1 to find the location. If the bottom scanning electrode is below the bottom edge of the scapula, it is too low. The bottom edge of the scapula may be easily palpated.

Interpretation

There are many layers of muscles at this site. Contributions from trapezius (inferior fibers), rhomboids, longissimus, semispinalis, and multifidus muscles may determine the sEMG readings. These muscles have two functions: (1) to stabilize or move the thoracic spine and (2) to stabilize or move the scapula. In the free-sitting posture (no back support), these muscles may be very active. This is one of the few sites where higher levels of activation are expected during free sitting than during free standing. Pain in the midback or neck is commonly associated with elevations or asymmetries at this site.

T-10 Paraspinal Muscles

Placement

The scanning electrodes are placed so that they run parallel to the spine. They are approximately 3 cm out from the vertebral ridge. The vertical placement along the spine may be counted down from T-1, if the spinal processes are prominent. One can palpate for the ribs, and place the scanning electrodes slightly above where the rib cage disappears. Another method is to take approximately one half the distance between the L-3 placement and the bottom of the scapula.

Interpretation

There are many layers of muscles at this site. The primary contributors appear to be the longissimus and multifidus muscles. There is a possibility of contributions from latissimus dorsi and serratus posterior. The primary function of these muscles is postural support and stabilization of the spine. Because this is the region of the back where lateral bending is possible, this site may reflect this action. These muscles play a role in rotation of the back. Protective guarding and splinting patterns or asymmetries are commonly observed in this region for back pain patients. This phenomenon appears to be augmented in patients who have had surgery (particularly fusions) on the lower back. Posture strongly affects this site, and elevations or asymmetries may not be observed until the patient has assumed the standing posture.

This region seems to correlate most highly with the total amount of muscular energy observed in a scan. If a "key muscle" were to be selected that is indicative of general muscle tension, this would be the muscle.

L-3 Paraspinal Muscles

Placement

The scanning electrodes are placed so that they run parallel to the spine and approximately 3 cm out from the vertebral ridge. The iliac crest (top of the pelvic girdle) is used as the landmark to guide the placement. The practitioner should palpate for the iliac crest. Once this has been found, the practitioner should draw an imaginary horizontal line across the back toward the spine, placing the lower scanning electrodes at this level.

Interpretation

There are many layers of muscles at this site. The muscles thought to contribute most heavily to the sEMG recording are the iliocostalis lumborum and multifidus. The major function of these muscles is postural support—the stabilization of the trunk during standing. In addition, they are extensors of the lower back; they come into action with an eccentric contraction during forward bending (flexion) and in concentric fashion during the return to the upright position. Protective guarding/splinting may be seen at this site in some patients with chronic low back pain. The site is strongly affected by posture, and the sEMG recordings may radically shift as the patient goes from sitting to standing. During quiet standing, only minimal muscle activity in the low back region is needed as long as the patient is over his or her center of gravity. If one shifts slightly off the center of gravity (by leaning forward a little), these muscles come into play. It is important for the practitioner to note whether surgery has been conducted in this region. If so, the surgeon may have removed or denervated some of the muscles or in some way altered the neuromuscular structure. Needle EMG may be done to assess for denervation. Although the effect of denervation on sEMG potentials has not been adequately studied, practitioners should exercise caution in their interpretation of data in a region where surgery has been conducted.

Abdominal Muscles

Placement

The scanning electrodes are placed approximately 3 cm to the left or right of the umbilicus (belly button). The scanning electrodes are placed on opposite sides of the umbilicus. The direction of the electrodes is vertical, and they run parallel to the muscle fibers of the rectus abdominis.

Interpretation

These muscles play a role in the stabilization, elevation, and rotation of the pelvis. They are commonly underdeveloped as a result of lack of use. They may be covered with a thick layer of fat. If this is true, the recordings are lower due to the attenuation of the signals by the adipose tissue. Asymmetries may be noted in patients with low back pain, but this is very uncommon. Elevations may be noted in patients with pain of abdominal origin.

High Frontalis

Placement

The scanning electrodes are placed in the center of the forehead; 1 to 1½ inches above the eyebrows, just below the hairline.

Interpretation

This placement provides a general recording from the frontalis muscle group. The advantage of this placement is that it separates out the potential cross-talk from the corrugator muscle group. Therefore, it provides a cleaner sample of frontalis muscle activity.

Lateral Neck/Scalene

Placement

The scanning electrodes are placed in the hollow on the side of the neck, which is formed by the sternocleidomastoid anterior to it, the upper trapezius posterior to it, and the collarbone below it. The electrodes run parallel to the scalene muscle.

Interpretation

The scalene muscle is well known for its stabilizing influence on the neck. It plays an active role in lateral bending and is an ancillary muscle of respiration. Practitioners should observe the sEMG signal for spontaneous signs of respiration. Large excursions are considered pathognomonic. Abnormalities at this site could play a role in thoracic outlet syndromes.

Capitis Site

Placement

The muscles just below the base of the cranium are scanned. Because these muscles are in the hairline, the practitioner must pay particular attention to site preparation. The hair must be parted, a very vigorous alcohol abrade must be done, and an ample amount of electrode paste must be used. If the hair is too thick or coarse, it may not be possible to scan this site. The scanning electrodes are placed parallel to the spine, just lateral to the spinal process over the muscle belly.

Interpretation

Interpretation of high sEMG values at this site should be interpreted with extreme caution, because elevations may be due to poor impedance values. If high sEMG values are recorded, the practitioner should examine the site after the electrodes are removed to see how well the electrode paste penetrated the hair. The practitioner should then scan the site a second time to see if the same values are obtained. Exceptionally low values indicate electrode paste bridging.

This site is an extensor of the head when both sides are activated and is a synergist in lateral flexion and rotation when activated unilaterally. Therefore, head position should be noted whenever this site is monitored.

Anterior Deltoid*

Placement

The scanning electrodes are placed so that they run parallel to the muscle fibers in the anterior deltoid group. The scanning electrodes are placed on the anterior medial surface of the upper arm, just below the shoulder joint. The upper scanning electrode is placed approximately 3 cm below the clavicle bone, with the lower electrode going laterally at approximately a 25-degree angle from vertical, so as to follow the muscle fibers.

Interpretation

This muscle group plays a role in the flexion, horizontal adduction, and medial rotation of the humerus or upper arm.

Posterior Deltoid*

Placement

The scanning electrodes are placed so that they run parallel to the muscle fibers. When the patient's arms are hung to the side, the scanning electrodes are placed on the posterior lateral surface of the upper arm, just lateral to the shoulder joint. The upper scanning electrode is placed 3 to 5 cm below the spine of the scapula, with the lower electrode going laterally at approximately a 25-degree angle from vertical to follow the orientation of the muscle fibers.

Interpretation

The posterior deltoid group provides extension, horizontal abduction, and lateral rotation of the humerus or upper arm. Low sEMG recordings are often noted with multidirectional shoulder instability and chronic anterior subluxation or dislocation of the shoulder.

Pectoralis Major*

Placement

The scanning electrodes are placed so that they run parallel to the middle fibers of this rather large and flat muscle group. The electrodes are placed below the clavicle and above the breast and nipple, with the scanning electrodes running almost parallel to the ground.

Interpretation

The primary function of this muscle group is the adduction and medial rotation of the humerus or upper arm. Activation patterns have also been noted in post–myocardial infarction patients who continue to have a fear of a future myocardial infarction.

Biceps*

Placement

With the patient's arms hung to the sides, the scanning electrodes are placed on the anterior surface of the humerus in a vertical plane, so that the scanning electrodes run parallel to the muscle fibers. They are placed over the muscle belly, approximately two thirds of the distance between the shoulder and the elbow.

Interpretation

The primary function of this muscle is the flexion of the elbow and supination of the forearm.

Triceps*

Placement

With the patient's arms hung to the side in the standing posture, the scanning electrodes are placed on the posterior lateral surface of the upper arm. The scanning electrodes are placed over the belly of the muscle, approximately half the distance between the shoulder and the elbow. The electrodes are oriented in a vertical plane so as to follow the fibers of the muscle.

Interpretation

The primary function of this muscle is to extend the elbow.

Wrist Extensors*

Placement

The scanning electrodes are placed on the middle of the dorsal forearm about 6 cm down from the elbow. Asking the patient to engage in a wrist extension will help clarify the muscle belly. The scanning electrodes are placed over the muscle belly in a vertical plane so that they follow the muscle fibers. This site may be scanned with the patient in either standing or sitting postures. In the standing posture, the patient's arms should hang naturally at the sides. During sitting, the patient should rest the arms on the lap or some other surface.

Interpretation

This muscle group causes an extension of the wrist and fingers. It may be indicated in lateral epicondylitis or arm pain in general (such as from carpal tunnel syndrome). Elevations at this site in patients with pain conditions away from the arm may indicate an overall emotional arousal problem that involves the neuromuscular system. Elevations are also noted with lack of adequate scapular stabilization.

Wrist Flexors*

Placement

The electrodes are placed on the anterior surface of the forearm, approximately 6 cm from the elbow. The muscle belly is easily identified by having the patient flex the wrist. The electrodes are placed over the muscle belly in a vertical direction (while the patient is standing), such that the scanning electrodes follow the muscle fibers.

Interpretation

The primary function of this muscle group is to flex the wrist and fingers. EMG elevations may be noted in medial epicondylitis or carpal tunnel syndrome. Elevations are also noted with lack of adequate scapular stabilization.

Gluteus Maximus*

Placement

The scanning electrodes are placed in the center of the posterior surface of the buttock. The scanning electrodes are oriented laterally at approximately a 25-degree angle off vertical, so that the electrodes follow the direction of the muscle fibers.

Interpretation

This very powerful muscle is used primarily in rising from sitting, going up stairs, and running. Its primary function is the forceful extension of the hip and lateral rotation of the extended hip.

Vastus Medialis and Vastus Lateralis*

Placement

For vastus medialis, the scanning electrodes are placed on the medial aspect of the thigh, at approximately a 55-degree angle, immediately above the patella. For the vastus lateralis, the scanning electrodes are placed on the lateral surface of the lower third of the thigh, approximately 6 cm above the kneecap. The scanning electrodes are oriented laterally at approximately a 20-degree angle from vertical, so as to run parallel to the muscle fibers.

Interpretation

These large, strong muscles stabilize the knee. In patients presenting for evaluation of total knee replacement, significant reductions in sEMG recruitment are noted in these muscles and the other quadriceps muscle groups. Asymmetries between the lateral and medial aspects have been noted in patients with patella femoral pain.

Rectus Femoris*

Placement

The scanning electrodes are placed on the medial anterior surface of the thigh, approximately

half the distance between the hip and the knee. The scanning electrodes are placed in a vertical plane from the ground so that the electrodes follow the muscle fibers.

Interpretation

The primary function of this very strong muscle is the extension of the knee and an assistive role in the flexion of the hip. This muscle helps to bring the leg forward during walking.

Hamstring*

Placement

The scanning electrodes are placed on the medial posterior aspect of the thigh, about half the distance between the hip and the knee. The electrodes are placed in a vertical plane relative to the ground so that they run parallel to the muscle fibers.

Interpretation

These muscles primarily extend the hip and flex or rotate the knees.

Gastrocnemius*

Placement

The scanning electrodes are placed medially, on the upper half of the posterior aspect of the calf. There are two rather large muscle bellies. Palpate the muscle to identify the muscle belly. Place the scanning electrodes in a vertical plane relative to the ground so that they run parallel to the muscle fibers.

Interpretation

These muscles assist in the flexion of the knee and play a major role in plantar flexion (pointing of the toe).

Soleus

Placement

The scanning electrodes are placed on the lateral, posterior side of the lower leg. Because this muscle lies underneath the gastrocnemius, the practitioner must attempt to monitor it from the lateral or outside portion of the lower third of the calf, where the gastrocnemius begins to narrow in its width. The electrodes are oriented in a near vertical plane relative to the ground, with the electrodes running parallel to the muscle fibers.

Interpretation

This muscle is a very strong plantar flexor. It is actually the only muscle a person needs to stand in an erect posture (all other muscles should remain quiet while the person hangs on the ligaments). The practitioner should expect to see sEMG activity when the patient is standing.

Tibialis Anterior

Placement

The electrodes are placed about a third of the distance from the knee to the ankle, lateral to the tibia on the anterior surface of the lower leg. The electrodes are oriented in a vertical plane relative to the ground, so that they follow the muscle fibers.

Interpretation

The primary action of this muscle is the dorsiflexion of the ankle and inversion of the foot. This muscle lifts the foot during swing through as part of normal gait. Paralysis may cause "foot drop." Patients with poor foot control (ie, excessive pronation) use this muscle excessively in an attempt to control the foot or ankle, which may contribute to the development of shin splints.

Digastric/Suprahyoid

Placement

The scanning electrodes are placed under the chin, so that they run in an anterior/posterior direction, approximately 1/2 inch to the left or right of the middle of the chin, following the muscle fibers of the digastric muscle. The patient must not raise the head so as to help the practitioner with this placement. The practi-

tioner should ask patients to sit comfortably and should provide no specific instructions regarding the position of the mandible. Men with beards cannot be scanned at this site.

Interpretation

This muscle is part of a group of muscles called the suprahyoids. Their primary function is to elevate the hyoid bone during swallowing where the mandible is stable, or to open the jaw when the hyoid is stable. It is an important muscle to assess in patients with temporomandibular joint problems.

Posterior Temporalis

Placement

The scanning electrodes are placed slightly above the ear, toward its posterior flap. The electrodes are oriented downward at approximately a 45-degree angle relative to the ground. Electrodes should be clearly above the mastoid process and below the hairline.

Interpretation

This muscle, like the anterior temporalis, plays a role in elevating and stabilizing the mandible. Because of its more posterior location, the vector of force also includes the retraction of the jaw. This is an important muscle group to consider in patients with temporomandibular joint dysfunction.

Paraspinal Muscles (C-2, C-6, T-2, T-4, T-8, L-1, L-5)

Placement

The scanning electrodes for these muscles are placed so that they run parallel to the spine, approximately 2 to 3 cm out from the vertebral ridge over the belly of the paraspinal muscle. These muscles may be visually seen in some individuals but may need to be palpated in others. The vertical placement for each site is as follows:

- *C-6 placement:* For the cervical region, it is probably best to start at the bottom and move upward. The electrode placements go from easy to more difficult. The C-6 electrodes are placed so that the lowest scanning electrode is directly across from the C-7/T-1 prominence.
- *C-2 placement:* This is a very important, yet very difficult site to scan. The potential problems lie with the hairline. The most accurate method for vertical placement is to count up 5 vertebrae from the C-7 prominence and place the middle of the scanning electrode opposite this spinous process. An alternate rule is to place the lower electrode for the C-2 scan at the spot where the upper scanning electrode was for the C-4 scan. The residue left behind should help guide this placement, but the practitioner should avoid problems with the bridging of electrode paste.

  Placing electrodes at the hairline can be problematic. Make certain that the abrade for the site is rough and adequate, particularly around the hairline. If the patient's hairline is too low, so that the upper scanning electrode clearly reaches into a thick patch of hair, this will push scanning technology to its limits. If the scanning electrode that reaches into the hairline does not make a good, clean contact with the skin (scalp), this poor contact will artificially drive up the sEMG readings as a result of interference with the differential amplifier. When this occurs, the practitioner must decide if a high reading is real sEMG or just instrument noise.

  As an alternate means of monitoring the area, the practitioner can place the electrodes at an oblique angle, just below the mastoid process, rather than up into the hairline. This arrangement might better reflect the activity of the group of muscles that cross the atlas/axis joint. Practitioners who use this concept should give it a different label, such as "capitus," to differentiate it from the C-2 configuration.
- *T-4 placement:* To locate this site, simply count down four vertebrae from the C-7/

T-1 prominence and place the space between the active electrodes directly across from the vertebral prominence.
- *T-8 placement:* It is typically very easy to count down from the C-7/T-1 prominence, placing the space between the active electrodes directly across from the vertebral prominence. The location of this site is approximately where a women's bra strap would run.
- *L-1 placement:* To locate this site, count down 13 vertebrae from the C-7/T-1 prominence. Another method is to use the iliac crest to determine the L-3 vertebra (see the L-3 placement in the original scan site descriptions), and count up two vertebrae from that point.
- *L-5 placement:* To locate this site, count down 17 from the C-7/T-1 prominence or 2 down from the L-3 vertebra determined using the iliac crest method described above. This site is typically below the belt line.

Interpretation

When monitoring from the paraspinal muscles, there are many layers of muscles to consider: longissimus, spinalis, semispinalis, and multifidus may contribute to the signal. All of these muscles play a substantial role in stabilization of the spine. In addition, when both the right and left aspects are activated, extension of the spine occurs. Unilateral contractions of one side lead to either rotation or lateral bending of the spine.

Some chiropractors believe that an asymmetry in sEMG at one level indicates a rotated or subluxated vertebra at that level. This may or may not be true. An unpublished pilot study on 25 chiropractic patient records for sEMG (neutral posture) and radiographic findings (using the Gonsted method) indicated that the relationship between asymmetry in sEMG and vertebra rotation/subluxation varied from level to level. The strongest relationships were found at sites of the greatest spinal instability: the axis and L-5 levels. At the axis, 21 of 25 patients showed abnormal radiographic findings. Of the 23 who were scanned at this site, 9 (39%) showed significant sEMG asymmetries. Of those with sEMG asymmetries, 6 (67%) had concomitant radiographic evidence. At L-5, 18 of the 25 patients showed radiographic evidence. Of the 22 who were scanned at this site, only 6 (27%) had clinically significant asymmetries. Of those with asymmetries, 5 (83%) had concomitant X-ray findings. At the T-1 paraspinals, only 4 abnormal X-ray findings were identified for the 25 patients. Of the 14 patients scanned at that site, only 4 (29%) had clinically significant sEMG asymmetries. Of those 4, only 1 (25%) had a concomitant X-ray finding. At a similar site, T-7, there were 4 patients with abnormal X-rays, and of the 14 patients receiving an sEMG scan at

this site, only 2 (14%) were asymmetrical. Both of these patients (100%) had abnormal radiographic findings. From this brief study, it may be concluded that it is too simplistic to say that an sEMG asymmetry at a given level indicates a rotated or subluxated vertebral body. X-ray evidence of rotation is not always associated with asymmetrical sEMG activity. In addition, when clinically significant asymmetries of sEMG activity are noted, they are not always associated with radiographic evidence of rotation. In addition to rotation, practitioners should consider other diagnostic concepts such as scoliosis, pain displays of splinting/guarding, functional problems, hypermobile and hypomobile segments, and emotional displays.

REFERENCES

1. Stedman TL. *Stedman's Medical Dictionary*. 25th ed. Baltimore: Williams & Wilkins; 1990.

2. Cram JR, Engstrom D. Patterns of neuromuscular activity in pain and non-pain patients. *Clin Biofeedback Health*. 1986;9:106–116.

3. Iacona C. Muscle scanning: caveat emptor. *Biofeedback Selfregul*. 1991;16:227–241.

4. Haynes S. Muscle-contraction headache: Psycho-physiological perspective in etiology and treatment. In: Haynes S, Gannorn W, eds. *Psychosomatic Disorders: A Psychophysiological Approach to Etiology and Treatment*. Westport, CT: Greenwood Press; 1981.

5. Dolce JJ, Raczynski JM. Neuromuscular activity and electromyography in painful backs: psychological and biomechanical models in assessment and treatment. *Psychol Bull*. 1985;97:502–520.

6. Travell J, Simons D. *Myofascial Pain and Dysfunction: A Trigger Point Manual, I and II*. Baltimore: Williams & Wilkins; 1983.

7. Donaldson S, Skubick D, Clasby B, Cram J. The evaluation of trigger-point activity using dynamic EMG techniques. *Am J Pain Manage*. 1994;4:118–122.

8. Cram JR, Steger JC. Muscle scanning and the diagnosis of chronic pain. *Biofeedback Selfregul*. 1983;8:229–241.

9. Kessler M, Cram JR, Traue H. EMG muscle scanning in pain patients and controls: a replication and extension. *Am J Pain Manage*. 1993;3:20–28.

10. Cram JR. *Clinical EMG for Surface Recordings, I*. Poulsbo, WA: J&J Engineering; 1986.

11. Cram JR, Lloyd J, Cahn T. The reliability of EMG muscle scanning. *Int J Psychosom*. 1990;37:68–72.

12. Kaplan RH, Saccyzzo DP. *Psychological Testing: Principles, Applications and Issues*. Monterey, CA: Brooks/Cole; 1989.

13. Ahern DK, Follick MJ, Cocurcil JR, Laser-Wolston N. Reliability of lumbar paravertebral EMG assessment in chronic low back pain. *Arch Phys Med Rehab*. 1986;76:762–765.

14. Thompson JM, Rolland EP, Offord KP. EMG muscle scanning: stability of hand held surface electrodes. *Biofeedback Selfregul*. 1989;14:55–61.

15. Cram JR, Kall R. *The CAM Scan Software*. Nevada City, CA: Clinical Resources; 1990.

16. Callet R. *Soft Tissue Injury and Disability*. Philadelphia: FA Davis; 1977.

17. Donaldson S, Donaldson M. Multi-channel EMG assessment and treatment techniques. In: Cram JR, ed. *Clinical EMG for Surface Recordings, II*. Nevada City, CA: Clinical Resources; 1990:143–174.

18. Cram JR. Diagnostic frameworks for surface EMG. *Biofeedback Selfregul*. 1988;13:123–137.

19. Lewit K. *Manipulative Therapy in Rehabilitation of the Locomotor System*. Boston: Butterworth Heinemann; 1991.

20. Donaldson S, Skubick D, Donaldson M. *Electromyography, Trigger Points and Myofascial Syndromes*. Calgary, Alberta: Behavioral Health Consultants; 1991.

21. Hollingshead WH. *Functional Anatomy of the Limbs and Back*. Philadelphia: WB Saunders; 1976.

22. Basmajian JV. *Muscles Alive*. 3rd ed. Baltimore: Williams & Wilkins; 1974.

Chapter Questions

1. The muscle scanning procedure requires:
   a. a scanning head
   b. abrading the site
   c. electrode paste
   d. holding the electrodes motionless
   e. all of the above

2. Typically, one must stay on the site for how long before it becomes stable?
   a. 2 seconds
   b. 10 to 20 seconds
   c. 2 minutes
   d. 5 minutes

3. Which of the following is *not* one of the pitfalls of muscle scanning?
   a. bridging of electrode paste (values too low)
   b. excessive resistance (values too high)
   c. excessive variability (too long at the site)
   d. excessive movement during range of motion

4. Which of the following is *not* one of the general clinical concepts associated with muscle scanning?
   a. site of activation/inhibition
   b. level of symmetry
   c. impact of posture
   d. degree of reciprocal inhibition

5. During muscle scanning, what approach should be used in positioning the patient's posture?

   a. Place the patient in the ideal posture.
   b. Allow the patient to assume his or her natural posture.
   c. Ask the patient to sit or stand up straight.
   d. Always study the end range of motion of a posture.

6. The muscle scanning assessment of the static component of the neuromuscular system provides information about which of the following?
   a. hyperactive muscles
   b. antalgic postures
   c. trigger points
   d. a and b

7. During a muscle scan, an antalgic posture (protective guarding) is noted when:
   a. the activation is greater during standing than sitting
   b. the activation is on the ipsilateral side of the pain
   c. the activation is on the contralateral side of the pain
   d. both a and c

8. During a muscle scan, muscle splinting is noted when:
   a. the activation pattern is greater during sitting than standing
   b. the activation pattern is on the ipsilateral side of the pain
   c. the activation is on the contralateral side of the pain
   d. the activation is greater standing than sitting
   e. both a and b

CHAPTER 7

Emotional Assessment and Clinical Protocol

MUSCLES AND EMOTIONAL DISPLAY

Along with posture and movement, another key attribute of muscles is emotional display. In fact, one can conceptualize emotional display as muscle activation patterns that are but one step removed from intentional movement (e-motion). When muscle activation associated with emotions occurs, more energy is sent into the neuromuscular system, taking up the "slack" in the system and increasing the tonic or resting level. This emotional bracing or increased tonus may also affect the quality of movement.[1,2] Professional athletes certainly know how emotional arousal can unintentionally alter levels of exertion and change the timing associated with coordinated movement. In addition, it is not uncommon for a patient to react to stressful events in a stereotypic fashion. "Individual response stereotypy"[3] is the tendency for an individual to respond to a variety of stressors with a similar physiologic response. This tendency was first noted in the early 1960s, when some individuals were always observed to respond to a stressful event by, say, speeding up their heart rates or by tensing their shoulder muscles. Within the neuromuscular system, emotional arousal and associated stereotypy have been studied for the facial muscles,[4] the postural muscles,[5] and the muscle spindle.[6]

The procedure used to study the emotional reactivity of the body is called *stress profiling*. Throughout the history of psychophysiology, researchers have looked for the psychophysiological correlates to emotions.[7–9] Researchers hoped that this technique would help them to determine the individual's emotional state without having to rely upon the patient's self-report. As investigations have moved into applied clinical research, the questions have been directed more at how to identify individuals who are at risk for a particular disorder. Haynes has considered this question, looking at both the reactivity and recovery of the individual's physiology to a stressor.[10] This chapter reviews the procedures used in stress profiling. For a more complete description of stress profiling in assessment of psychological and medical disorders, refer to *Biofeedback: A Practitioner's Guide* edited by Mark Schwartz.[11]

THE FACIAL MUSCLES

One form of emotional display is found on the human face, creating the movements of the skin that are recognizable around the world.[4] Muscle scanning of the cephalic muscles may reveal some of the rudimentary aspects of these facial displays. However, the wide frontalis placement in the atlas in Part II provides an excellent barometer of negative emotional displays. Such emotional displays are most prominently seen on the upper face or forehead. For this reason, the wide frontalis placement is commonly used in stress profiling. Figure 7–1 shows surface electromyography (sEMG) activation in the

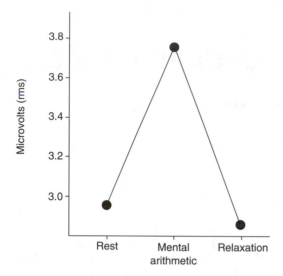

Figure 7–1 Surface EMG response of frontalis muscles during stress profiling. *Source:* JR Cram, EMG Biofeedback and the Treatment of Tension Headaches: A Systematic Analysis of Treatment Components, *Behavior Therapy,* Vol 11, pp 699–710, Copyright © 1980 by the Association for Advancement of Behavior Therapy. Reprinted by permission of the publisher.

frontalis muscles in headache patients during a simple stressor such as "serial sevens" (ie, counting backwards from 1000 by sevens).

Normative data have been collected on healthy subjects of different ages. In the reference base reported in Table 7–1, the resting and stress values are presented for the facial and shoulder muscles and for two autonomic nervous system (ANS) indicators. It is very common to monitor sympathetic activation along with the central nervous system (CNS) patterns of the neuromuscular system. The sEMG recordings for this normative sample were conducted using an Autogen 1700 with a 100 to 200 Hz band-pass filter and wide placements on the frontalis and upper trapezius sites. Beaton, Egan, and Mitchell studied 46 healthy adults from 18 to 75 years of age.[12,13] Although they studied the data across three age spans, they found no significant differences as a function of age.

THE TRUNK MUSCLES

Emotional impact on the neuromuscular system may also be seen in the postural muscles. Simple visual observation of depressed patients indicates stooped shoulders, while anxious patients may have their shoulders markedly elevated. Whatmore[2,14] has verified this phenomenon using sEMG recordings. The sEMG activation of the trunk muscles may take on a general form, affecting all muscles and generally taking up the slack in the system as a whole. This is what Whatmore referred to as *bracing*. In addition, the trunk muscles may show a high level of specificity. In Figure 7–2, the sEMG recordings of the right and left trapezius muscle groups using the cervical trapezius placement from the electrode atlas are shown for a patient who injured the right upper quarter during a fall down some stairs. This patient presents with headache and right upper quarter pain. Only the right cervical trapezius lead initially responds to the stressor, following by a very poor recovery pattern (return to baseline).

Table 7–1 Surface Electromyography and Autonomic Nervous System Values during Stress Profiling Procedure

Physiological Measure	Rest Mean	Rest Standard Deviation	Stressor (Serial Sevens) Mean	Stressor (Serial Sevens) Standard Deviation
Wide frontalis sEMG (µv)	2.58	0.63	3.2	0.86
Wide trapezius sEMG (µv)	3.30	0.69	3.75	0.51
Hand temperature (°F)	83.95	0.28	83.4	0.32
Skin conductance (mohm)	9.05	0.41	12.0	0.78

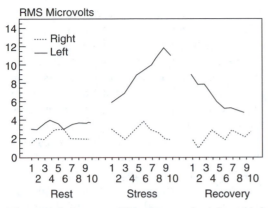

Figure 7–2 Stress profiling response in right and left trapezius of a patient with injury to the right trapezius. *Source:* Reprinted with permission from JR Cram, Surface EMG Recordings and Pain Related Disorders: A Diagnostic Framework, *Biofeedback and Self-Regulation,* Vol 13:127, © 1988, Plenum Publishing.

The effects of stress can result in emotional displays from the neuromuscular system that involve the muscles of the face and shoulders. Some suggest that these muscles have phylogenetically evolved from the gills of the fish and are "hard wired" for emotional displays.[15] The emotional nature of the gills of the fish is best represented in the threat displays of the Siamese fighting fish. When threatened, these fish instinctively enlarge their gills to appear much larger than they really are and to frighten off the intruder. When this theory is extended to the human species, it suggests that the head and neck muscles have a genetic predisposition for reacting to stressful events with activation patterns. Anatomists[16,17] have studied the facial muscles extensively, finding that these muscles have direct anatomical connections to the lower centers of the brain (ie, the facial nerves of the pontine nucleus). Given this strong connection to the reptilian brain, they have concluded that the facial muscles should be considered an autonomic organ.

Flor et al have also demonstrated the specific effects of emotions on the muscles of the low back.[18] They studied the right and left aspects of the erector spinae muscles in a group of low back pain patients, a group of general pain patients (ie, pain other than low back), and a group of healthy control subjects. Each group was presented with various types of stressors. The findings, presented in Figure 7–3, clearly show that only the low back pain patients demonstrated an emotional response (activation pattern) in the left erector spinae muscles, and only during stressors relevant to the patient's condition. In other words, while the serial sevens subtraction task evoked an activation response, the task of describing their pain and its impact on their lifestyles evoked the largest response. This study strongly suggests the need to study the relationship of personally relevant stressors to painful states.

RELATIONSHIP OF EMOTIONAL AROUSAL TO MUSCLE ACTIVATION

The effects of stress may be observed throughout the neuromuscular system.[5] On rare

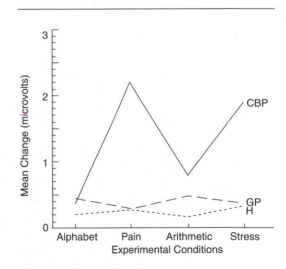

Figure 7–3 Surface EMG activation patterns in the left erector spinae muscles for three groups of patients during four levels of stressors: (1) saying alphabet; (2) describing their pain; (3) doing serial sevens mental arithmetic; and (4) describing the impact of pain on their lives. H = healthy controls; GP = general pain control group (ie, pain other than in the torso); CBP = chronic back pain patients. *Source:* Reprinted with permission from H Flor, D Turk, N Birbaumer, Assessment of Stress-Related Psychophysiological Reactions in Chronic Back Pain Patients, *J Consult Clinic Psychol,* Vol 53, No 3, p 359, © 1985.

occasions emotional activation may affect the entire neuromuscular system, but it is typically reflected in patterns of activation of specific muscles. These muscles are usually involved in the patient's symptom complex. For example, if the patient reports a painful neck, the muscles of the neck or upper back have a higher probability of being activated during a stress profiling procedure than those of the lower legs.

How does stress find its way into the muscles? The more traditional formulations suggest that emotional stress facilitates a shift in the balance of the hypothalamic system toward an ergotropic (or sympathetic) dominance. This, in turn, activates the limbic/autonomic circuits mentioned above and increases the efferent outflow to the muscles.[19] In their recent study, McNutty and colleagues suggested a more specific mechanism by which stress finds its way into the neuromuscular system: via autonomic innervation of the muscle spindle.[6] In this study, the researchers demonstrated that stressful events increased activation of fine wires placed in tissue thought to be muscle spindles. The intrafusal muscle fibers are known to be innervated by[19] and stimulated to contract[17] via the sympathetic nervous system. Hubbard and Berkoff[20] have demonstrated that activity from the tissue into which McNutty and colleagues inserted their fine wires was not blocked by agents that block acetylcholine, yet was blocked by sympathetic blocking agents. Thus, autonomic nervous system activation through the muscle spindle may play a role in pain-related disorders. Such a mechanism may affect the general resting tone of the extrafusal muscle fibers from the muscle group of origin, as well as increasing the muscles' responsivity to stressful events. Or, as Hubbard and Berkoff have argued, excessive activation of the muscle spindle itself may provide a pathway for nociception and thus play a role in the perpetuation of painful states.

RELIABILITY OF STRESS PROFILING

How consistent are these individual response stereotypes to stressful events? Three studies have attempted to answer this question. Walters et al[21] have demonstrated that approximately half of the patients continue for two weeks with the same stereotypic response patterns (they continue to respond to a variety of stressors in the same way, such as increased frontal activity). The other half of the subjects fell more into some form of "stimulus stereotypy." This indicates that they tended to respond physiologically to slightly different stressors in slightly different ways. For example, during the first assessment, they might have responded with increased frontal activity to mental stressors, while at two weeks they may have responded with increased trapezius activity to a loud noise. In a second study, Arena and Hobbs[22] found approximately the same percentage of response stereotypy (42%), with 20% of the remaining subjects showing stimulus specificity. The intraclass correlation coefficient for the wide frontal placement was 0.87, with observations taken on four occasions distributed across four weeks. This suggests a strong level of persistence in the type of response pattern. The third study, by Voas,[23] sampled from a broad set of muscle groups (including lower leg muscles, forearm muscles, trapezius, masseter, and frontalis) under three conditions (rest/relaxation, mental arithmetic, and stress/frustration) over the course of 9 days. His findings demonstrate that one cannot generalize the findings from one site to another, or from one condition to another. For example, he found the lower leg muscles to have the lowest level of reliability across all conditions (0.15 to 0.48). The forearm muscles showed the greatest reliability during the active tasks (0.59 to 0.93), with lower levels of reliability during quiet activities (0.17 to 0.46). Trapezius and masseter muscles showed the greatest consistency during mental arithmetic (0.69 to 0.87), with much lower correlations during the other tasks (0.23 to 0.39). Only the wide frontal placement showed consistently high test-retest correlations across all tasks (0.80 to 0.91). This study suggests that the concepts of stimulus specificity are found in the trapezius and arm muscle groups, with response stereotypy occurring in the wide frontal placement.

THE STRESS PROFILING PROTOCOL

In conducting a stress profile, the first thing the practitioner must consider is which muscle sites to monitor. One general rule of thumb is to monitor sEMG activity at the site of pain complaint. Two thirds of the time, the resting muscle tone at the site of pain may look normal,[10] but the possibility of referred pain patterns[24] may still exist. The neuromuscular component at the painful site may not be ruled out until one has observed the effects of perturbation on the muscle(s) being monitored. Thus, the practitioner should not draw any conclusions regarding a myogenic component of pain based on resting tone alone. The practitioner would be wise to see how the painful site reacts to stress of a mental stressor before coming to conclusions. If the site reacts easily to the stressor or has a poor rebound or recovery, this may potentially explain the myogenic origin of the patient's pain. In addition, the practitioner may want to select and study muscle sites away from the reported site of pain. The selection of these sites could be based on the findings of the muscle scan study or upon the knowledge of which muscle sites could harbor potential trigger points that could refer to the area of described pain.

Next, the practitioner should select a "stressor" to be used to create the perturbation of the emotional system. One standard stressor is a mental arithmetic task termed "serial sevens." Here, the patient is asked to perform a mental arithmetic task in which he or she is to count backward from 1000 by sevens. In other words, the patient is to take the number 1000 and subtract 7, take that total (993) and subtract 7 from it, take that total (986) and subtract 7 from it, and so forth. The patient is instructed to do this out loud, and as quickly and accurately as possible. The astute practitioner encourages the patient to stay on task and go quickly, while tracking the patient's responses and pointing out any errors. For some patients, this is an excellent stressor and the practitioner can observe this from the physiological response in the sEMG or autonomic nervous system channels. For other pa-

tients, this task is too difficult and they simply give up. The practitioner must monitor the mental arithmetic process of the patient to capture the timing of this event. For other patients, the task may be too easy and they will not react to it. If the task is too easy, one might consider administering another test such as the Pace Serial Arithmetic Test (PSAT). This is a serial arithmetic task that all subjects will eventually find stressful and fail. If the task is too hard, the practitioner may want to explore other potential stressors. An alternative standardized stressor might include the introduction of a sudden sound that startles the patient. Here the practitioner might stand outside the patient's view and suddenly slam a book down on a hard surface. The unexpected noise acts as the stressor. Other options include playing the patient an audiotape that presents a series of environmentally stressful sounds (eg, phones ringing, cars honking, dogs barking, babies crying).[25] Or, as Flor and colleagues[18] did, the practitioner might make the stressor relevant to the patient by asking the patient to describe the pain or the impact of the pain on his or her life.

Once the practitioner has selected the muscle sites to monitor and the appropriate stressor for the patient, the practitioner should follow some sort of standardized single subject protocol. Typically, such a procedure uses an A-B-A type of design. Here, the practitioner runs a baseline sEMG reading (condition A), introduces a stressor (condition B), and completes the assessment with a recovery phase commonly termed the postbaseline recording (return to condition A). In practice, however, most practitioners usually conclude the stress profile with a combination of return to baseline while the patient is encouraged to engage in some form of relaxation. Thus, the patient's relaxation skills are tested "under fire." The design of such a protocol is presented in Exhibit 7–1.

PATTERNS OF ACTIVATION AND RECOVERY

The psychophysiological assessment protocol is examined for three elements: (1) initial resting

Exhibit 7–1 Typical Design of a Stress Profile

Baseline (A)	Stressor (B)	Recovery/Relaxation (A)
2–4 minutes (or until stable)	3–5 minutes (or until there is some sort of physiological response)	5–10 minutes minimum (or until there is recovery)

baseline levels; (2) level of response to the stressor; and (3) ability of the emotional component of the muscular system to recover to prebaseline levels.

Baseline Levels

An assessment for some of the resting baseline values may be roughly determined by comparing the resting values for the site of placement to that of the electrode atlas benchmark values or those presented in the group norms listed earlier in this chapter. If elevations in the resting levels are noted, they could influence the ability of the system to react to the stressor. This is due to the "law of initial value,"[26] which states that physiological systems operate within certain limits or boundaries. If the person is near the ceiling of a given system, that system has less room for "reactivity" than when the prestimulus levels are toward the bottom end of the range.

Level of Response to the Stressor

Next, the practitioner examines the patient's level of response to the stressor. If multiple sites are monitored, the practitioner examines the sEMG signals for which sites react first and which sites react with the strongest sEMG activation. There is approximately a 50/50 chance of seeing a significant physiological reaction to a stressor. In a meta-analysis of a variety of stressors on diverse populations of subjects, Haynes[10] found that 45% of the studies showed nonsignificant reactivity to a stressor. To increase the probability of finding significant clinical results, the practitioner should study more than one por-

tion of the neuromuscular system, study sites of painful complaint as well as sites away from the pain (ie, trigger points for referred pain), or use personally relevant stressors.

To determine reactivity to a stressor, one would want to see if the activation pattern during stress exceeds the natural variations in the resting tone for a given site. Many computerized physiological monitoring systems generate information on a patient regarding the mean level of sEMG activity for the site, as well as the variability of the signal. Taking the mean level of the prebaseline activity and adding the standard deviation to it will indicate if the stressor had a mild impact on the muscle site that is above the ambient variations of its resting tone. The practitioner should note that it is normal for the neuromuscular system to react to emotional stress with increased activation. In fact, the success of the stress profiling protocol depends upon this. This is the validity check that indicates if the neuromuscular system is actually stressed. What is abnormal, however, is for one aspect of the system to react more strongly than another. A headache patient with dull bifrontal headache, for example, may be within "normal" sEMG limits for the cephalic and neck muscles at rest, but react more strongly with the frontal musculature during a stressful event. The certainty of this type of conclusion is enhanced by examining the means and standard deviations for each muscle group during the stressful event. Taking the mean and both adding and subtracting the standard deviation to this mean will provide an average range of operation for the sEMG channel that is used. If the means for either of the muscles falls *within* the range of the other muscle, then the conclusion about one muscle reacting more than the other would be weakened. If the mean of one muscle falls *outside* the range of the other muscle, however, the conclusion is strengthened and clinically significant. If the standard deviation is doubled before it is added or subtracted to the mean and the mean is still outside the range of the other muscle, this suggests a "moderate" reactivity; in this case, the conclusion is not only clinically significant but also statistically significant. In either event, when one muscle group reacts to a greater extent than another muscle group, this finding must be considered in the etiology of pain. This conclusion, however, is strengthened when hyperreactivity is coupled with poor recovery to prebaseline levels.

Recovery to Prebaseline Levels

Finally, the pattern of stress profiling is examined for the level of recovery. Here, one would expect the recovery pattern to return to the prebaseline levels. When the recovery phase remains one standard deviation above the initial baseline level, this is considered mildly elevated; when it remains two standard deviations above baseline level, this is considered moderately elevated. Lack of recovery is important because it can change the biochemistry of the muscle. For example, 10% to 50% of maximum voluntary isometric contraction (MVIC) is known to reduce the blood flow to a muscle significantly.[27,28] Prolonged reduction of blood flow leads to the buildup of lactic acid, which stimulates the chemoreceptors in the muscle that signal pain. Ischemia also leads to an increase in the release of bradykinins, prostaglandins, and serotonin,[29] which brings about an increased sensitization of pain reception at a local level. If the reactive muscle group activates frequently and is followed by only a partial recovery, each reactivity cycle could lead to a gradual buildup of lactic acid over the course of the day; this could result in a dull, bilateral headache that is felt toward the latter part of the day.

Table 7–2 provides an example of these comparisons. In this example, the mean sEMG level of both muscles is within the range of the other muscle during the prebaseline phase. During the stressor, muscle A shows a mild reaction. When the mean sEMG level of muscle A during stress is compared to the range of its own prebaseline phase, the stress mean is greater than the first standard deviation for the prebaseline period. For muscle B, the stress mean is greater than the second standard deviation of the prebaseline period, suggesting a moderate level of reactivity. In addition, the mean for the reactivity of muscle B is outside the range of the second standard deviation for the reactivity of muscle A, strongly supporting the notion that muscle B reacted more strongly to the stressor than did muscle A. Finally, muscle A recovered quickly from the stressor, and the recovery mean for muscle A is within the range of the prebaseline values for muscle A. Muscle B, on the other hand, did not recover well; the mean for the recovery phase for muscle B is greater than the range of the second standard deviation for the prebaseline phase. In addition, the recovery mean for muscle B is outside the second standard deviation range for the recovery phase of muscle A. This finding provides substantial evidence that the recovery patterns of muscles A and B are different.

The lack of recovery to prebaseline levels reflects a dysregulation of the homeostasis of the body. In a normal muscle system, a return to baseline is expected. Because muscle reactivity potentially leads to a change in the pH balance of the tissue (lactic acid), delayed recovery to prestress levels increases the probability of this metabolic imbalance. How long should it normally take to recover from a stressor? Arena and Hobbs[22] suggest that 6 minutes is adequate for the facial muscle reactivity but inadequate for hand temperature. The 10-minute time frame suggested in Exhibit 7–1 is usually more than adequate for both the central nervous system and autonomic nervous system components. To define the recovery process better, one might measure the length of time it takes for the muscle activity to return to within 5% of its prebaseline levels following the cessation of the stressful event.

Table 7–2 Surface Electromyography Data Obtained from Two Muscle Sites during a Stress Profiling Procedure in Which There Is a Differential Reaction to Stress and Recovery

Condition	Muscle A				Muscle B			
	Mean	SD	No. SDs	Range	Mean	SD	No. SDs	Range
Prebaseline	2.3	1.7	1	0.6–3.0	2.5	1.5	1	1.0–4.0
			2	0.0–5.7			2	0.0–5.5
Stressor*	4.1	2.5	1	1.6–6.6	12.3	5.2	1	7.1–17.5
			2	0.0–9.1			2	2.1–13.4
Recovery*	2.5	1.8	1	0.7–4.3	7.3	2.3	1	5.0–9.6
			2	0.0–6.1			2	2.7–11.9

*Indicates difference between muscle A and muscle B or between the various conditions within a given muscle.

REFERENCES

1. Jacobson E. Electrophysiology of mental activities. *Am J Psychol.* 1932;44:77–94.

2. Whatmore G, Kohli D. *The Physiopathology and Treatment of Functional Disorders.* New York: Grune & Stratton; 1974.

3. Engel BT. Stimulus response and individual-response stereotypy. *Arch Gen Psychiatry.* 1960;2:305–313.

4. Ekman P, Friesen WV. *Unmasking the Human Face.* Englewood Cliffs, NJ: Prentice-Hall; 1972.

5. Goldstein B. Electromyography: A measure of skeletal muscle response. In: Greenfield S, Sternbach R, eds. *Handbook of Psychophysiology.* New York: Holt, Rinehart & Winston; 1972.

6. McNutty W, Gevertz R, Berkoff G, Hubbard D. Needle electromyographic evaluation of a trigger point response to a psychological stressor. *Psychophysiology.* 1994;31:313–316.

7. Lacey J, Lacey B. Verification and extension of the principle of autonomic response-stereotype. *Am J Psychol.* 1958;71:50–73.

8. Lader MH, Mathews AM. A physiological model of phobic anxiety and desensitization. *Behav Res Ther.* 1968;6:411–421.

9. Malmo RB, Shagass C. Physiologic studies of reaction to stress in anxiety and early schizophrenia. *Psychosom Med.* 1949;11:9–24.

10. Haynes S. Muscle-contraction headache: Psycho-physiological perspective in etiology and treatment. In: Haynes S, Gannorn W, eds. *Psychosomatic Disorders: A Psychophysiological Approach to Etiology and Treatment.* Westport, CT: Greenwood Press; 1981.

11. Schwartz M, ed. *Biofeedback: A Practitioner's Guide.* New York: Guilford; 1987.

12. Beaton R, Egan K, Mitchell P. Frontalis and trapezius electromyographic activity in healthy non-patients and in clinical headache samples. *Am J Clin Biofeedback.* 1984;7:3–12.

13. Egan KJ, Beaton R, Mitchell P. Autonomic indicators in healthy non-patients and in clinical headache samples. *Am J Clin Biofeedback.* 1984;7:31–41.

14. Whatmore G, Ellis R. Some neurophysiologic aspects of depressed states. *Arch Gen Psychiatry.* 1959;1:70.

15. Skubick D, Clasby R, Donaldson CCS, Marshall W. Carpal tunnel syndrome as an expression of muscular dysfunction in the neck. *J Occup Rehab.* 1993;3:31–43.

16. Horst GJ, Copray JCVM, Lein RSB, Van Willgren JD. Projections from the rostral parvicellular reticular formation to pontine and medullary nuclei in the rat: involvement in autonomic regulation and orofacial motor control. *Neuroscience.* 1991;40:735–758.

17. Paloheimo M. Quantitative surface electromyography (qEMG): applications in anesthesiology and critical care. *Acta.* 1990;93(suppl):34.

18. Flor H, Turk D, Birbaumer N. Assessment of stress-related psychophysiological reactions in chronic back pain patients. *J Consult Clinic Psychol.* 1985;53(3):359.

19. Santini M, Ibata Y. The fine structure of thin unmyelinated axons within muscle spindles. *Brain Res.* 1971;33:289–302.

20. Hubbard D, Berkoff G. Myofascial trigger points show spontaneous needle EMG activity. *Spine.* 1993; 18: 1803–1807.

21. Walters WF, Williamson DA, Bernard BA, Blouin DC, Faulstich ME. Test-retest reliability of psychophysiological assessment. *Behav Res Ther.* 1987;25:213–221.

22. Arena JG, Hobbs SH. Temporal stability of psycho-physiological response profiles: Analysis of individual response stereotypy and stimulus response specificity. In: *Proceedings of the 23rd Annual Meeting of the Association for Applied Psychophysiology and Biofeedback.* Colorado Springs, CO; 1992.

23. Voas RB. *Generalization and Consistency of Muscle Tension Levels.* Dissertation. Reviewed in Goldstein IB. Electromyography: A measure of skeletal muscle response. In: Greenfield S, Sternbach R, eds. *Handbook of Psychophysiology.* New York: Holt, Rinehart & Winston; 1972.

24. Travell J, Simons D. *Myofascial Pain and Dysfunction: A Trigger Point Manual, I and II.* Baltimore: Williams & Wilkins; 1983.

25. Thomas A. *The Psycho-Physical Assessment.* Nevada City, CA: Clinical Resources; 1993.

26. Wilder J. The law of initial value in neurology and psychiatry. *J Nerv Ment Dis.* 1957;125:73–76.

27. Bonde-Peterson F, Mork AL, Nielson E. Local muscle blood flow and sustained contraction of human arm and back muscles. *Eur J Appl Physiol.* 1975;34:43–50.

28. Mortimer JT, Kerstein MD, Magnusson R, Petersen H. Muscle blood flow in the human biceps as a function of developed muscle force. *Arch Surg.* 1971;103:376–377.

29. Robard S. Pain in contracting muscles. In: Crue BL, ed. *Pain Research and Treatment.* New York: Academic Press; 1975.

Chapter Questions

1. When a patient responds to a variety of stressful events in the same physiological way (eg, always increasing muscle tension in the forehead), this is called:
   a. response stereotypy
   b. stimulus response specificity
   c. stress profiling
   d. stress profile response specificity

2. The law of initial values states that when the prestimulus level of physiological activity is near the ceiling level for that system, the magnitude of the stress response will be:
   a. larger than normal
   b. limited because of the lack of room to respond
   c. smaller than normal
   d. enhanced as a result of the ceiling effect

3. Negative emotions are found primarily on the:
   a. upper face
   b. neck
   c. back
   d. legs

4. Stress responses can find their way into:
   a. the face
   b. the muscle spindle
   c. an injured area
   d. all of the above

5. The term *serial sevens* refers to:
   a. adding by sevens
   b. multiplying by sevens
   c. subtracting from 1000 by sevens
   d. none of the above

6. In stress profiling, one would interpret:
   a. initial baseline data
   b. level of reactivity
   c. recovery data
   d. all of the above

CHAPTER 8

Dynamic Assessment

DYNAMIC EVALUATION OF THE NEUROMUSCULAR SYSTEM

The dynamic evaluation of the neuromuscular system is a much broader, more generic, and older procedure than the static evaluation or stress profiling techniques. It has been used in kinesiologic studies for decades. One of the oldest clinical studies of pain that used surface electromyography (sEMG) as its primary descriptive tool was conducted by Price et al[1] in the 1940s. Floyd and Silver[2] provided a nice base of information about the back during the 1950s. And Basmajian and DeLuca's book, *Muscles Alive*,[3] served as a foundation of sEMG work and stimulated broad interest in electromyography.

The use of dynamic sEMG in the clinical assessment of various syndromes entails examining how the muscular energy is used to support the body against gravity, how it is used to do work through movement, and how often it rests. Practitioners want to examine the muscles not only to determine disordered movement patterns, but also to note how these movements are affected by prior baseline levels and how the movements might disturb the ability to return to resting levels. In dynamic assessment procedures, muscles are monitored using attached electrodes that "float" above the skin. Information about exact placement of electrodes to monitor from a specific muscle group can be obtained in the electrode atlas (Part II). The specific sets of muscles to monitor are primarily determined by the nature of the patient's complaint. The static assessment may help to provide clues about where the disturbances in resting tone might lie. In dynamic assessment, usually four to eight channels of sEMG are monitored to allow the practitioner to study the right and left aspects of two opposing muscle groups. For example, in patients with neck problems, the sternocleidomastoid and cervical paraspinals might be examined during flexion, extension, rotation, and lateral bending of the neck. The practitioner should ask the patient to go through the desired movements several times and in verbally guided and paced fashion. In this way, the sEMG tracings of the movement can be easily examined for the quality of the movement. The electrode atlas in Part II provides some templates of sEMG recording from a variety of muscles and movements. Practitioners can compare these templates to their patients' movements. The sEMG record can be examined for some key elements. Issues pertaining to the amplitude of sEMG activation are extremely important, as are issues pertaining to timing and rest. Kasman[4] has developed two figures that describe these issues. Figure 8–1 depicts the issues pertaining to amplitude, and Figure 8–2 presents the issues pertaining to timing. These features are briefly reviewed in the sections that follow.

THE "TONIC BASELINE" AMPLITUDE

The level of muscular energy present prior to and following a movement can be the marker for

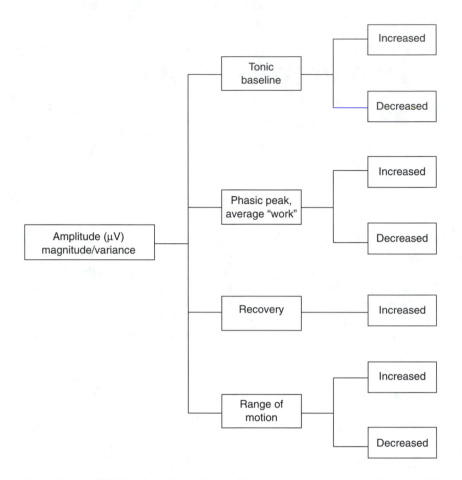

Figure 8–1 Aberrant sEMG activity: Issues in amplitude. *Source:* Reprinted with permission from G Kasman, *Surface EMG in Physical Therapy: Applications in Chronic Musculoskeletal Pain,* © 1995, Movements Systems.

dysfunction. Figure 8–1 identifies two "tonic baseline" components: tonic baseline and recovery. In the absence of voluntary movement, abnormal muscle tone (an elevated or depressed tonic level) reflects a dysregulation in posture and/or emotional tone. In a neutral posture—one where the body alignment is at its theoretical ideal—the weight of the body should stack on the bones and hang on the ligaments with little muscular involvement. Elevations in the tonic baseline state may be caused by increased emotional tone or postural disturbances, as described in previous chapters. Usually, elevated resting tone must be treated in some way before disor-

dered movement can be addressed. If one describes the elevated resting baseline as the "noise" in the neuromuscular system, then it is best to reduce that noise before trying to refine timing issues.

RECOVERY OF BASELINE LEVELS FOLLOWING MOVEMENT

When surface electrodes are attached, the practitioner can assess for the impact of movement upon postural resting tone. This is termed *recovery*. The patient is asked to engage in a movement (eg, abduction of the shoulder), fol-

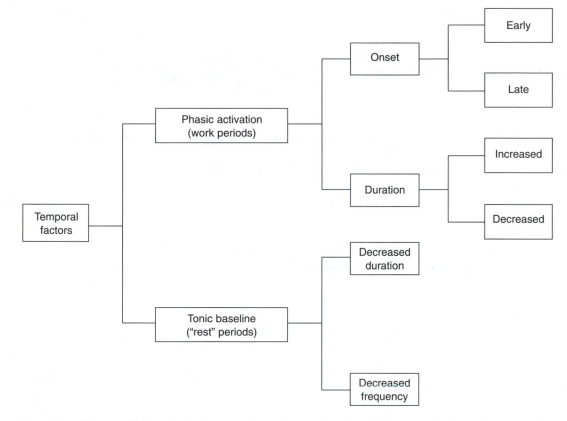

Figure 8–2 Aberrant sEMG activity: Issues in timing. *Source:* Reprinted with permission from G Kasman, *Surface EMG in Physical Therapy: Applications in Chronic Musculoskeletal Pain*, © 1995, Movements Systems.

lowed by a return to the neutral position. As in stress profiling, it is important to establish a stable resting baseline prior to a movement. Then, the practitioner should introduce the movement and examine how well the muscles return to the prebaseline level following the movement. The movement can be regarded as a mechanical stressor on the postural system, and the practitioner assesses how well the postural network recovers following this movement/ stressor. Ettare and Ettare[5] have created a therapeutic protocol based upon training individuals to recover successfully following various movements and in a variety of postures.

When a muscle fails to recover to prebaseline levels following movement, it is termed *postmovement irritability*. What is the mechanism associated with the lack of recovery? One explanation is that irritable muscles harbor a trigger point that disturbs the resting tone. Hubbard and Berkoff[6] have presented some very interesting data that suggest that the trigger point may reside within the muscle spindle. According to the theory, the trigger point may be a muscle spindle in "spasm," and this is the palpable "pea-like" tissue noted in a trigger point examination. When a muscle spindle is disturbed, it sends out impulses to the spinal cord and reflexively activates the motor unit from which it is housed. This activation could create the taut band, along with more general activation of the muscle as a whole and increased resting tone. The individual who exhib-

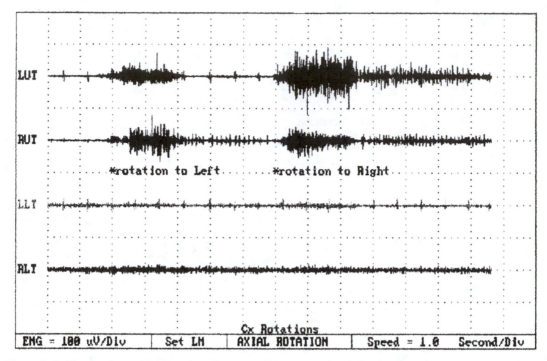

Figure 8–3 Abnormal raw sEMG tracing of upper and lower trapezius during head rotation. Note postmovement irritability, along with "long hairs" suggestive of trigger point. *Source:* Copyright © Clinical Resources, Inc.

its a poor recovery following movement is rarely consciously aware that the muscle is still active.

Observe the recruitment pattern shown in Figure 8–3. Failure to recover following movement is noted by comparing the thickness of the postcontraction and precontraction tracings. In the postcontraction tracing, note the frequent "solitary" excursions that rise above and fall below the common width of the tracing. It looks as if the tracing needs a "haircut," because it has so many straggly ends. These "long hairs" probably represent a disturbance in the muscle spindle and therefore the potential presence of a trigger point within the muscle. When the muscle is examined and treated for trigger points, the appropriate resting tone returns. In addition, it may be necessary to train the patient regarding how to terminate a movement pattern appropriately. It is helpful to eliminate this postmovement irritability before attempting to retrain and refine dynamic movements. Again, think of this post-

movement irritability as a source of noise within the system that hinders the acquisition of refined motor skills.

ASSESSMENT OF TRIGGER POINTS

Considerable research on this topic has been conducted, and the exemplary research by Fishbain et al documents the important role of trigger points in pain-related work.[7] Among the 283 consecutive admissions to a comprehensive pain center that these authors studied, a primary organic diagnosis of myofascial pain syndrome was assigned to 85% of the cases. In a related study of 164 chronic neck and headache patients,[8] 55% of the cases had a primary diagnosis of myofascial pain. Given its prevalence, it is wise for a practitioner working with muscles to become familiar with myofascial pain. The most comprehensive text on this topic may be found in a two-volume set by Travell and Simons.[9] For an update on the area, consider a recent review by Simons.[10]

Assessment and treatment of trigger points should help to normalize muscle function. In fact, it may be impossible to retrain a disordered movement pattern using sEMG feedback without first eliminating trigger points within the muscle. The anatomical foundation of trigger points is still being explored, but its diagnostic criteria have become clearer. The clinical features associated with the presence of a trigger point are given in Table 8–1.

Treatment of trigger points is achieved either through ischemic pressure applied directly to the trigger point, dry needling of the trigger point, or the application of a coolant spray during stretching of the affected muscle. For further information on this topic, consult Travell and Simons.[9]

RANGE OF MOTION

During dynamic movement, the practitioner should visually examine the movement for the range of motion (ROM). Differences in the symmetry of the movement pattern could help to explain patterns of symmetry or asymmetry of sEMG recruitment. Assessment of ROM may also provide valuable information regarding me-

Table 8–1 Clinical Features Associated with the Presence of a Trigger Point

Clinical Concept	Description
History	The patient has a history of spontaneous localized pain associated with acute overload or chronic overuse of the muscle. The pattern of described pain provides valuable clues about the location of the potential trigger point.
Palpable band	A cord-like band of fibers is palpable. The band assists in locating the tender points.
Spot tenderness	This involves a very tender and very small spot that is found in the band. Sensitivity of the band is directly related to the amount of pressure applied.
Jump sign	Pressure on the spot of tenderness causes the patient to react physically to the pain with a spontaneous exclamation or movement.
Pain recognition	Pressure on the spot induces at least some of the pain of which the patient complains, and the patient recognizes it as his or her pain.
Twitch response	The local twitch response is a transient contraction of the fibers of the taut band associated with a trigger point. It can be elicited by vigorous snapping palpation of the taut band. This criterion is possible only in sufficiently superficial and accessible muscles.
Elicited referred pain and tenderness	The trigger point refers pain in a pattern that is characteristic for that muscle. Often, this pain is not local; some 85% of the pain is referred to some distant site. Adequacy of the amount of pressure may determine whether referred pain patterns are discovered.
Restricted range of motion	Full-stretch range of motion of the affected muscle is restricted by pain. This restriction is relieved by the release of the taut band through the inactivation of the trigger point.
Muscle weakness	Clinically, the patient is unable to develop normal strength on static muscle testing when compared to an unimpaired homologous muscle group. Surface EMG findings show greater peak amplitudes on the affected side during repeated movements.

chanical impediments to sEMG retraining. It may be necessary to institute manual therapies prior to dynamic sEMG training for such training to be effective.

ISSUES PERTAINING TO THE WORK PEAK

Symmetry of Recruitment

Along with the range of motion, the practitioner should concurrently examine the recruitment pattern for its amplitude, paying particular attention to the amplitude of the maximum recruitment or peak(s). In many cases, the practitioner should monitor the right and left aspects of homologous muscle groups and inspect for the level of symmetry of the peak contractions. The following rule should apply: *During symmetrical movements, such as forward flexion of the trunk, expect to see a symmetrical recruitment pattern from homologous muscle pairs.* Donaldson and Donaldson[11] have described lack of symmetry at the peak of movement in cervical and lumbar flexion studies as commonly associated with injury and/or pain. These authors collected data on healthy subjects and pain patients during forward flexion of the neck and trunk, and determined that a 20% difference in peak values is within the normal range. Differences above that are less common and should be considered abnormal. As a result of the natural variation in these normalized percentage asymmetry scores, differences greater than 20% should be of interest, and differences of 40% or greater should be considered *clinically significant*. This is because the average level of asymmetry for the pain population was slightly greater than 40%.

Donaldson and Donaldson introduced the concept of the hypoactive site.[11] In their symmetry model, the side that evidenced the least recruitment would be labeled as *hypoactive*. Similarly, the site with the most activity would be considered *hyperactive*. It is important to note that *hyper-* and *hypoactive* are merely relative terms. The terms do not refer to a referential da-

tabase, and these authors did not use a statistical basis to obtain these labels. In fact, the so-called hypoactive site is usually in the same range of peak amplitudes as those seen in healthy subjects. It is the asymmetry that is considered the red flag. In addition, Donaldson and Donaldson reported that it is commonly the hypoactive site that is the injured one. Using flexion extension injury to the cervical region associated with motor vehicle accidents as an example, these authors suggest that the hypoactive site is likely to be the side to have experienced the hyperextension injury. This injury is thought to alter the sensitivity of the muscle spindle. These authors argue that the injured site falls into a "disuse" pattern secondary to pain; following the injury, protective guarding does not allow the muscle spindle to come back "on-line." The hyperactive side takes over the workload for the protected side and becomes overused. This overuse pattern commonly results in the development of a trigger point in the overused muscle. In one study of recruitment patterns of the upper trapezius and cervical paraspinals during forward flexion and reextension of the head, Donaldson et al[12] demonstrated increased activation during the reextension phase of the movement pattern in muscles that harbor a trigger point.

Cocontractions

Issues concerning peak work values may also be observed during asymmetrical movements, such as rotation or side bending. The following rule applies: *During an asymmetrical movement, such as rotation, the recruitment pattern from homologous muscles should be asymmetrical.* In the rotation of the head, for example, one would expect the sternocleidomastoid to activate so that primarily the left sternocleidomastoid is active during the right rotation, while primarily the right sternocleidomastoid is active during left rotation. Abnormal findings are noted when this synergy pattern breaks down and there is a coactivation of the right and left aspects of a muscle group during an asymmetrical movement. This coactivation is called a *cocon-*

traction. Here, the prime mover is not allowed to do its work efficiently because of excessive activation of the opposing or antagonistic muscle group. Tracings from normal and abnormal recruitment patterns may be seen in Figures 8–4 and 8–5. In assessing any movement pattern, the practitioner should be alert to the patient's active ROM. Asymmetrical recruitment is commonly accompanied by an asymmetrical ROM. When this is observed, further investigation of the recruitment patterns is suggested. For example, the clinician could ask the patient to do the movement so that it has symmetry in ROM at the smaller end of the ROM; then the practitioner would observe to see whether there is a separation of muscle function or whether the cocontraction persists. While respecting the patient's comfort zone, the practitioner should have the patient increase the ROM in a symmetrical fashion; the practitioner would then observe at what point the excessive activation kicks in.

ISSUES PERTAINING TO TEMPORAL FACTORS

Flexion/Extension

Temporal factors have to do with timing. Does the recruitment pattern come on too soon or too late? Does it last too long, or is it too short? A good clinical example of timing issues is the study of forward flexion and return to midline of the trunk. Figure 8–6 shows a normal recruitment pattern for the erector spinae site at the third lumbar vertebra (L-3), while Figure 8–7 shows an abnormal one. Here, timing is as important as amplitude. The normal recruitment pattern for this movement should show recruitment during both the eccentric and concentric

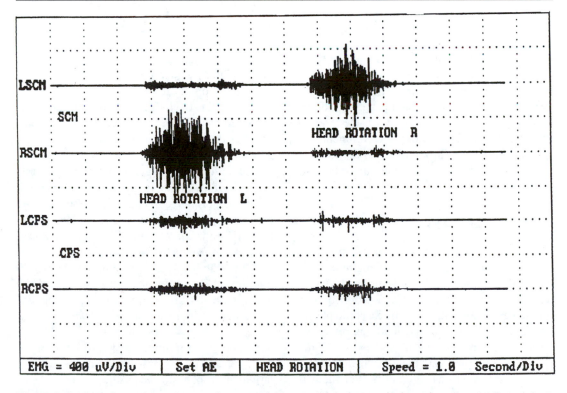

Figure 8–4 Normal recruitment pattern for sternocleidomastoid during cervical rotation. *Source:* Copyright © Clinical Resources, Inc.

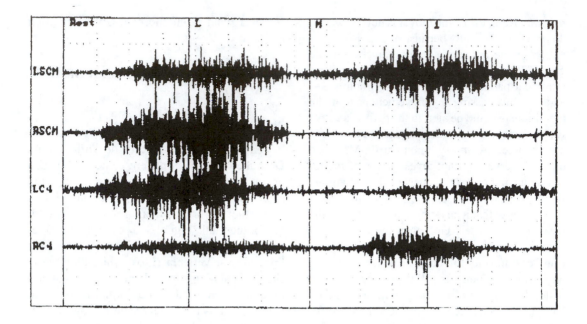

Figure 8–5 Abnormal recruitment pattern for sternocleidomastoid during cervical rotation. Note cocontraction during the right rotation (right portion of EMG). *Source:* Copyright © Clinical Resources, Inc.

phases, but there should be a greater level of recruitment during the concentric phase of the work (return to midline). In addition, during the last 45 degrees of flexion and hang, one should observe a flexion-relaxation of the erector spinae muscles. The abnormal recruitment pattern in Figure 8–7 shows a lack of the flexion-relaxation response during the hang phase of trunk flexion.

Agonist/Antagonist/Synergy Issues

Evaluation of timing issues is complex and usually requires examination of multiple muscles under various conditions. Surface EMG relationships may change as a function of isometric versus concentric versus eccentric phases of work, or over repeated loadings or movements. In a complex system, the practitioner should examine agonist/antagonist reciprocation versus cocontractions to determine if there is agonist/synergist balance in the movement. The practitioner should assess whether a muscle re-

cruits at the right time or whether it comes on early or late; whether, once it is recruited, its duration is appropriate for the task; whether the work period is too long or too short; whether the muscle gets a chance to rest between repetitions; whether those rest periods occur often enough; and whether they are long enough.

The following paragraph provides a simple example of the timing issues the practitioner will confront. For an examination of these issues in greater depth, see the electrode atlas section (Part II) and *Clinical Applications in Surface Electromyography* by Kasman et al.[13]

In the stabilization of the shoulder during abduction, Will Taylor[14,15] has argued that the lower trapezius is the major stabilizer during this movement. Figure 8–8 demonstrates a fairly typical synergy pattern; there is a relative balance between the upper and lower trapezius, with the lower trapezius showing a slightly larger burst pattern. According to Taylor, the general rule is that the ratio between the upper and lower trapezius (upper trapezius/lower tra-

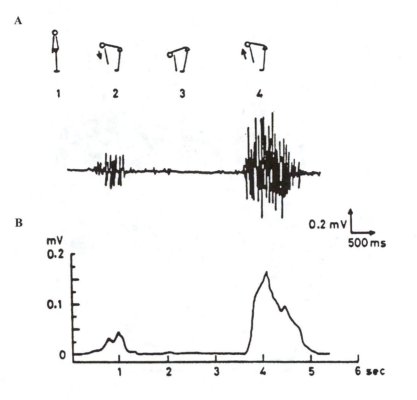

Figure 8–6 Normal flexion and reextension pattern at L-3 for the trunk. (**A**) Tracing reflects a fine-wire recording from the erector spinae; (**B**) tracing reflects an RMS (root mean square) display from concurrent surface electrodes. *Source:* Reprinted with permission from T Sihvonen, J Partanin, H Osmo, and Soimakalio, Electric Behavior of Low Back Muscles during Lumbar Pelvic Rhythm in Low Back Pain Patients and Healthy Controls, *Archives of Physical Medicine and Rehabilitation,* Vol 72, pp 1080–1087, © 1991, WB Saunders Company.

pezius) should be less than 1.0. Figure 8–9 shows an exaggeration of lower trapezius dominance; the lower trapezius muscle groups show a strong burst of activity, while the upper trapezius site remains relatively quiet. In the normal body, however, such synergy is rarely seen and would probably disturb the glenohumeral rhythm of the shoulder. Figure 8–10 demonstrates a recruitment pattern where the upper trapezius dominates over the lower trapezius during this movement. The tracing is grossly abnormal. Here, the weight of the arms would be transferred to the neck instead of being borne on the thorax. The examination of the movement and stabilization of the shoulder and arm as depicted here is greatly simplified. A more comprehensive study of shoulder movement and stabilization would require that one consider more than simply the relationship of the upper and lower trapezius, and that one study more movement patterns than abduction. With more channels of sEMG available, the practitioner could consider other muscle groups such as serratus anterior; supraspinatus/upper trapezius; infraspinatus; anterior, posterior, and middle deltoids; and the clavicular aspect of pectoralis. Recruitment patterns associated with abduction, flexion, scaption (abduction halfway between the frontal and sagittal planes), shoulder elevation, internal rotation, external rotation, and real and varied life activities could be examined. Amplitude and timing issues will vary, depend-

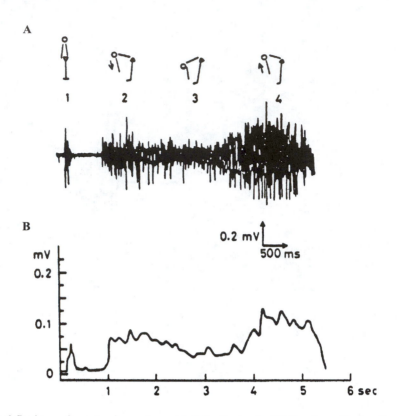

Figure 8–7 Abnormal flexion and reextension pattern at L-3 for the trunk. (**A**) Tracing reflects a fine-wire recording from the erector spinae; (**B**) tracing reflects an RMS (root mean square) display from concurrent surface electrodes. *Source:* Reprinted with permission from T Sihvonen, J Partanin, H Osmo, and Soimakalio, Electric Behavior of Low Back Muscles during Lumbar Pelvic Rhythm in Low Back Pain Patients and Healthy Controls, *Archives of Physical Medicine and Rehabilitation,* Vol 72, pp 1080–1087, © 1991, WB Saunders Company.

ing upon which muscle groups are monitored and under what movement conditions. The electrode atlas (Part II) provides information about what some of the synergy patterns would look like.

THE ISSUE OF REST

As a result of the current level of computerized technology readily available to the practitioner, timing issues pertaining to recruitment are easier to examine than timing issues pertaining to rest. Yet, in order for the neuromuscular tissue to remain healthy, it needs to rest from time to time. Sustained contractions of moderate intensity (ie, 50% of maximum voluntary con-

traction) for relatively short periods of time (a minute or two) will lead to muscle fatigue and eventually to a failure point. The physiology of this phenomenon is discussed in Chapter 2, and the electrophysiology is discussed in Chapter 3. During real and varied life activities, there is usually a rhythm to work. On a macro level, the human body is limited by the basic rest activity cycle (BRAC)[16] of approximately 90 minutes of work. This should then be followed by a 20-minute rest period. In a normal, healthy body that is allowed to self-regulate, this 2-hour rhythm is reflected as natural fluctuations in such things as the neuroendocrine system, arousal levels, and attentional processes. Human cortisol levels fluctuate, as do body tempera-

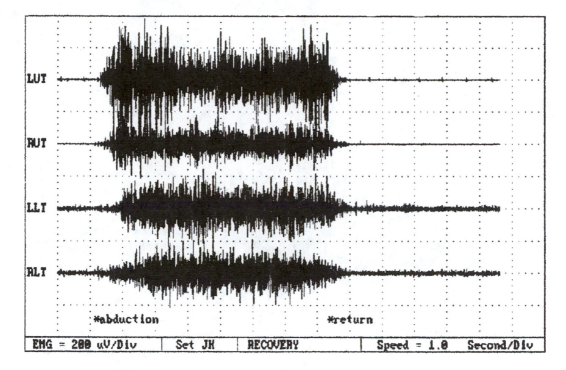

Figure 8–8 The "nearly-normal" relationship of upper and lower trapezius during abduction to 90 degrees. It is mildly abnormal with an asymmetry in left upper trapezius to right upper trapezius, with left upper trapezius hyperactive. *Source:* Copyright © Clinical Resources, Inc.

tures, brain rhythms, and mentation. Unfortunately, many of us have lost touch with these natural body rhythms and attempt to stay aroused or active or to remain productive.

Scandinavian researchers[17,18] have been studying micromomentary rest or "EMG gaps" that occur during the work cycle. Visually, Taylor[14] has presented this concept in Figure 8–11. Here, he has superposed four 1.5-minute tracings of the right upper trapezius while the patient undergoes four separate conditions. (1) The first tracing is taken while the patient is at rest (arms in the lap), with the baseline resting levels appearing quite low. (2) The second tracing is taken while the patient undergoes stress profiling. Here, there is a slight increase in the sEMG levels. (3) The third tracing shows sEMG activity while the patient is typing. Here, there are periodic and momentary drops in the sEMG activity below 5 microvolts throughout the tracing.

These brief drops are the "EMG gaps." (4) The fourth tracing is taken while the person is typing while simultaneously undergoing a stressful event. A comparison of this tracing to the third tracing indicates that not only does the level of sEMG activity rise, but also the EMG gaps disappear. This places the patient in a form of "double jeopardy"; the patient has increased metabolic demands due to increased levels of activation, but the mechanism for profusion of the muscular tissue—rhythmic and interspersed rest—is missing. The buildup of retained metabolites (lactic acid) is very likely.

Another method for examining the sEMG record for interspersed rest is the *probability amplitude distribution* discussed in Chapter 3. Briefly, the occurrence of discrete amplitude "bins" of the sEMG are plotted for a given unit of time. In Figure 8–12, the probability amplitude distribution for a patient with right-sided

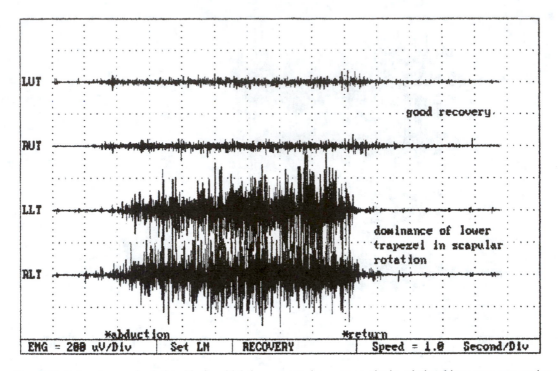

Figure 8–9 An abnormal relationship in which lower trapezius overrecruits in relationship to upper trapezius during abduction to 90 degrees. Courtesy of Will Taylor, Blue Hills, Maine.

neck and headache pain is displayed. The distribution curve represents a 20-minute period of typing. Note that the left upper trapezius (LUTr) shows a clear bimodal distribution with a work peak in the 9 to 10 microvolt range and a nice, strong rest peak in the 2 to 3 microvolt range. This distribution looks "normal." The amplitudes of work are relatively quiet, and there is ample rest. The right upper trapezius (RUTr), however, shows a work peak in the 22 microvolt range and a much smaller rest peak (50% smaller) in the 2 to 3 microvolt range. Although the work amplitude is strikingly higher in the affected right upper trapezius compared to the left upper trapezius, the smaller levels of rest may account for the tension myalgia in the right side of this patient's neck.

The second example provides a much clearer picture of the phenomenon and is presented in Figure 8–13. Here a 20-minute recording from the right and left upper trapezius during typing is taken on a patient with left-sided carpal tunnel syndrome. Note that the left upper trapezius takes the form of a unimodal distribution with a work peak around 11 to 12 microvolts, with no distinct rest peak. The right upper trapezius shows a work peak in the 6 to 10 microvolt range, with a very solid rest peak in the 3 to 4 microvolt range. Here, because the work peaks are nearly the same, the primary difference is in the presence or absence of a rest peak.

RELIABILITY OF DYNAMIC SURFACE ELECTROMYOGRAPHY ASSESSMENTS

The reliability of sEMG recordings is a complicated issue. An excellent discussion of the issues and potential solutions is presented in a recent article by Knutson et al.[19] The issues are complicated by the type of contraction studied

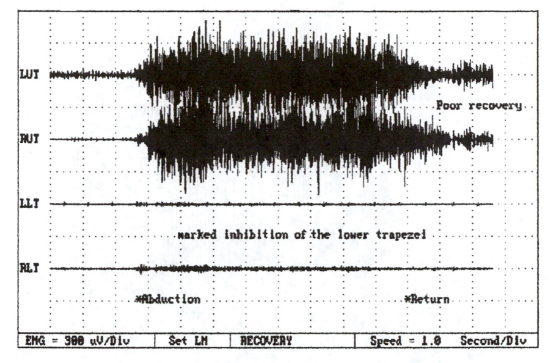

Figure 8–10 A "grossly abnormal" recording of the relationship between upper and lower trapezius during abduction to 90 degrees, in which upper trapezius dominates over lower trapezius. *Source:* Copyright © Clinical Resources, Inc.

(isometric versus open chain), level of contraction (10% versus 80% maximum voluntary contraction), type of statistic utilized (Pearson, internal consistency coefficient, or coefficients of variation), same versus multiple days, etc. Major questions include how consistent these recordings should be as one performs the same movement several times on the same occasion, and from one occasion to another. Donaldson has studied the reliability of the peak amplitude during forward flexion of the neck over five repetitions (personal communication). The correlations between the first movement peak and the other four movement peaks was relatively low (<0.40). However, the correlation between the second to fifth movement peaks was very high (>0.90). This suggests that the first movement pattern of an assessment is an unreliable measure that should always be thrown out, and the third repetition represents a reliable estimate of the recruitment pattern for the patient.

Knutson et al[19] reviewed nine studies that assessed reliability of sEMG recordings within the same day on a variety of muscles and found the Pearson correlations to be between 0.77 and 0.98. Mathiassen et al[20] reported coefficients of variation (CV) to be around 6% to 14% for a series of studies on upper fibers of trapezius conducted on the same day. The within-day reliability values are quite respectable. Knutson reviewed five studies that assessed reliability across days and found Pearson correlations as high as 0.92 and as low as 0.32. Mathiassen et al reported a CV of 23% to 25% in upper trapezius recordings across days.[20] Thus, variability of findings increases as time between recordings increases.

Ahern and colleagues[21] have investigated the reliability of sEMG over an extended period of time using dynamic assessment procedures. In this study, these researchers found initially high test-retest correlations on day 1. But, as they re-

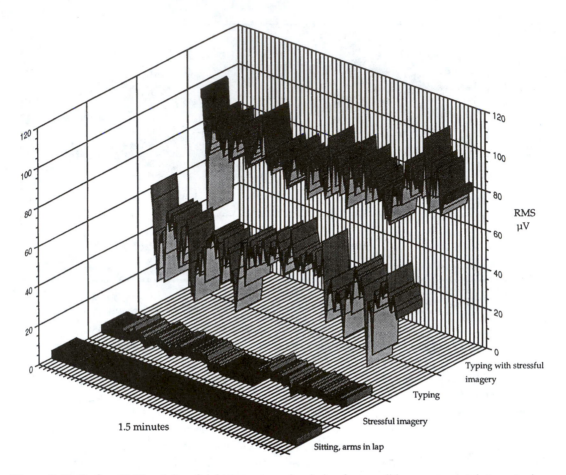

Figure 8–11 Surface EMG activity of right upper trapezius during four conditions: rest, mental stress, typing, and typing while under stress. The micromomentary rest phenomenon may be observed during a typing task. These brief periods of rest are represented by momentary drops in the sEMG activity. Courtesy of Will Taylor, Blue Hills, Maine.

assessed a small sample of individuals at longer and longer time intervals, they found the test-retest correlations to fall off substantially. This finding may be restricted to sEMG patterns observed in the population they studied—"normal" backs. And perhaps this finding is a signature of health; one could argue that because the neuro-muscular system is a fluid and dynamic one, high test-retest correlations for days, months, or years would be found only in pathological populations. Chronic back pain patients, for example, might show higher test-retest scores over time because of their pathology. One might want to

consider sEMG as a "state" rather than a "trait" measure, changing in response to the task and the environment. Highly consistent and persistent bracing or postural patterns of activation or habitual movement patterns might indicate an emerging or expressed pathology.

ASSESSMENT OF THE PELVIC FLOOR

Surface EMG recordings help in the assessment and treatment of urinary and fecal incontinence, as well as pelvic floor pain such as vulvodynia and vulvar vestibulitis. The scope of

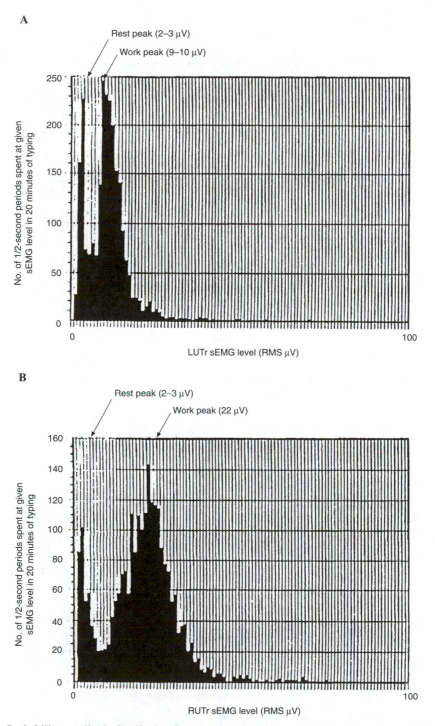

Figure 8–12 Probability amplitude distribution for (**A**) left and (**B**) right upper trapezius during a typing task for a patient with chronic neck and headache pain primarily on the right side. Note change of scale for LUTr and RUTr. Courtesy of Will Taylor, Blue Hills, Maine.

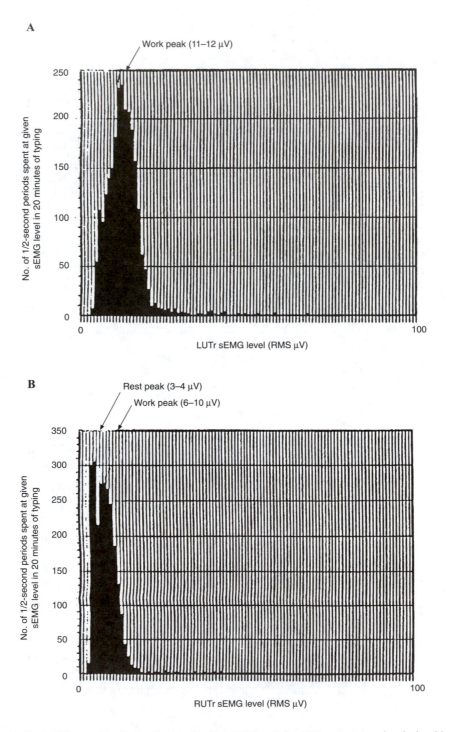

Figure 8–13 Probability amplitude distribution for the left (**A**) and right (**B**) upper trapezius during 20 minutes of typing for a patient with left-sided carpal tunnel syndrome. Note absence of rest peak on the left upper trapezius. Courtesy of Will Taylor, Blue Hills, Maine.

these problems is immense; it is estimated that 80% of the geriatric population is incontinent[22] and 15% of all women suffer from some sort of pelvic pain disorder.[23]

The same assessment protocol is used for all of these conditions. Consistent with the functions of the pelvic floor musculature (sexual, sphincteric, and supportive), and in order to look at recruitment and endurance, three types of contractions are studied using different durations[24] (see Figure 8–14). Six attributes of sEMG are examined (see Table 8–2). Once the electrodes are in place and the patient is comfortably placed in the reclining position, the practitioner records a resting level for 3 to 5 minutes and checks the level of resting tone. It should be low and with good stability. Next, in each of six 5-second periods, the patient is asked to create a strong, brief contraction (called a "flick") in the middle of the epoch. The practitioner examines these sEMG recordings for latency of recruitment, amplitude, and fatigue. This is followed by a rest period of approximately 15 seconds. Next, a series of ten 10-second periods is studied in which the patient alternates between resting and contracting. The patient is asked to make a full contraction and hold it for 10 seconds, and then to stop the contraction and rest for 10 seconds. This is examined for the ease of recruitment and derecruitment, the amplitude of contraction, and the presence of any fatigue. This is followed by a 10-second rest period. Finally, the patient is asked to contract fully and hold for as long as possible over a 60-second period. The practitioner examines this sEMG recording for amplitude and the rate of fatigue. This recording is followed by a resting baseline, which the practitioner examines for its amplitude and stability.

A normal recruitment pattern for a 10-second hold can be seen in Figure 8–15. Initially, the resting tone is low; there is a crisp recruitment to a high amplitude; and at the cessation of the 10-second hold, the sEMG level falls off rapidly and returns to a low resting tone level. In Figure 8–16, an abnormal recruitment pattern is presented. Here, the patient exhibits an elevated and unstable resting baseline. When the patient is asked to contract completely for 10 seconds, a low amplitude/poor recruitment is seen, followed by fatigue (indicated by the declining amplitude over time). Upon cessation of the recruitment, the release is not crisp, but slow. Finally, postbaseline levels remain elevated and variable.

Table 8–2 gives the criteria for examining attributes of sEMG recordings from the pelvic floor.[25] These recordings are based upon Flexiplus sEMG instrumentation (see Table 3–1 for benchmark equivalence). Comparison of the hit rate for 55 "nonmorbid" subjects (no pain, no incontinence) to 32 vulvar vestibulitis patients is presented. The percentage of these two cohorts meeting the diagnostic criteria is given. Some of the sEMG attributes distinguish the two groups better than others. The level of variability seems

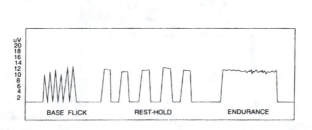

Figure 8–14 Normal patterns of sEMG recruitment observed during assessment of the pelvic floor. *Source:* Reprinted with permission from J Corocos, S Drew, and L West, Urinary and Fecal Incontinence, *Electromyography: Applications in Physical Therapy,* © 1992, Thought Technology.

Table 8–2 Surface Electromyography Attributes/Criteria for Comparisons of Normal Subjects (Nonmorbid) and Patients with Vulvar Vestibulitis

sEMG Attribute	*Criterion (sEMG Value)	Nonmorbid Subjects (N = 55)	Vestibulitis Patients (N = 32)
1. Resting baseline (supine posture)	>2.0 µV (RMS)	18%	71%
2. Contraction amplitude (averaged over 6 occasions)	<17.5 µV (RMS)	13%	65%
3. Postcontraction resting baseline variability (6 occasions)	>0.2 µV (RMS)	21%	93%
4. Recruitment time	>0.2 second	1%	3%
5. Derecruitment time	>0.2 second	6%	86%
6. Mean spectral frequency during contraction (6 occasions)	>115 Hz	12%	69%

*Based upon Flexiplus sEMG and intravaginal sensors. All values represent the criterion cutoff used in determining the percentage of correct classification.

Source: Copyright © Marek Jantos, PhD.

to be the most sensitive indicator, suggesting that the pelvic muscles are quite "noisy" in that population. Inability to cease the contraction, which suggests irritability in the neuromuscular system, is also an indicator. Contractile ampli-

tudes and resting baselines also separate out the two groups.

The assessment criteria also suggest potential biofeedback treatment opportunities. These are discussed in Chapter 9.

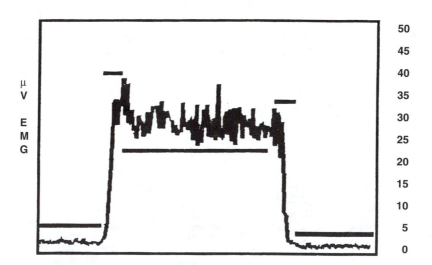

Figure 8–15 A normal recruitment pattern recorded from the pelvic floor using an intravaginal recording electrode. *Source:* Copyright © Marek Jantos, PhD.

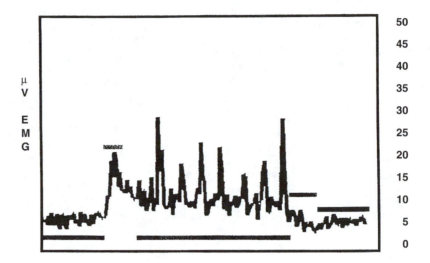

Figure 8–16 An abnormal recruitment pattern recorded from a patient with vulvar vestibulitis. *Source:* Copyright © Marek Jantos, PhD.

REFERENCES

1. Price JP, Clare MH, Ewerhardt RH. Studies in low backache with persistent spasm. *Arch Phys Med.* 1948; 29:703–709.

2. Floyd WF, Silver P. The function of the erector spinae muscles in certain movements and postures in man. *J Physiol.* 1955;129:184–203.

3. Basmajian JV, DeLuca C. *Muscles Alive.* 5th ed. Baltimore: Williams & Wilkins; 1985.

4. Kasman GS. *Surface EMG in Physical Therapy: Applications in Chronic Musculoskeletal Pain.* Seattle, WA: Movements Systems; 1995.

5. Ettare D, Ettare R. Muscle learning therapy: a treatment protocol. In: Cram JR, ed. *Clinical EMG for Surface Recordings, II.* Nevada City, CA: Clinical Resources; 1990:197–234.

6. Hubbard D, Berkoff G. Myofascial trigger points show spontaneous needle EMG activity. *Spine.* 1993;18: 1803–1807.

7. Fishbain DA, Goldberg M, Meagher BR, Steel R, Rosomoff H. Male and female chronic pain patients categorized by DSM-II psychiatric diagnostic criteria. *Pain.* 1986;26:181–197.

8. Fricton JF, Kroening R, Haley D, Siegert R. Myofascial pain syndrome of the head and neck: a critical review of clinical characteristics of 164 patients. *Oral Surg.* 1985;60:615–623.

9. Travell J, Simons D. *Myofascial Pain and Dysfunction: A Trigger Point Manual, I and II.* Baltimore: Williams & Wilkins; 1983.

10. Simons D. Clinical and etiological update of myofascial pain from trigger points. *J Musculoskeletal Pain.* 1996;4:97–125.

11. Donaldson S, Donaldson M. Multi-channel EMG assessment and treatment techniques. In: Cram JR, ed. *Clinical EMG for Surface Recordings, II.* Nevada City, CA: Clinical Resources; 1990:143–173.

12. Donaldson S, Skubick D, Clasby B, Cram J. The evaluation of trigger-point activity using dynamic EMG techniques. *Am J Pain Manage.* 1994;4:118–122.

13. Kasman G, Cram J, Wolf S. *Clinical Applications in Surface Electromyography.* Gaithersburg, MD: Aspen Publishers; 1997.

14. Taylor W. Patterns of sEMG. Presented at meeting of the Surface EMG Society of North America; 1993; Boston.

15. Taylor W. Dynamic EMG biofeedback in assessment and treatment using a neuromuscular reeducation model. In: Cram JR, ed. *Clinical EMG for Surface Re-*

cordings, II. Nevada City, CA: Clinical Resources; 1990:175–196.

16. Shannahoff-Khalsa D. Lateralized rhythms of the central and autonomic nervous system. *Int J Psychophysiol.* 1991;11:225–251.

17. Veiersted KB, Westgaard RH, Andersen P. Electromyographic evaluation of muscular work pattern as a predictor of trapezius myalgia. *Scan J Work Environ Health.* 1993;19:284–290.

18. Veiersted KB, Westgaard RH. Work related risk factors for trapezius myalgia. *Int Arch Occup Environ Health.* 1990;62:31–41.

19. Knutson LM, Soderberg GL, Ballantyne BT, Clarke WR. A study of various normalization procedures for within-day electromyographic data. *J Electromyogr Kinesiol.* 1994;1:47–59.

20. Mathiassen SE, Winkel J, Hagg GM. Normalization of surface EMG amplitude from the upper trapezius muscle in ergonomic studies: a review. *J Electromyogr Kinesiol.* 1995;5:197–226.

21. Ahern DK, Follick MJ, Cocurcil JR, Laser-Wolston N. Reliability of lumbar paravertebral EMG assessment in chronic low back pain. *Arch Phys Med Rehab.* 1986;76:762–765.

22. Portnoi VA. Urinary incontinence in the elderly. *Am Fam Physician.* 1981;23:151–154.

23. Goetsch MF. Vulvar vestibulitis: Prevalence and historic feature in a general gynecologic practice population. *Am J Obstet Gynecol.* 1991;164:1609.

24. Glazer HI, Rodke G, Swencionis C, Hertz R, Young A. Treatment of vulvar vestibulitis syndrome with electromyographic biofeedback of pelvic floor musculature. *J Reprod Med.* 1995;40:283–290.

25. White G, Jantos M, Glazer H. Towards establishing the diagnosis of vulvar vestibulitis. In press.

Chapter Questions

1. Resting baseline of muscle tone is primarily affected by:
   a. posture
   b. emotional tone
   c. kinematics
   d. a and b

2. When a muscle fails to return to baseline following a movement, it is called:
   a. dysfunctional
   b. irritable
   c. hypoactive
   d. hyperactive

3. During a symmetrical movement, one would expect to see:
   a. an asymmetrical activation pattern
   b. a symmetrical activation pattern
   c. a symmetrical activation pattern for homologous muscle groups
   d. an asymmetrical activation pattern for homologous muscle groups

4. During an asymmetrical movement, one would expect to see:
   a. an asymmetrical activation pattern
   b. a symmetrical activation pattern
   c. a symmetrical activation pattern for homologous muscle groups
   d. an asymmetrical activation pattern for homologous muscle groups

5. Symmetrical movement is to asymmetrical recruitment as asymmetrical movement is to:
   a. irritability
   b. cocontraction
   c. flexion-relaxation
   d. synergy

6. The probability amplitude distribution of sEMG should be:
   a. bimodal
   b. unimodal
   c. curvilinear
   d. multiphasic

7. In assessing vulvodynia, which sEMG attribute best separates out normal subjects from patient populations?
   a. amplitude of contractions
   b. resting baseline amplitudes
   c. resting baseline variance
   d. spectral frequency

8. A "flick" consists of a short, brisk contraction. For which disorder is it commonly used?
   a. upper quarter pain
   b. incontinence
   c. vulvodynia
   d. b and c only

9. In incontinence assessments, fatigue is noted by:
   a. an increase in amplitude
   b. a decrease in amplitude
   c. an increase in blood flow
   d. an increase in urine flow

10. How much asymmetry is considered to be within the normal range?
    a. 5%
    b. 10%
    c. 20%
    d. 50%

11. The erector spinae muscles are expected to _____ during full-trunk flexion.
    a. cocontract
    b. turn off
    c. recruit
    d. become hypoactive

12. During abduction of the arms to 90 degrees, what should be the ratio of sEMG activity for the upper and lower trapezius?
    a. approximately 1 to 1
    b. 2 to 1
    c. 1 to 2
    d. none of the above

13. Which of the following is not a sign of a trigger point?
    a. jump sign
    b. taut band
    c. muscle weakness
    d. referred pain
    e. all of the above

CHAPTER 9

Treatment Considerations and Protocols

AN OVERVIEW OF TREATMENT

Once the clinical assessment has been completed, the formation of treatment plans and the setting of goals are the next order of business. Whenever possible, the practitioner should place the patient's particular dysregulation pattern into the context of emotional, postural, and movement components. Once all three elements are considered, a treatment plan is developed. If the practitioner proceeds through all three elements of treatment, it is recommended to start with relaxation, then postural treatment, and then movement. The area of interest and expertise of the practitioner and the nature of the patient's dysfunction will determine the extent that each element is emphasized. Exhibit 9–1 provides a partial list for the scope and sequence associated with surface electromyography (sEMG) treatments.

Treatment using sEMG falls within an educational model. In the most general sense, biofeedback entails providing patients with information concerning their physiology—in this case, muscle activity. In the world of physical medicine this is called *neuromuscular reeducation*. The sEMG feedback is used to teach the patient how to normalize his or her muscle function. The approaches given below are suggestions for how to optimize the learning experience. Two cases are considered: (1) dysfunction of the up-

per and lower trapezius and (2) dysfunction of the cervical muscles.

Relaxation

If a patient's dysfunction has emotional, postural, and movement components, the practitioner should begin with quieting or relaxation therapies. Although relaxation work is not a necessary ingredient for all successful sEMG therapy protocols, it is advisable to teach patients how to become quiet before attempting to teach them how to self-regulate the neuromuscular-musculoskeletal system. By *downtraining* the neuromuscular system, one reduces the "noise" in the system. This is done before initiating a dynamic, uptraining phase; it allows the patient to begin the reeducation process with a quiet nervous system, which allows the patient to attend to the proprioception associated with the sEMG feedback signal and facilitates the learning process. Another potential source of noise in the learning process is behavioral or socioemotional issues (ie, significant pain displays). If these issues are clearly present, the practitioner should address them before moving on to more physical components of sEMG treatments. Dynamic relaxation should also be considered. Micromomentary rest periods can be learned or at least encouraged. Longer rest periods, such as being able to return the muscle to a

Exhibit 9–1 A Partial List of Scope and Sequence for Treating the Neuromuscular System Using sEMG Feedback

1. Reduce excessive resting tone.
  • possible relaxation strategies to lower emotional tone
    – progressive relaxation
    – autogenics therapy
    – guided imagery
    – breath work
  • possible dynamic relaxation strategies to fine-tune the movement system
    – muscle learning therapy
    – recovery training
    – Feldenkrais method
 	
2. Make postural corrections.
  • Cuing and sEMG feedback
    – physical prompting
    – sEMG training
  • stretching
    – sEMG guided stretches
3. Develop recruitment and timing synergies.
  • isolation training
  • discrimination training
  • coordinated recruitment/synergy training
4. Promote generalization through activities of daily living.

low level of activity following its use, is a form of dynamic relaxation and may be a key to successful treatment.

Posture

Postural aspects of dysfunction should be considered next. These may relate significantly to the emotional or movement components of dysfunction, and it may be impossible to separate out posture as a separate component. Movement, for example, cannot occur without posture. And postural correction will not be retained if it is strongly linked to emotional elements, because the emotional display tends to dominate over volitional control of posture in the long run. If movement patterns are based upon a faulty posture, they seldom have the correct agonist/antagonist/synergist relationships. Correcting the limitations placed on a movement by faulty postures greatly enhances any movement-oriented exercise.

Movement

The movement component of dysfunction is superimposed on the emotional and postural components. Provided that the muscle and connective tissues have not been altered, the fluidity of movement depends upon the presence of well-regulated emotional tone along with proper postural alignment. Movement is directed by many aspects of our being; it cascades down through the complex neural network described in Chapter 2. The idea for the movement originates in the frontal lobes; the prefrontal cortex sets the general plan for the movement; the motor cortex tunes the finer aspects of the movement; and the cerebellum integrates the movement with the other senses, sets the postural tone through its control of the collateral gamma motor activity, and provides the final link in the actual execution of the movement. Segmental and suprasegmental reflex arcs from the muscle spindle, Golgi tendon organs, Ruffini's corpuscles, and free nerve endings impinge upon the descending information at a spinal tract level, bringing about the output for the final common pathway—the lower motor neuron. Disease in any aspect of this very complex system alters this recruitment pattern and resultant movement. The job of the practitioner is to understand and tease apart this puzzle, to determine which part of the system has gone awry, and to work with those aspects of the problem that can be corrected. This may involve joint mobilization, stretching exercises, isolation training for specific muscle groups, integrating the solitary muscle into correct agonist/antagonist/synergist relationships with other muscles, and finally shaping the movement pattern to fit the patient's lifestyle.

Generalization of Training

It simply is not enough to teach the patient to relax in one posture or move through one plane of motion. Cram and Freeman[1] demonstrated that sEMG relaxation-based feedback to the frontal muscles does not spontaneously generalize to the neck or shoulder, nor does it generalize from the reclining posture to the standing posture. In addition, posturally based sEMG feedback to the upper back while standing does not generalize to the seated posture. These authors found the same to be true for the erector spinae muscle group. In other words, you reap what you sow. When practitioners conduct sEMG training in one posture, there is no guarantee that it will spontaneously generalize to another posture. This lack of generalization applies to quieting the neuromuscular system as well as to learning how to turn it on and coordinate it. Therefore, the practitioner must use strategies that allow patients to generalize their newly acquired motor skills to new settings. For this reason, practitioners should encourage patients to demonstrate their sEMG abilities during activities of daily living.

Relaxation Strategies

The muscular system is typically 50% of an individual's body weight, and it consumes a major amount of a person's metabolic resources. Thus, it is reasonable to assume that the muscles could reflect or influence other aspects of the body system. The fine art of relaxation has been passed down through the ages. Even the ancient yogis embedded relaxation into their yoga posture rituals, recognizing its role in learning to control one's life.[2] During the early 1900s, Edmund Jacobson became well known for his use of general relaxation in the treatment of a variety of functional or "psychosomatic" disorders.[3] At the same time that Jacobson was intro-

ducing his treatment in the United States, a German named Wolfgang Luthe[4,5] developed a series of autogenic phrases or formulae that patients could be taught as a means to treat a variety of psychosomatic disorders. Unfortunately, these relaxation techniques were replaced with Valium during the 1950s as the cultural model shifted to "better living through chemistry." During the 1960s, Wolpe[6] reintroduced Jacobson's technique to American psychology in an abbreviated form known as *progressive relaxation*. This technique was used as the relaxation component for a psychological procedure called systematic desensitization. A little later, George Whatmore, a student of Jacobson, published *The Physiopathology and Treatment of Functional Disorders*.[7] In this work, Whatmore detailed his adaptation of Jacobson's techniques in which he used sEMG instrumentation as part of the relaxation-based training. During the 1970s, relaxation protocols flourished with the publication of hundreds of relaxation-based, guided-imagery tapes. One of the most prolific producers of these tapes was psychiatrist Emmett Miller.[8] There has been some fine-tuning of these imagery tapes for medical uses. For example, Hank Bennett,[9] using language very specific to the human body, produced an audiotape entitled *Preparation for Surgery*, which has been shown to reduce blood loss during surgery, reduce the need for narcotic analgesia following surgery, and reduce the number of days of required hospitalization significantly.

Progressive Relaxation Training

Relaxation training is a verbally mediated event in which the practitioner helps the patient change his or her physiology through the use of actions. For Jacobson, the model was one of tensing and releasing various muscle groups. The therapist instructs the patient about how to tense and release muscles in isolation, with an emphasis upon downtraining.

A typical beginning session works on the upper extremity. The patient is instructed to progress up the forearm, one arm at a time, through the following muscles:

1. *Wrist extensors:* "Lift the wrist up, tensing the muscle responsible for this up here on your upper arm until you can feel the tension in that muscle. Then let go of that tension quickly. Let your wrist drop, and feel the tension leave your arm. Relax that muscle completely for the next minute."

2. *Wrist flexors:* "Next, push your wrist down. Tense the muscles making that movement happen until you can feel them on the bottom of your arm. Then suddenly let go of that tension. Feel the tension leave the muscle, letting the arm relax as completely as it can for the next minute."

3. *Biceps:* "Next, bend your arm up at the elbow, tensing the muscle of your upper arm until you can clearly feel the tension in that muscle. Then suddenly let it go. Feel the tension leave your upper arm as you let it relax as completely as you possibly can for the next minute."

4. *Triceps:* "Next, let your arm go straight, tensing the muscle responsible for the movement so that you can feel the tension on the back of your upper arm. Then let it go quickly, feeling the tension leave that muscle as you relax to the best of your ability for the next minute."

Figures 9–1 and 9–2 show the effects of progressive relaxation over a course of sessions. In Figure 9–1 the tensing and releasing of each specific muscle group affects other sites as well. There is an overgeneralization of the muscular effort to multiple sites, resulting from the patient's moving the extremity in order to feel and sense a particular site. The patient is treated, using a combination of sEMG feedback and progressive relaxation procedure. Figure 9–2 shows that by the third session the patient demonstrates a good ability to make very specific small isometric contractions at the various sites without the excessive spillover of muscular efforts seen in Figure 9–1.

Progressive relaxation training involves several components. Initially, the patient is asked to move the joint associated with the muscle as he or she intentionally tenses the muscle to the point of tension perception. As training progresses across sessions, the practitioner encourages the patient to become more aware of tension at lower levels of activation. Toward the end of training, the patient is able to activate and sense a specific muscle group without moving the associated joint. It takes a very relaxed muscle and a fair amount of training for the patient to sense a brief burst of isometric tension in a muscle. In the 1960s, Whatmore demonstrated that sEMG instrumentation and feedback made this task much easier.[7] Second, the practitioner must teach the patient to "let go" of tension. The above example suggests that practitioners teach the patient to let go quickly. Jacobson used the term "zero down" to describe what it means to let go of muscle tension quickly and completely. It is the relaxation component that has the greatest therapeutic effect. "Tense with will, relax and feel." The "relax and feel" is at least twice as important as tensing the muscle. Third, a long period of quiet time and relaxation follows each tension cycle. The ratio of tension to relaxation should be 1 to 5. Fourth, opposing pairs of muscles are systematically activated. This is to maintain a healthy balance in the neuronal pool of spinal segments that control these muscles. At a segmental and suprasegmental level, the output from the Golgi tendon organ and muscle spindles provides collateral excitatory or inhibitory influences on related contralateral or opposing lower motor neurons (see Chapter 2). Finally, the practitioner progresses from one muscle group to another, working through the various kinetic chains. The second session might work on the arms and then add in the muscles of the shoulder and upper back. The third session might work on the arms, the shoulder, and the head and neck. As the therapy progresses, the patients become more and more adept at activating only the muscles that they intend to activate. For more elaborate and specific information on this technique, the original

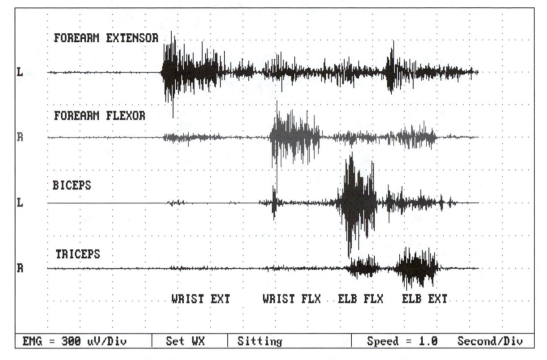

Figure 9–1 Surface EMG recordings from forearm extensors and flexors (wide placement), biceps, and triceps are shown during voluntary activation of each site. Note the lack of specificity of activation, as there is spillover of muscular effort to multiple sites. *Source:* Copyright © Clinical Resources, Inc.

work of Edmund Jacobson, *You Must Relax,*[3] is highly recommended.

Briefer adaptations of Jacobson's protocols are available.[6] Typically, they reduce the specificity of the contraction by asking the patient to cocontract the agonist/antagonist muscles (eg, "Make a fist and feel the tension throughout your entire forearm"). The focus is upon feeling large contractions, and there is no effort to recognize the smaller "efforts." In addition, those protocols use a shorter, 15-second relaxation phase. These briefer relaxation protocols are appropriate and adequate if the patient is already fairly relaxed or has some rudimentary relaxation skills, and if the practitioner wishes to induce a lighter level of relaxation.

Autogenics Therapy

Autogenics therapy (AT) uses words and images without action. It is a form of self-hypnosis.

The patient learns to use very specific self-suggestions or phrases to affect his or her physiology. AT approaches six different domains:

1. heaviness—neuromuscular relaxation
2. warmth—vascular dilatation
3. slow and regular heartbeat—cardiac regulation
4. slow and regular breath—respiratory regulation
5. abdominal warmth—visceral relaxation
6. cooling the forehead—cooling the brain

The structure of the therapy is very specific. It begins with setting the correct posture. The therapy can be done while the patient is lying, reclining, or sitting. In the lying posture, the head is supported by pillows, the palms are down, and the feet are slightly apart. In the reclining posture, the feet are on the ground, the arms are positioned on the armrests of the chair with the palms down, and the head is supported

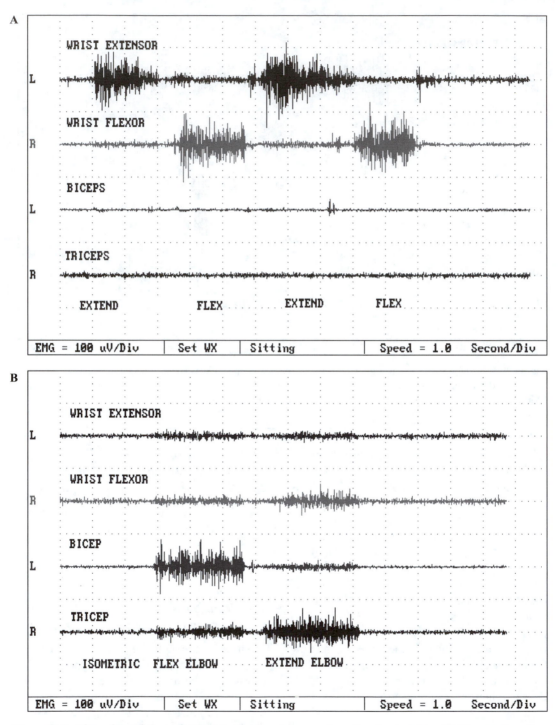

Figure 9–2 After a few sessions of sEMG feedback and progressive relaxation training, sEMG recordings from forearm extensors and flexors (wide placement), biceps, and triceps sites are shown during voluntary activation of each site. (**A**) Isolated wrist extensor and flexor activity, (**B**) isolated bicep and tricep activity. *Source:* Copyright © Clinical Resources, Inc.

in some way. In the sitting posture, the feet are on the ground, the arms are in the lap (palms down), and the torso is slumped forward with the head in the fully flexed posture.

The patient is encouraged to use *passive volition*. That is, the person is encouraged to focus on the body part in question, use phrases suggested, yet have a casual attitude about the outcome of the effort. It is more like wishing for something to happen, rather than making it happen. It is helpful to begin the exercises with a verification phase, one where the patient is asked to close his or her eyes and mentally visualize the part(s) he or she is going to work on. Then the practitioner gives phrases. This is followed by a minimum of a 30-second observation period by the patient. Finally the exercise is terminated by asking the patient to move the part(s) of interest vigorously, breathe out heavily, and open his or her eyes. This procedure is explored for each autogenic phrase or set of phrases, and the patient is asked to note any discharges that result from the procedure. These discharges are thoughts, feelings, or physical sensations associated with the autogenic phrase.

The autogenic phrases are repeated to the patient, and the patient thinks the phrases himself or herself, five or six times over the course of 30 to 60 seconds per phrase. During the first visit, the practitioner usually begins with one phrase and goes through the entire cycle. On subsequent visits, the practitioner adds more phrases to the patient's suggestions, making the training sessions longer and deeper. The standard autogenic phrases are as follows:

- My right (left) arm is heavy.
- My right (left) leg is heavy.
- My right (left) arm is warm.
- My right (left) leg is warm.
- Both my arms (legs) are heavy.
- Both my arms (legs) are warm.
- I am at peace.
- My heart beat is slow and regular.
- My breathing is slow and regular.
- It breathes me.
- My abdomen (solar plexus) flows warmly.
- My forehead is cool.

For a more in-depth review of autogenic training, see Luthe's *Autogenics Therapy: Autogenic Methods*, volume 1. In addition, there is a tremendous amount of literature available on the physiological effects of this technique. The reader is referred to volume 4 of the *Autogenics Therapy* series for an in-depth review of this literature.[5] The effects of AT appear to be quite specific. The suggestions of heaviness appear to bring about reductions in sEMG activity, suggestions of warmth bring about increased hand temperature, suggestions of slowness of the heart and breath seem to slow both systems, and suggestions of coolness of the forehead appear to lower the temperature of the upper face. If practitioners want to work on quieting down a particular organ system or part of the body, it appears that they should direct their language in very specific ways to those body parts and organs.

Guided Imagery

Guided imagery is a much broader concept than AT. It is a form of self-hypnosis, in which patients are encouraged to think, visualize, hear, feel, and/or smell their way into a relaxed and comfortable space. Guided imagery procedures attempt to begin with a state of general relaxation. The script by Thomas[10] provided in Exhibit 9–2 is directed toward this generic sense of relaxation. From there, many practitioners may overlay a particular therapeutic theme for the patient. For example, a tape may be specifically designed to assist the patient in drifting off to sleep.[11] The images used for sleep differ significantly from those used to cope with pain.[12] One of the best tapes with a specific application area has been authored by Bennett[9,13,14] on preparing the patient for surgery. Like the language for AT, the language for this tape has been selected for its desired effect. For example, the surgical preparation tape uses a very specific approach to suggestions, which make the suggestions quite believable, if not commonplace. It then uses language that asks the body to take the physiologically correct action to minimize the trauma of surgery. And, strange as it may seem, the ap-

Exhibit 9–2 Guided Imagery Script for General Relaxation

Now relax and let all stressful memories fade away . . . for the next 20 minutes you can just relax as you listen to suggestions on how to allow yourself to be calm . . . as you begin this period of relaxation let your body get as comfortable as you can . . . if you need to adjust anything, do it now . . . be sure that you can breathe easily . . . keep your eyes gently closed . . . this is your time to forget all cares and worries . . . give yourself permission to use this time to simply be . . . to let go of tension . . . to relax . . .

"Now allow your mind to drift far, far away . . . away from your everyday life . . . away from all your anxieties, worries, and responsibilities . . . let your mind drift to a place where you can feel safe, comfortable, and tranquil . . . as this happens just passively listen to suggestions for relaxation . . . don't try to make anything happen . . . just let it happen . . . just let your muscles relax all by themselves . . . suggest to your muscles that they may take a vacation now . . . the chair will hold you . . .

"Now focus on your breathing . . . become aware of your breathing . . . let it be deep, and abdominal . . . let it be slow, and regular . . . let the air come in through your nose and go directly to your abdomen . . . feel your stomach muscles expand as you breathe in . . . let your stomach muscles relax as you breathe out . . . just let your breathing be calm . . . and take no effort at all . . . inhale and exhale . . . inhale and exhale . . . calm, and placid, and tranquil . . . with no cares nor worries . . . just think about relaxing every muscle in your body . . . from the top of your head to the tips of your toes . . . just let the air breathe for you . . . as you focus your attention elsewhere . . .

"Let your attention focus on your face and head . . . let the muscles in your forehead relax . . . imagine all those tiny muscles becoming smooth and relaxed . . . let the muscles around your nose relax . . . let the muscles around your eyes relax . . . let the muscles in your jaw relax . . . let your teeth part slightly . . . let the muscles in your eyelids relax . . . allow your eyelids to find a place that is just right for them to rest comfortably . . . now let this relaxation spread into the temple

area . . . allow your temples to relax . . . as your temples relax you may even be able to feel your ears letting go . . . and dropping with gravity ever so slightly . . . notice how good that feels . . . remember to keep your breathing slow, deep, and regular . . . maybe you can even feel the slight tug of gravity on your face and head . . . more and more calm . . . more and more serene with each breath you take . . . feeling your body becoming heavier and heavier . . . now let the muscles in your throat just let go entirely . . . let them relax . . . let all the muscles in your throat just let go completely and relax . . . maybe you can imagine that all the muscles from the neck up have become loose . . . and soft . . .

"Now just think about relaxing all the muscles in your shoulders . . . imagine the back of your neck and your shoulders . . . feel all the muscles in the back of your neck and shoulders becoming very loose and very slack . . . just let all the muscles in your neck and shoulders sink deeper and deeper into the chair . . . each time you exhale you may notice the contact of your body with the surface it is on . . . feeling the surface beneath you, becoming more and more comfortable . . . let this relaxation flow down your spinal column . . . let all the muscles from the base of your head all the way down to your tailbone relax . . . let them be smooth, and soft . . . loose, and slack . . . feel the comfort of the chair as it holds you . . . let go of the tension as that wonderful feeling spreads into your chest and abdomen . . . feel all your abdominal muscles become smooth, and soft . . . loose, and slack . . . keep your breathing slow, and deep . . . let all your internal organs be soft, and comfortable . . . and now your arms . . . feel your arms let go . . . and become heavy, and soft . . . loose, and slack . . . just let your arms and hands be heavy, and warm . . .

"Let all the tension in the muscles of your entire body relax . . . and now focus on your hips and buttocks . . . let those large muscles be at ease . . . smooth, and soft . . . loose, and slack . . . let the large muscles in your thighs relax . . . and the joints of your knees . . . let the calves of your legs

continues

Exhibit 9–2 continued

relax . . . going very loose and slack . . . and now your feet . . . let them relax . . . perhaps you can imagine that the joints in each and every toe relax . . . as you feel more and more calm . . .

"Now we are going to spend 10 more minutes visualizing a pleasant experience . . . just passively follow the suggestions and enjoy yourself . . . as you begin this next period of relaxation allow your body to feel comfortable . . . now let yourself focus again on your breathing . . . once again becoming aware of your breathing . . . let it be deep . . . and abdominal . . . let it be slow . . . and regular . . . feel your abdomen expand as you breathe in . . . feel your abdomen relax as you breathe out . . . just let your breathing be still . . . and make no effort at all . . . inhale and exhale . . . inhale and exhale . . . calm . . . relaxed . . . tranquil . . . no cares . . . no worries . . . just think about relaxing every muscle in your body . . . just let the air breathe for you . . . as you focus your attention elsewhere . . .

"Now I am going to 'paint' a picture with words . . . listen to the words and see the picture in your mind's eye . . . allow this 'voice picture' to be vivid and real . . . see the colors . . . taste the tastes . . . feel the feelings . . . smell the smells . . . and hear the sounds . . . as I describe the scene, let it be real for you . . . as if you were really there . . . allow your mind to roam freely . . . maybe you can discover new places I may not even describe . . . that would be OK . . . this can become your picture . . . let it develop all on its own . . .

"Now imagine you are on a wonderful vacation . . . with no cares . . . with no worries . . . with no one to be responsible to . . . completely free from your daily pressures and expectations . . .

"You are walking along the beach; it is midsummer . . . it is warm and comfortable . . . it is late afternoon . . . this perfect summer day . . . the sun is a blazing golden yellow in the brilliant blue sky . . . the sun shines down and warms you . . . as you casually walk along you can feel the hard-packed sand beneath your bare feet . . . feel the warmth of the sand . . . feel the dampness of the sand . . . wiggle your toes in the sand . . . isn't it wonderful? . . . as you continue to walk you can hear the sound of the surf on the beach . . . the gentle rhythm of the waves lapping in and out . . . in and out . . . hear the distant cry of a gull as it soars through the sky . . . you look toward the sound . . . the sky is a beautiful deep blue . . . it is filled with fluffy white clouds . . . see the clouds slowly moving and changing their shapes . . . you feel overcome with a feeling of peace and tranquility . . . it is a lazy day that reminds you of many wonderful experiences from your past . . .

"You come to a small mound of pure white sand . . . you find a comfortable place to sit . . . you feel alone and still . . . now you lie back and watch the wispy clouds as they float by . . . you drift, and dream that warm summer day . . . you feel the warmth of the sand beneath you . . . you feel the warmth of the sun as it shines down on you . . . you continue to enjoy this wonderful place for what seems like hours . . . allowing your mind the freedom to wander as it wishes . . . you enjoy this stillness . . . this warmth . . . this quiet . . .

"Now you slowly sit up again . . . as you look toward the sea . . . the sun is beginning to set in the west . . . it reflects in beautiful patterns off the sea . . . colors dance and skip in all directions . . . along the horizon there is a sparkling glimmer where the sky touches the water . . . you can see a sailboat, its sails billowing in the wind . . . you can almost feel yourself on that sailboat piercing through the sea . . . there is a gentle ocean spray . . . it is cooling and refreshing . . . you are aware of the fresh smell of the salt in the spray . . . there is a light residue on your lips . . . you can taste it if you lick your lips . . . with each movement of the sun as it slowly sets you find yourself becoming more and more relaxed . . . all your senses are merging with the calm environment around you . . . you allow yourself to enjoy this wonderful time . . . with no cares . . . no worries . . . no uneasiness . . .

proach works. Patients tend to bleed less, use less medication following surgery, have fewer complications, and be discharged earlier. Practitioners who want more information on what types of images seem to work with what types of disorders should refer to Barber's article on this topic.[15]

Breath Work

Respiration should be considered as part of the comprehensive view of the neuromuscular network. After all, it is the muscles that bring the air into our bodies. When breathing is done efficiently, the diaphragm is predominantly involved. When respiration becomes inefficient and disordered, it begins to overuse the ancillary muscles of respiration such as the sternocleidomastoid, scalene, or upper trapezius. This may be seen in Figure 9–3. In the case of upper back or neck pain, it is essential to consider inappropriate breathing patterns as part of the assessment. If these are noted, training in appropriate respiratory patterns is indicated. In addition, training of the respiratory system can be one of the avenues for teaching the patient general relaxation. Such training reduces the metabolic demands on the breath and increases the mechanical efficiency of the upper back in general.

Teaching a relaxed respiratory pattern involves teaching the patient to breathe abdominally. This can be done several ways. The easiest, noninstrumented method involves placing a small (5-pound) sandbag or small phone book on the patient's abdomen as he or she lies in a well-supported supine posture. Figure 9–4 shows this procedure. Next, the practitioner asks the patient to invite his or her breath down into the abdomen, while pressing up against the weight of the sandbag or book. As the patient exhales, he or she then lets the weight fall. The patient is asked to let his or her body tell him or her how fast or slow he or she should breathe. As the patient increases the tidal volumes (the amount of air breathed), it is not uncommon for the respiration rate to fall and for the patient to report feelings of relaxation. If the patient notes sensations of

arousal or anxiety associated with this procedure, the practitioner might suspect a hyperventilation syndrome and the breathing disorder will need to be treated somewhat differently.[16] If all goes well with supine abdominal breathing, the practitioner should make sure that it generalizes to other postures. The practitioner should observe the patient's ability to breathe abdominally in the sitting and standing postures. Further training may be needed for specific postures. Patients should be encouraged to practice the abdominal breathing in the various postures.

The practitioner may want to use sEMG to monitor the ancillary muscles of respiration during training in abdominal breathing. Electrodes attached to the scalene, sternocleidomastoid, or trapezius muscle groups would provide information concerning excessive use of these muscles. Thresholds can be set that encourage the patient to practice breathing while keeping these muscles relaxed.

Treating patients with respiratory anomalies may be quite complex. If simple training in abdominal breathing does not correct the problem or makes matters worse, the practitioner may want to consult a respiratory therapist. For further information on teaching patients how to breathe correctly, see Rama and colleagues' *The Science of Breath*[17] or Fried's *The Breath Connection*.[16]

Generalization of Relaxation Training

In relaxation training, there are issues relating to the transfer of training effects from one muscle group to another, from one posture to another, and from one situation to another. Several studies have shown that relaxation-based sEMG feedback directed toward one muscle group does not necessarily generalize to other muscle groups.[1,18,19] In addition, Cram and Freeman[1] found that relaxation effects do not generalize from the sitting posture to the standing posture. Although there are no formal studies on the generalization of relaxation skills from the clinic to the home or office setting, it would be safe to assume that such generalization does not sponta-

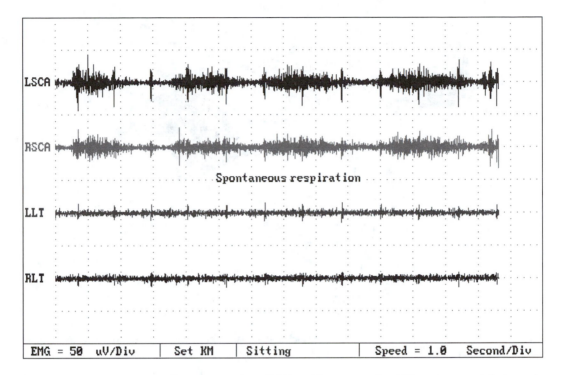

Figure 9–3 Surface EMG recordings from scalene (SCA) and lower trapezius (LT) are presented during quiet sitting. The pattern of rhythmic activation is associated with respiration and the inappropriate use of the ancillary muscles. Courtesy of Will Taylor, Blue Hills, Maine.

neously happen. It appears that the central nervous system is fine-tuned for specificity in the learning of physiological regulation. The practitioner must enhance and promote generalization rather than expect it. For example, to transfer skills from one posture to another, the practitioner should train in both postures.

DYNAMIC RELAXATION STRATEGIES

Relaxation training does not need to occur only in the quiet, recumbent posture. It is possible to teach a patient to turn off the muscular system quickly following its use or simply to move in a more relaxed and synergistic fashion. Two such therapies are described below: Muscle learning therapy developed by Ettare and Ettare[20] and the Feldenkrais method.[21] These are not the only such therapies to consider. Other possible avenues to quiet, relaxed movement in-

clude Tai Chi, the Alexander technique, Aston patterning, and other techniques.

Muscle Learning Therapy

This unusual sEMG training technique has been described in detail by Ettare and Ettare.[20] Its essence and beauty lie in the emphasis on teaching the patient, from the first day, to quiet the muscles following their use. Rather than using the Jacobson technique of an isometric contraction of a specific muscle, a change of posture and/or a functional movement is the perturbation that precedes the practice of relaxation. Dynamic relaxation is defined here as the ability to voluntarily quiet or *derecruit* the muscles following movement.

The system is intentionally a regional one. Electrode placement recommendations are presented in the electrode atlas section of this book

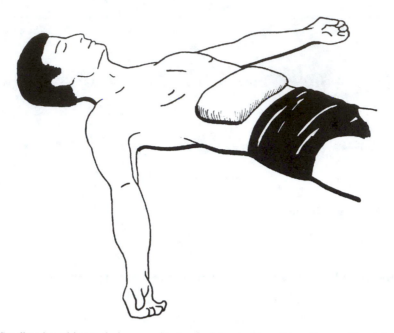

Figure 9–4 Sandbag breathing technique used to teach abdominal breathing. *Source:* Reprinted with permission from Swami Rama et al., *The Science of Breath,* © 1990, Himalayan Press.

and are represented by the widely spaced, non-specific recording at: cervical trapezius (wide); cervical dorsal (wide); and dorsal lumbar (wide).

During the assessment phase, the protocol for the upper back and neck entails having the patient go from sitting, to standing, to walking, to standing, and back to sitting (see Figure 9–5). During training, the practitioner should have the patient go from sitting to standing; once the patient is standing, the practitioner should find ways in which the patient can quiet the upper quarter as much and as quickly as possible. Next, the patient is trained to lower the sEMG levels to a "normal" resting level (below 2 microvolts using a J&J M-501), following the change in activity. This may entail postural changes, stretching, and intentionally learning to "let go." Finally, the patient is encouraged to recognize the sensations of released tension as soon as the sEMG amplitude has dropped. The goal is to transfer the awareness of tension from the biofeedback displays to proprioception. By the end of several visits of training, the sit, stand,

walk, stand, sit protocol is transformed into the sEMG recordings shown in Figure 9–6.

Ettare's rich protocol has several variations on the theme of using controlled relaxation to facilitate transfer of skills. For example, there is sit-stand training, sit-stand training with reverse counting; blind sit-stand training; typing; walking; sit-walk-sit; and stand-to-lying. An excellent description of this protocol, including a 12-session description, may be found in Ettare and Ettare.[20]

Recovery Training

Recovery training is a variation of the Ettare protocol, in that the goal is to teach the patient how to turn off his or her muscle after it has been intentionally activated. As noted in Chapter 8, muscles may be subject to postcontraction irritability. Here the muscle continues to remain active, even though the patient has intentionally ceased the activity. Figure 9–7 illustrates a mild example of this phenomenon following the

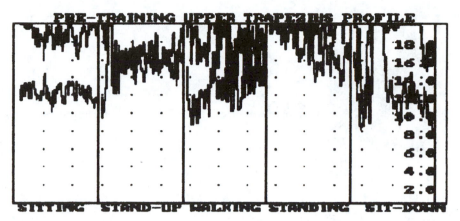

Figure 9–5 Typical pretraining guarding or hypertonic profile for upper trapezius. This represents a 20-second epoch. *Source:* Copyright © 1990, JR Cram, *Clinical EMG for Surface Recordings: Volume 2*, Clinical Resources, Inc.

movement of abduction. There is a 2-second period in which the muscle remains active following the return of the arms to the sides of the body. In more extreme examples, the persistent activity may last for several minutes following the termination of the action.

As with the Ettare protocol, sEMG biofeedback training can be directed toward teaching the patient how to turn off the recruitment as quickly as possible following the activating event. Figure 9–8 provides an example of how this might look after just a few trials of feedback. Once the patient is able to do this with visual

feedback, the practitioner should ask the patient to close his or her eyes, practicing without external feedback and tuning into proprioceptive feedback instead. Generalization to other postures may be important as well. The level of asymmetry in Figure 9–8 is large enough (approximately 40%) to be of clinical interest. Working on issues pertinent to symmetry of recruitment might be the next therapeutic task at hand.

Quieting exercises may also be conducted using isometric contractions. Here, one would want to begin with small efforts and gradually

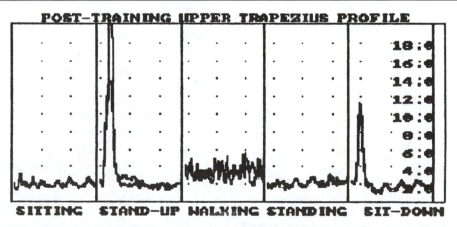

Figure 9–6 Typical posttraining profile for upper trapezius using the Ettare model of treatment. *Source:* Copyright © 1990, JR Cram, *Clinical EMG for Surface Recordings: Volume 2*, Clinical Resources, Inc.

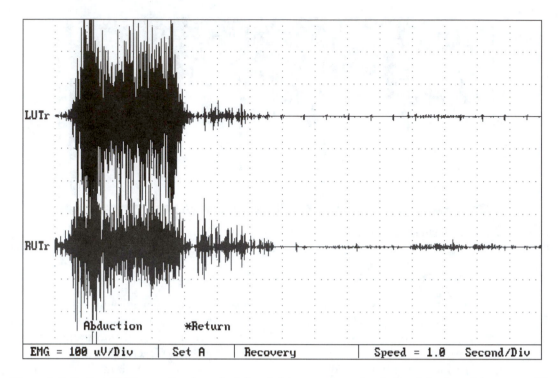

Figure 9–7 Surface EMG recording from the left and right upper trapezius during abduction of the arms to 90 degrees and return. Note the persistent activity for 2 seconds following the return of the arms to the sides. Courtesy of Will Taylor, Blue Hills, Maine.

move to larger and larger efforts. The training increases the patient's awareness of the muscle of interest by teaching him or her how to turn it on and off. This training takes some of the "noise" out of the neuromuscular system.

The Feldenkrais Method

Moshe Feldenkrais developed another excellent technique to teach dynamic relaxation, which is currently taught around the world by his students. For more in-depth reading, there are several books available on this topic.[21,22] Surface EMG biofeedback and Feldenkrais movement exercises complement each other. The Feldenkrais movement strategies provide a structure for instructing the patient and encouraging normalized movement patterns, while the sEMG feedback documents that these patterns

are recruiting the desired muscles, at the desired amplitude, and with the desired timing. The movement exercises are used to correct asymmetries, cocontractions, and poor timing of recruitment.

The cornerstone of the therapy is to teach the patient to engage in gentle movement patterns that facilitate the normal recruitment of muscle. The practitioner should instruct the patient as follows:

1. Ask the patient to make small movements. The patient should do only what is comfortable and easy, without pushing himself or herself. Do not encourage the movement pattern to the point of pain.
2. Encourage the patient to reduce any unnecessary movement. According to Feldenkrais, less muscular effort will bring the patient more physical benefit.

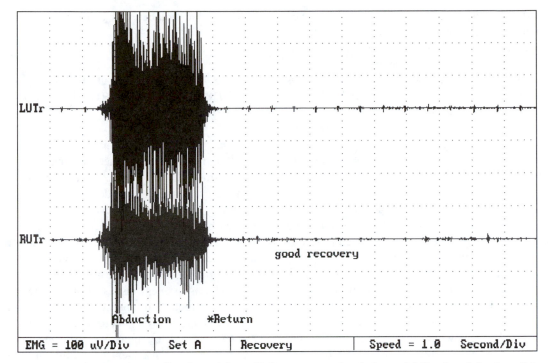

LUTr

RUTr

good recovery

Abduction   *Return

| EMG = 100 uV/Div | Set A | Recovery | Speed = 1.0   Second/Div |

Figure 9–8 Surface EMG recording from right and left upper trapezius during and following abduction of the arms to 90 degrees. Here the patient is intentionally trying to quiet the muscles as quickly as possible following the cessation of the movement. Courtesy of Will Taylor, Blue Hills, Maine.

His theory is that the brain can detect differences more easily when the senses are less stimulated. Slow, small, and easy movements allow the nervous system to detect any unnecessary muscular effort.

3. Encourage the patient to do each movement slowly—to take time to sense and feel what the patient is doing. By doing the movement slowly, he or she will be able to detect any unnecessary effort and strain. Feldenkrais states that once the patient becomes aware of this extra effort, the nervous system will automatically attempt to reduce it.

4. Encourage the patient not to try too hard. Learning of new movements will be enhanced if the patient forgets about competing or trying to succeed. Trying too hard is one of the ways in which the patient introduces excessive effort into the movement.

5. Allow the patient to go at his or her own rate. The rate at which the muscles and nervous system change is different for each person.

6. Make certain that the patient rests between each movement. The patient should return to the neutral position and stop there for several seconds before going on to the next movement. Also, allow the patient to stop and rest for a half minute or so every few minutes. After the patient has done an entire sequence of movements, allow the patient to rest before introducing a new movement, or even a repetition of the same movement.

There are many Feldenkrais movement patterns to choose from. Movement exercises to add flexibility to the neck region are described below. The patient can do these exercises sitting or lying. The instructions below are given for the sitting position. The practitioner should begin by having the patient rotate the head as far as it is comfortable to the left and to the right. The patient should note how far it is that he or she turned. The exercises described below are to the left. But once the patient has done the left aspect, he or she should follow through with the right aspect.

1. Using the six pointers above, ask the patient to rotate the head to the left while keeping the eyes fixed forward. Do this two or three times.
2. Ask the patient to allow the eyes to lead the rotation as they would normally do. Do this a couple of times.
3. Ask the patient to rotate the shoulders to the right while he or she is rotating the head to the left. Do this two or three times.
4. Ask the patient to rotate the shoulders in the direction of the head turn, like he or she would normally do. Do this a couple of times.
5. Ask the patient to push the right knee forward. Have the patient observe any tension felt in the torso. Encourage the patient to find the natural rotation of the torso associated with this knee push. See if the patient can find his or her way into rotating not only the torso, but also the shoulders and head. Do this rotation two or three times.
6. Conclude by asking the patient simply to rotate the head to the left, and see if it is any farther than it was before the patient started Step 1.

The simple rotational patterns described above can bring about more normalized recruitment patterns in the sternocleidomastoid and C-4 paraspinal muscles. These are relatively simple exercises to give the patient as part of the home exercise program. Patient-oriented books[22] and audiotapes[23] are available commercially.

SURFACE ELECTROMYOGRAPHIC FEEDBACK AND NEUROMUSCULAR REEDUCATION

These protocols place dynamic sEMG feedback training into an active neuromuscular training paradigm. Once specific deficits are noted from the assessment, these deficits may be addressed by working with the muscle itself and also with the central nervous system. This therapy guides the efforts of the practitioner and patient in the restoration of muscle function.

The dynamic sEMG can go awry in many ways. The assessment issues of amplitude, recovery, symmetry, timing, cocontraction, agonist/antagonist/synergy, and rest are explored in Chapter 8. During treatment, it may be necessary to address any of these elements within the context of a full physical, postural, emotional, and dynamic movement perspective.

Some of the strategies associated with neuromuscular reeducation are reviewed below. Specific treatment approaches to the various syndromes detailed in Chapter 8 are developed in depth in *Clinical Applications in Surface Electromyography* by Kasman et al.[24] The descriptions below introduce readers to some of the general clinical concepts associated with the use of sEMG for treatment.

Correction of Simple Postural Dysfunctions

As was noted earlier, posture is the basis upon which movement is made possible. Dynamic movement patterns are frequently improved as a function of postural change. Thus, the practitioner must consider posture and postural correction as part of any dynamically oriented work. Once a postural dysfunction is noted, it is best approached by placing the sEMG electrodes over the postural muscles of interest and assisting the patient in finding his or her way into the "correct" posture. If muscle shortness somewhere in the musculoskeletal system limits one's ability to obtain the correct posture, stretching is necessary. If muscle weakness prevents the patient from obtaining or maintaining the correct posture, strengthening exercises are in order.

Middaugh and colleagues[25] have presented a chapter on problems associated with the neck and shoulder region. Monitoring from the upper trapezius and suboccipital sites, they have demonstrated that a head-forward posture is associated with increased activation of the upper trapezius muscle group. In addition, they have demonstrated that this is frequently normalized when the head is placed in proper alignment above the shoulders. These authors commonly use the suboccipital as a feedback site for uptraining the endurance of these muscles, in order to facilitate the normal posture of the head. Because placement of electrodes into the hairline is difficult, temporal mastoid placement found in the atlas with specific reference to the cervical site location is recommended. Once these electrodes are in place, the therapist instructs the patient how to retract the head back over the neck ("turkey tuck") while observing the sEMG recruitment pattern. A strong burst of activity should be noted during the tuck, followed by a return to prior resting tone. A 10-second recruitment followed by a 50-second rest, with five repetitions, is a good starting place and provides a basis for an easy home program to follow between visits.

Surface Electromyographic–Guided Stretching

A reeducation program might require stretching shortened muscles before they can be retrained. Stretching can be done with or without instrumentation. There are clinical books on the topic by Travell and Simmons,[26] McKenzie,[27] and Lewit,[28] along with a book for laypersons by Andersen.[29]

Practitioners who work with patients who have cervical or upper quarter pain may notice restrictions in movement in one or more planes. Such restrictions are commonly associated with exaggerated stretch reflexes during active and passive range of motion. These exaggerated stretch reflexes may impede progress when uptraining a normal recruitment pattern. When the practitioner uses sEMG feedback during stretching, the goal is to teach the patient to place the muscle on stretch while keeping the stretch receptor drive on the alpha motor system as low as possible (ie, at an RMS level as low as possible). In this way, the practitioner maximizes the patient's ability to quiet the gamma motor system, thus allowing it to recalibrate to a lower level of activity while simultaneously lowering the stretch receptor threshold.

To use sEMG as part of a stretching program, the practitioner should place electrodes over the muscle that he or she plans to stretch. Then, the practitioner should ask the patient to place that muscle gently on stretch, moving to lengthen it. Many times, these stretches are guided by gravity, and other times they are assisted by the patient. The patient should stay in the stretched position for at least 20 to 60 seconds. During this time, the patient should breathe into the stretch (ie, take a deep breath) and then relax into the stretch for at least three respiration cycles. The practitioner should suggest that with each breath, the patient should relax more completely into the stretch. The sEMG feedback should guide the patient to lower the levels of sEMG activity associated with each breath into the stretch. Audio feedback is extremely helpful here. This way the patient can hear the amplitude of the muscle activity without looking at a screen. If an audio threshold is available, the practitioner could systematically shape lower and lower levels of sEMG activity by gradually changing the threshold to lower levels of sEMG. The goal is to be able to go to full range of motion passively, without recruiting sEMG. Figure 9–9 shows a 30-second stretch to relax for the cervical paraspinals. Notice how they began with a mild asymmetry. By the end of the stretch, the amplitudes are much lower and more symmetrical.

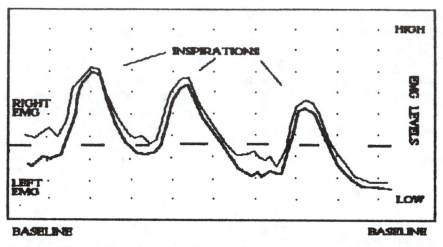

Figure 9–9 Surface EMG recordings from the right and left C-4 paraspinals as the patient breathes into the stretch. *Source:* Copyright © 1990, JR Cram, *Clinical EMG for Surface Recordings: Volume 2*, Clinical Resources, Inc.

SURFACE ELECTROMYOGRAPHIC FEEDBACK: DEVELOPMENT OF RECRUITMENT AND TIMING SYNERGIES

Once a recruitment pattern is noted for abnormalities in amplitude or timing and the practitioner has a sense of why the recruitment is abnormal, he or she may choose to *uptrain* the muscles for a correct recruitment pattern. Knowing what is normal is sometimes tricky; this knowledge develops from hours of clinical experience. The practitioner must also consider which muscles to monitor and under what movement conditions. Although the tracings given in the electrode atlas provide a basis for such knowledge, the practitioner should remember that the atlas provides only a limited set of examples of possible recruitment patterns and is not intended to be exhaustive. Practitioners are encouraged to use their own knowledge of the neuromuscular system to explore sEMG and movement.

Isolation Training

The uptraining process is a matter of working on quality rather than quantity of the recruitment pattern. Uptraining typically begins by teaching

the patient to isolate a particular muscle group. If the abnormal recruitment pattern is one where one muscle group literally is not pulling its weight, sEMG feedback would be directed toward bringing that muscle group back on-line. Commonly, this is seen in a cocontraction pattern during an attempted effort to activate a specific muscle. As can be seen in Figure 9–10, the patient is able to recruit and isolate the right lower trapezius readily, but the attempt to isolate the recruitment of the left lower trapezius is met with low levels of recruitment on the left and a cocontraction on the right.

Consider a case where the lower trapezius is severely inhibited during simple abduction of the arms to 90 degrees, while the upper trapezius overrecruits during the same movement (see Figure 8–10). The sEMG uptraining is directed toward the lower trapezius muscles. During training, the practitioner should pay attention to the posture of the rib cage and suggest that the patient lift the sternum if he or she is slouching. The patient is then asked to isolate the recruitment of only the left aspect of the lower trapezius. The practitioner instructs the patient on how best to attempt to recruit this muscle using isometric muscle-testing protocols. In this case, the patient is asked to press the elbow either into the palm of the therapist or the arm of the chair.

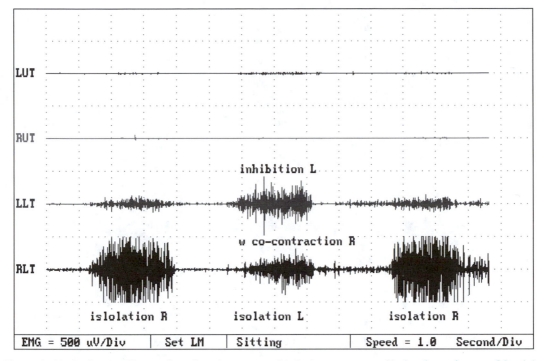

Figure 9–10 Surface EMG recordings from lower trapezius during an attempted isolated recruitment of the right and left muscles. Note the cocontraction present during the attempted recruitment of the left lower trapezius. Courtesy of Will Taylor, Blue Hills, Maine.

The patient must create just enough effort in the right lower trapezius to show a small burst pattern on the screen, but only for the left trapezius. There should be no overflow recruitment to the left lower trapezius or either upper trapezius (see Figure 9–11). If the patient puts out a muscular effort for left lower trapezius that begins to recruit other muscles, the patient is encouraged to cease the muscular effort at the time when the other muscle site(s) become active. As the patient gets better at isolating the particular muscle, he or she is asked to increase gradually and sustain the amplitude of the isolated recruitment. If at any time there is a spillover of recruitment to other sites as the patient increases the amplitude, he or she is asked to cease the muscular effort (see Figure 9–12).

As a general strategy, Donaldson's 10-50-5 model (10 seconds of activation, followed by 50 seconds of rest, for five repetitions) of training is used.[30] As the patient gets better at doing the left aspect of lower trapezius, he or she is asked to do

the same for the right aspect. Placing a template of the desired movement up on the screen for the patient to copy with his or her own muscular efforts may accelerate acquisition of the desired recruitment pattern.[31] Sometimes this can be done by having patients do the recruitment pattern on the side that they have already learned the desired pattern, followed by the other side that they are learning. The memory from the learned side can serve as the template.

Discrimination Training

Once the patient has demonstrated an ability to recruit the desired muscle while being guided by the visual or audio feedback associated with the sEMG recording, the practitioner must help the patient transfer the guidance to proprioceptive cues. The practitioner can ask the patient to close his or her eyes, conduct the isometric contraction, and then open the eyes and peek out at the results. By doing this, the patient begins to transfer the

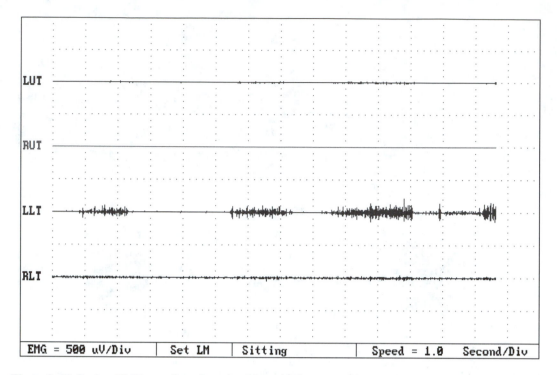

Figure 9–11 Surface EMG recordings from the right and left upper and lower trapezius during attempts at small, isolated efforts for the left lower trapezius. Courtesy of Will Taylor, Blue Hills, Maine.

isolation skills to his or her own internal sensations. There are variations on this process that can aid in such concepts as scaling. Here, the practitioner asks the patient to practice producing 100 microvolts of recruitment, then 50 microvolts, and then 25 microvolts. After the patient practices, the peeking exercise is instituted again. But now, the patient relies on proprioceptive cues for whether a muscle is activated and for much recruitment. In the case of lower trapezius isolation, both the right and left aspects of lower trapezius are passed through this discrimination task.

Coordinated Recruitment

Once the lower trapezius muscles are isolated using isometric contractions, the patient is asked to engage them during the coordinated dynamic movement of abduction. Remember, the tar-geted sEMG goal is to recruit the lower trapezius along with the upper trapezius during abduction of the arms. Therefore, the patient is asked to initiate the abduction of the arms, with an intentional effort to engage the lower trapezius. If the upper trapezius muscles come to grossly dominate during the movement, the abduction movement is stopped at less than 90 degrees and the arms are returned to the sides. The patient's recruitment pattern is gradually shaped across successive attempts at abduction using this technique, until there is a relatively balanced activation of the upper and lower trapezius during 90 degrees of this movement. This may entail having the patient raise the rib cage with a sternal lift prior to attempting the movement, or it might simply involve suggesting that the patient activate the lower trapezius muscles prior to initiating the movement. Again, it is helpful to

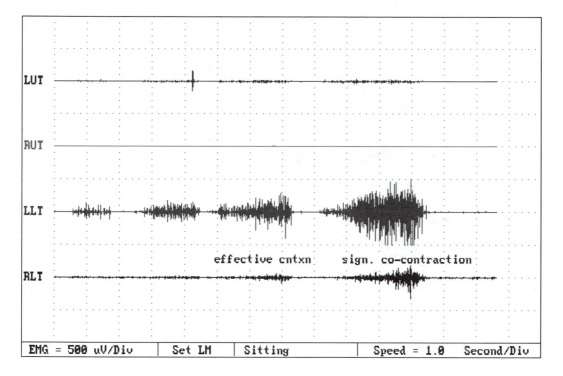

Figure 9–12 Surface EMG recordings from the right and left upper and lower trapezius during increasing efforts to recruit and isolate the left lower trapezius. Note that by the fourth attempted recruitment, the patient begins to cocontract the right trapezius along with the left. Courtesy of Will Taylor, Blue Hills, Maine.

use computer screen templates for the patient to copy using his or her own muscular efforts.

Functional/Daily Activities

The patient's newly acquired ability is then tested in both the sitting and standing postures. It is very important to begin the process of generalizing the newly learned recruitment pattern to varied environments and tasks. Forward flexion of the arms may be studied as well. Here, the serratus anterior is monitored along with the lower trapezius, since the serratus anterior is better known for scapular stabilization during forward flexion of the arms. It is important to consider the work environment of the individual and to test for the generalization of appropriate lower trapezius activity in the various postures and activities associated with the patient's work.

AN EXAMPLE INVOLVING THE CERVICAL MUSCLES

Let's now examine a second example. Here, a cocontraction is noted during rotation of the head to the left (see Figure 9–13). After some trigger point work and stretching exercises, uptraining is initiated. Uptraining begins by teaching the patient to isolate the sternocleidomastoid muscle that shows the lowest peak amplitude. In this case, the right sternocleidomastoid underrecruits during left rotation. Thus, the sEMG-guided uptraining is directed at that side. The easiest way to isolate the right sternocleidomastoid is to have the patient rotate the head to the left. To augment this recruitment, if necessary, a slight extension at the end of the rotation to the left can be added. Through instructed movement strategies along with sEMG feed-

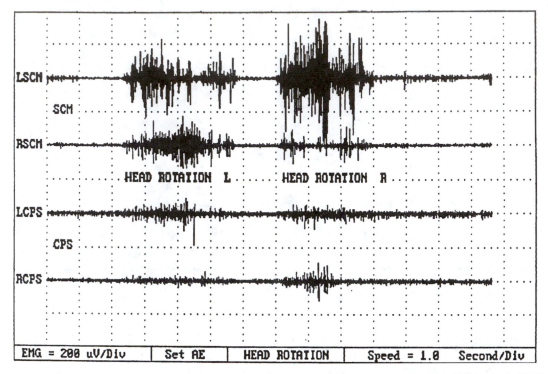

Figure 9–13 Surface EMG recordings from right and left sternocleidomastoid (SCM) and C-4 paraspinals (CPS) during rotation of the head prior to treatment. Note the cocontraction that occurs during rotation to the left. *Source:* Reprinted with permission from Donaldson et al, *Electromyography, Trigger Points and Myofascial Syndromes,* © 1991, Behavioral Health Consultants.

back, the patient is taught to isolate and activate the right sternocleidomastoid. Once the patient can selectively recruit the left sternocleidomastoid, he or she is asked to activate the muscle for approximately 10 seconds, then to rest for 50 seconds; the patient does five repetitions of the movement. The patient is asked to continue with this exercise regimen three times a day at home until the next office visit. The same protocol is used during the second visit. By the third visit, the patient should be able to engage in axial rotation without a cocontraction in the recruitment pattern (see Figure 9–14).

Once the desired recruitment pattern is obtained, the patient attempts to generalize the pattern. The practitioner should note if the recruitment is symmetrical in both the sitting and standing postures, and what the symmetry is like during other activities of daily living such as

reading, washing the dishes, or activities related to work.

SUMMARY FOR UPTRAINING

All uptraining protocols have several elements in common. First, postural and stretching considerations usually occur prior to or at the beginning of treatment. Second, uptraining begins with isolation training. Such training usually involves small, isometric contractions that attempt to avoid inappropriate recruitment of other muscles during the isolation. One may need to start with smaller movements and recruitment patterns and gradually increase the strength of the contraction. Motor copy strategies seem to accelerate the learning process. As isolation training becomes successful, the movement pattern is taken from the isometric contrac-

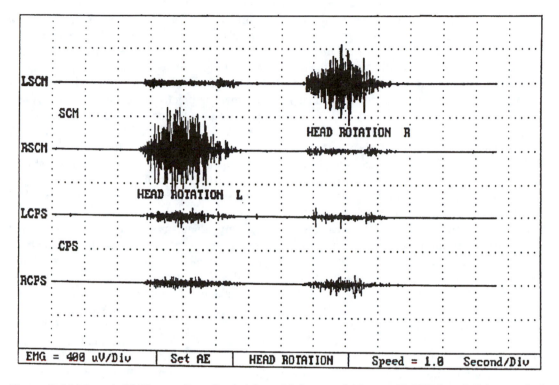

Figure 9–14 Normal sEMG recordings from right and left sternocleidomastoid (SCM) and C-4 paraspinals (CPS) during rotation of the head following three treatment sessions. *Source:* Reprinted with permission from Donaldson et al, *Electromyography, Trigger Points and Myofascial Syndromes,* © 1991, Behavioral Health Consultants.

tion to a coordinated dynamic movement. Third, generalization is facilitated by exploring the movement during different postures and during activities of daily living.

PELVIC FLOOR CONSIDERATIONS

Weakness and noise in the pelvic floor are thought to play a substantial role in incontinence and pelvic pain. A recent report from the U.S. Department of Health and Human Services Agency for Health Care Policy and Research[32] on urinary incontinence recommends that behavioral approaches, such as biofeedback, be attempted before consideration of surgical or other invasive procedures. For an excellent review of the issue of incontinence, see an article by Tries[33]; for the premier article on the treatment of pelvic pain, see Glazer et al.[34]

Surface EMG biofeedback procedures alone are not sufficient to treat incontinence. Diet and lifestyle must be considered, and a bowel and bladder monitoring program must be put into place. Vulvodynia cannot be approached without the appropriate concurrent medical treatment of the disorder. The cornerstone to sEMG treatment of both these disorders is training in isolating, strengthening, and controlling the pelvic floor muscles. Arnold Kegel knew this in the 1940s when he introduced the Kegel exercises. What biofeedback adds to the Kegel exercises, is the specificity of training effects. With Kegel exercises, the patient may inadvertently contract other muscles (such as the abdominals, buttocks, or thighs), leading to greater levels of fatigue and inappropriate pressure on the bladder itself. Through the use of feedback and trial-and-error learning, the patient quickly learns to isolate the pelvic floor muscles. Simultaneous monitoring of the abdominal muscles (or other mscles) can help shape the appropriate use of pelvic floor muscles. Here, the patient is instructed to contract the pelvic floor muscles but to stop the effort when the ancillary muscles (ie, abdominals) recruit as well.

The methods for assessing the pelvic floor, discussed in Chapter 8, may now be used to treat it. Treatment usually begins by teaching the patient to do "flicks." The patient is instructed to engage in short, strong contractions, resting briefly between each. These efforts are continued until there are signs of fatigue (reduced amplitude) or the recruitment spills over into ancillary muscles. Once this happens, a longer rest period is given and a different contraction strategy is initiated. The patient is encouraged to practice these finely tuned flicks or Kegel exercises frequently throughout the day. They are extremely useful in helping the patient to reduce stress incontinence associated with exertional efforts. Endurance training comes next. This is done with submaximal contractions held for increasing periods of time (eg, a 50% maximum voluntary isometric contraction starting at 10 seconds and working up to 30 seconds and finally to 60 seconds). These endurance exercises truly strengthen the support of the pelvic floor. Next, the speed of recruitment and derecruitment is practiced repetitively. The patient can attempt 1-second flicks, making certain that the sEMG quiets down following each effort. A variant to this approach is for the practitioner to instruct the patient to tense and release slowly over a 10-second period of time. The goal is to increase the patient's awareness of the pelvic floor muscles, while strengthening them and bringing them more and more under the patient's control. The total sEMG feedback training time is usually about 15 minutes. Additional session time is needed to review the bowel and bladder diaries and provide education concerning nutrition and lifestyle choices. Office visits for further training are typically carried out every 7 to 10 days, and many incontinent patients are "cured" by the third visit. Others need more time. Pelvic pain patients are typically offered approximately six sEMG feedback sessions.[34]

REFERENCES

1. Cram JR, Freeman C. Specificity in EMG biofeedback treatment of chronic pain patients. *Clin Biofeedback Health.* 1985;8:106–119.

2. Walters D. *The 14 Steps to Higher Awareness.* Nevada City, CA: Crystal Clarity; 1985.

3. Jacobson E. *You Must Relax.* New York: McGraw-Hill; 1976.

4. Luthe W, Schultz JH. *Volume 1: Autogenics Methods.* In: Luthe W, ed. *Autogenics Therapy.* New York: Grune & Stratton; 1969.

5. Luthe W. *Volume IV: Research and Theory.* In: Luthe W, ed. *Autogenics Therapy.* New York: Grune & Stratton; 1969.

6. Wolpe J. *The Practice of Behavior Therapy.* Elmsford, NY: Pergamon Press; 1973.

7. Whatmore G. *The Physiopathology and Treatment of Functional Disorders.* New York: Grune & Stratton; 1974.

8. Miller E. *Source Cassettes.* Stanford, CA: Source Cassettes; 1989.

9. Bennett H. *Preparation for Surgery* [audiotape]. Nevada City, CA: Patient Comfort Incorporated; 1995.

10. Thomas A. *The Psycho-Physical Assessment.* Nevada City, CA: Clinical Resources; 1993.

11. Barton B. *Relax to Sleep* [audiotape]. San Francisco: Crystal Clear Productions; 1994.

12. Miller E. *Changing the Channel on Pain* [audio cassette]. Stanford, CA: Source Cassettes; 1989.

13. Bennett HL, Disbrow E. Preparation for surgery and medical procedures. In: Golman D, Gurin J, ed. *Mind Body Medicine.* New York: Consumer Reports Books; 1994:401–428.

14. Disbrow EA, Bennett HL, Owings JT. Effects of preoperative suggestion on postoperative gastrointestinal motility. *West J Med.* 1993;158:488–492.

15. Barber TX. Changing "unchangeable" bodily processes by (hypnotic) suggestions: A new look at hypnosis, cognitions, imagining and the mind-body problem. In: Sheikh AA, ed. *Imagination and Healing.* Amityville, NY: Baywood Publishing; 1984.

16. Fried R. *The Breath Connection.* New York: Plenum; 1990.

17. Rama S, Ballentine R, Hymes A. *The Science of Breath.* Honesdale, PA: Himalayan Institute; 1990.

18. Alexander AB, Smith DD. Clinical Applications of EMG biofeedback. In: Gatchel RJ, Price KR, eds. *Clinical Applications of Biofeedback: Appraisal and Status.* New York: Pergamon; 1979.

19. Suarez A, Kohlenberg R, Pagano R. Is EMG activity from the frontalis site a good measure of general bodily tension in clinical populations? *Biofeedback and Self-Regul.* 1979;4:293–297.

20. Ettare D, Ettare R. Muscle learning therapy: a treatment protocol. In: Cram JR, ed. *Clinical EMG for Surface Recordings, II.* Nevada City, CA: Clinical Resources; 1990:197–234.

21. Feldenkrais M. *Body and Mature Behavior: A Study of Anxiety, Sex, Gravitation and Learning.* New York: International University Press; 1950.

22. Zemach-Berson D, Zemach-Berson K, Reese M. *Relaxercise.* San Francisco: Harper; 1990.

23. Reese M, Zemach-Berson D. *Relaxercise* [audiotape]. Berkeley, CA: Sensory Motor Learning Systems; 1986.

24. Kasman G, Cram J, Wolf S. *Clinical Applications in Surface Electromyography.* Gaithersburg, MD: Aspen Publishers; 1997.

25. Middaugh SJ, Kee WG, Nicholson JA. Muscle overuse and posture as factors in the development and maintenance of chronic musculoskeletal pain. In: Grzesiak RC, Ciccone DS, eds. *Psychological Vulnerability to Chronic Pain.* New York: Springer Publishing Co; 1994:55–89.

26. Travell J, Simons D. *Myofascial Pain and Dysfunction: A Trigger Point Manual, I and II.* Baltimore: Williams & Wilkins; 1983.

27. McKenzie R. *Treat Your Own Neck.* Low Hut, New Zealand: Spinal Publications; 1985.

28. Lewit K. *Manipulative Therapy in Rehabilitation of the Locomotor System.* Boston: Butterworth Heinemann; 1991.

29. Andersen B. *Stretching.* Bolinas, CA: Shelter Publications; 1980.

30. Donaldson S, Donaldson M. Multi-channel EMG assessment and treatment techniques. In: Cram JR, ed. *Clinical EMG for Surface Recordings, II.* Nevada City, CA: Clinical Resources; 1990:143–174.

31. Wolf S, LeCraw D, Barton L. Comparison of motor copy and targeted biofeedback training techniques for restitution of upper extremity function among patients with neurologic disorders. *Phys Ther.* 1988;69:719–735.

32. Agency for Health Care Policy and Research. *Urinary Incontinence in Adults: Clinical Practice Guidelines.* Rockville, MD: US Dept of Health and Human Services; March, 1992. AHCPR pub. 92-0038.

33. Tries J. Kegel exercises enhanced by biofeedback. *J Enterosomal Ther.* 1990;17:67–76.

34. Glazer HI, Rodke G, Swencionis C, Hertz R, Young A. Treatment of vulvar vestibulitis syndrome with electromyographic biofeedback of pelvic floor musculature. *J Reprod Med.* 1995;40:283–290.

Chapter Questions

1. If problems are noted in more than one area of the neuromuscular system (posture, emotion, and movement), in what order should they be approached?
   a. movement, emotion, posture
   b. posture, emotion, movement
   c. emotion, posture, movement
   d. emotion, movement, posture

2. Progressive relaxation training was developed by:
   a. Jacobson
   b. Schwartz
   c. Whatmore
   d. Luthe

3. During progressive relaxation the patient is taught to:
   a. make large tension contractions followed by relaxation of the muscle
   b. make small tension contractions followed by relaxation of the muscle
   c. relax without tensing first
   d. both a and b

4. In autogenics training, which key word is associated with muscular relaxation?
   a. warmth
   b. heaviness
   c. coolness
   d. slow and regular

5. Autogenics training utilizes:
   a. passive volition
   b. active volition
   c. quiet movement
   d. guided imagery

6. Guided imagery is a form of:
   a. self-hypnosis
   b. inner child work
   c. self-actualization
   d. self-analysis

7. During breath work, what goal would the patient have for the scalene muscles?
   a. increase their participation in quiet breathing
   b. decrease their participation in quiet breathing
   c. use to help breathe into the chest
   c. use to help breathe into the abdomen

8. What can be said concerning the generalization of relaxation effects?
   a. They automatically transfer from one muscle to another.
   b. They automatically transfer from one posture to another.
   c. Generalization must be cultivated to other muscles, various postures, and a variety of settings.
   d. Both a and b.

9. In muscle learning therapy, the patient is taught to:
    a. turn on specific muscle groups
    b. turn off the muscle following its use
    c. use specific muscles for real and varied life activities
    d. none of the above

10. The Feldenkrais method teaches the patient how to recruit muscles in their normal fashion. Which of the following is not one of the keys to teaching this concept?
    a. make large movements
    b. move slowly
    c. rest between movements
    d. reduce unnecessary movements

11. In treating simple postural dysfunctions, the practitioner may need to:
    a. teach correct postural alignment
    b. strengthen weakened muscle
    c. stretch shortened muscles
    d. all of the above

12. To use stretching effectively, one should go out onto stretch for a minimum of:
    a. 2 seconds
    b. 5 seconds
    c. 20 to 60 seconds
    d. it really doesn't matter how long you stretch as long as you can feel the stretch

13. Isolation training is used to:
    a. teach the patient how to turn on a specific muscle
    b. reduce the activity of a specific muscle
    c. reduce the range of motion of a joint segment
    d. quiet the mind

14. Discrimination training refers to:
    a. being able to know which muscles are working
    b. being able to know whether a muscle has been activated or not
    c. being able to discern large recruitment amplitudes from small recruitment amplitudes
    d. a and b
    e. a, b, and c

15. Donaldson's 10-50-5 rule pertains to:
    a. the number of repetitions of a recruitment sequence
    b. the amount of time spent on a series of three recruitments
    c. 10 seconds of contraction, followed by a 50-second rest, over 5 repetitions
    d. none of the above

16. Uptraining refers to:
    a. learning to stand in an upright posture
    b. learning how to uplift one's emotions
    c. learning to isolate and activate a specific muscle group
    d. learning how to lift up the arm during abduction

17. Surface EMG feedback to the pelvic floor is useful in the treatment of:
    a. urinary incontinence
    b. fecal incontinence
    c. vulvodynia
    d. all of the above
    e. a and b only

18. The sEMG assessment procedures commonly used to assess incontinence may also be used to treat incontinence.
    a. true
    b. false
    c. true for fecal incontinence only
    d. true for vulvodynia only

CHAPTER 10

Documentation

Clinical documentation is vitally important, for it allows practitioners to know what has been done. It provides a basis for analysis and the sharing of information with others; it allows for replication and comparison during future visits; and, in many cases, it provides the basis for insurance reimbursement. Documentation can be broken into the basic elements, which meet the medical-legal requirements, and supplementary elements, which are essential for research purposes or would be nice to document if time is permitting.

BASIC DOCUMENTATION

Documentation must cover at last four main items. A few years back, elements were referred to as SOAP: subjective, objective, assessment, and planning information.

The first layer of information represents the subjective—the self-report of the patient or the general status of the patient. The practitioner's records should reflect how treatments are affecting the patient. A practitioner who is primarily treating pain, for example, should consider having the patient rate the pain on a scale of 1 to 10 for each visit, and the practitioner should chart the patient's progress.

The second layer of information represents objective information. Surface electromyography (sEMG) provides a very powerful set of objective information to share with others. However, detailed information regarding the clinical

procedure should be given, so that a similarly trained individual could take a practitioner's notes and replicate the electrode setup and training procedure. If practitioners are using standard electrode placements, such as the ones listed in the atlas of this book, giving the muscle site name should be sufficient. If standard electrode placements are used, this convention should be documented in a policy and procedures manual for the Joint Commission on Accreditation of Healthcare Organizations, the Center for Accreditation of Rehabilitation Facilities, other accrediting agencies, and for general liability issues. It is preferable to state interelectrode distance if the practitioner has the option to use more than one set of interelectrode distances. If the sEMG instrument allows more than one band-pass filter selection, it is essential to specify which one is used. Even if the band-pass filter is fixed, incorporating this specification into the report provides the basis for other electromyographers to interpret findings correctly.

Once the electrodes are in place, the record of the sEMG study should be preserved. This can take the form of analogue tracings (strip charts/ screen dumps) or digital representations of the data (eg, mean, standard deviation, etc). Both graphic displays and digital representations should give some indication about the form of signal processing, such as "root mean square microvolts" (μV RMS), integral average (μV/sec), or microvolts peak to peak (μV pp). Analog graphs should contain information concerning the sensitivity of the graph (scale), along with the sweep speed. In more sophisticated reporting, a normalization procedure is commonly used. If used, the type and conditions under which the reference contractions were collected must be specified.

The next layer of information refers to the practitioner's assessment of the patient's information. Clinical diagnoses (or changes in diagnosis that have occurred over the course of treatment) are helpful. Comments about what works for the person and what does not can help to remind practitioners what has been tried. Information about obstacles to improvement is very important. The motivational attitude of the patient may be useful in understanding compliance issues. Some patients overdo it, while others underdo.

The last layer of information refers to the practitioner's treatment plan. Given all of the above information, where does the practitioner plan to go next? This information may help the related staff to provide continuity in care of the patient.

ASSESSMENT CONSIDERATIONS

Documentation associated with assessment typically includes a finer level of detail than documentation associated with treatment. As the assessment protocol unfolds, some descriptions regarding its findings might include:

- posture of the body/position of the limb
- resting baseline values
- movement peak amplitude obtained
- rate of change from baseline to peak (fast, slow, smooth, jagged)
- recovery from movement
  - postmovement baseline levels
  - rate of recovery (fast, slow, "descending" notch)
- concentric versus eccentric phase of the recruitment pattern (amplitude comparisons)
- isometric contractions
- comparison of one channel of activity to

another (Note: These comparisons may be made for homologous muscle groups with confidence. However, comparison between different muscle groups may be problematic because of a number of anatomical features, such as area of muscle bulk. Such comparisons should be made with caution. They are best done in muscles where the magnitude of relationships is already known—such as upper to lower trapezius or vastus medialis oblique to vastus lateralis. Normalized comparisons, of course, are preferred.)
  - appropriate isolated muscle activity without cocontractions for asymmetrical movements
  - appropriate cocontraction for symmetrical movements
  - appropriate activation and timing of agonist/antagonist groups for joint stabilization
  - relative signal magnitude at peaks during range of motion
  - relative timing of recruitment/derecruitment during the eccentric and concentric phases of the movement
- interpretation of the findings:
  - magnitude
    1. insufficient magnitude (inhibited/hypoactive) relative to the task or in relation to other synergists
    2. excessive magnitude (hyperactive) relative to the task or in relation to other synergists
  - timing
    1. delayed onset required for the movement
    2. premature onset for the required movement
    3. excessive duration for the particular phase of the movement
- recommendation for further assessment or treatment

Comparisons may be made between homologous recording sites from the involved versus uninvolved sides, or between a site and the normal template for that movement at that site (if available), or integrated and digitalized information may be compared to normative data. Using the protocol developed by Donaldson and Donaldson,[1] movement patterns should be conducted for at least three repetitions to ascertain stability. Typically, the first movement pattern is tossed out because it is frequently dissimilar to the other two repetitions. The third movement is usually kept because it is the most stable.

A sample text for Figure 10–1 might read like this:

> Nancy Smith. 36 years old. Female. Dx: Upper quarter pain.
>
> The patient presents with complaints of upper quarter pain (7 on 10-point scale), which is exacerbated with use of the left upper extremity. Recordings from upper, middle, and lower trapezius along with serratus anterior were taken during a simple shoulder elevation and release (see Scan 8). Initial baselines were observed to be within normal limits. Shoulder elevations show fairly equal symmetry, with some slowness to derecruit at the cessation of the movement, more on the left than the right. Left recruitment greater than right for lower trapezius and serratus anterior during shoulder elevation. Left lower trapezius shows spontaneous recruitment and irritability postmovement. Irritability suggests possible trigger point involvement. Assess and treat potential trigger point at next visit. Work on recovery training of sEMG.

A sample text for assessing abduction of the arms, while monitoring upper and lower trapezius, might read something like this:

> Nancy Smith. 36 years old. Female. Dx: Headache and neck pain.
>
> The patient presents with headache (4 on 10-point scale) and neck pain (5 on 10-point scale). Recordings from up-

per and lower trapezius were taken during abduction of the arms to 90 degrees. Resting baselines were low and symmetrical, around 2 to 3 µV RMS. Peak values were symmetrical but showed upper trapezius muscles to be 2X that of lower trapezius (20 µV versus 10 µV). Lower trapezius muscles appear to be hypoactive or inhibited, thus placing additional mechanical loads on the neck. Headache probably secondary to neck-related problems. Upper quarter sEMG training protocol indicated.

Some cases are more complicated. The case presented below would be greatly enhanced if the physical exam preceded the sEMG finding and if examination results were integrated into the interpretations and recommendations.

> Nancy Jones. 37 years old. Female. Dx: Left upper quarter pain.
>
> The patient presents with upper quarter pain, primarily on the left (8 on 10-point scale). Pain made worse with upper extremity work. Palpation exam indicates active trigger points at T-1. Head, neck, and shoulder posture fairly normal. Manual muscle testing indicates normal strength in cervical and upper trapezius muscles. Recordings from upper and lower trapezius were recorded during abduction and forward flexion of the arms to 90 degrees. Resting baselines show the right upper trapezius as mildly elevated (7.2 µV RMS), with all others within normal limits. During forward flexion, synergy pattern is within normal limits. During abduction, however, right upper trapezius is nearly 2X more active (45 µV RMS peak) compared to the left upper trapezius (25 RMS µV peak). Both lower trapezius muscles were inhibited, with the left lower being more severely inhibited (2.5 µV RMS peak) than to the

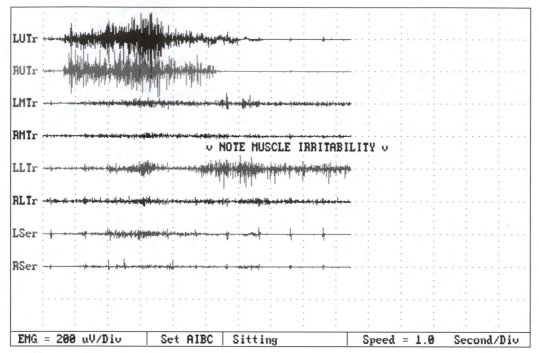

Figure 10–1   Surface EMG recording from upper trapezius, middle trapezius, lower trapezius, and serratus anterior during shoulder elevation. Note muscle irritability that emerges following the shoulder elevation. *Source:* Copyright © Clinical Resources, Inc.

right lower trapezius (12.5 µV RMS peak). During unilateral abduction, the right upper trapezius recruits for both left and right movements. This suggests a protective guarding pattern noted on the right, along with dyssynergy between upper and lower trapezius muscles, especially on the left. Left lower trapezius inhibited/hypoactive. Recommend neuromuscular retraining for shoulder muscles, with particular emphasis on uptraining the left lower trapezius.

TREATMENT CONSIDERATIONS

When sEMG is used as part of a biofeedback or neuromuscular reeducation program, it is very important to document the sites of electrode placement in order to allow replication of place-

ment during future visits. This is particularly true if the practitioner wants to compare the same sites over sessions. For consistent electrode placement, the practitioner should consider some of the following elements: use of standard electrode sites (see Part II); reference of anatomical landmarks; anatomical templates; or indelible marker.

Uptraining Considerations

Because the goal of uptraining is to maximize muscle output, the practitioner should note the highest µV level obtainable without feedback. Then the practitioner should document the highest level µV output observed during feedback. Sometimes as a variation, the average peak value for a training session is reported. If a threshold is used to provide an incentive for increasing the peak contraction, record what that threshold is or the percentage of time the patient reached and exceeded the threshold. Because the initial resting length of muscle or the posture associated with training can enhance or inhibit one's ability to recruit a muscle, these should be noted. If resting values are an issue, the effects of uptraining on resting values should be noted during a postbaseline period.

Below is an example of a brief chart note:

Nancy Jones

Visit 2. Patient reports pain levels are about the same. Uptraining/isolation training of lower trapezius conducted using standard upper and lower trapezius electrode placements and the wide (25–1000 Hz) filter during the seated posture. Initial resting levels (RMS μV) were RUTr = 7.9, LUTr = 2.5; RLTr = 1.3; LLTr = 1.5. Initial isometric peak contraction of RLTr = 9.2; LLTr = 2.6. Discrimination with eyes closed utilized. Ending isometric peak contraction RLTr = 14.7; LLTr = 7.9. Resting baseline at end of session for RUTr = 3.3. Intervention appears to bring a better balance to muscle synergies. Patient instructed to practice lower trapezius recruitment using 10-50-5 rule, three times a day. Continue isolation training on next visit.

Relaxation or Downtraining Considerations

The goal of downtraining is to minimize the sEMG output using relaxation protocols (ie, progressive relaxation, autogenics) or quiet movements (ie, Ettare protocols, Feldenkrais). Baseline levels should be recorded, along with the lowest level of sEMG activity achieved during the session. Because the ability to downtrain is acquired in a particular posture, one must attempt to generalize it to other postures through training in these alternate postures. Thus, the posture in which the training is conducted should be noted. Again, a threshold may be used to provide an incentive during training for low-

ering the sEMG levels. This threshold is usually lowered across time to help shape the desired behavior. If this feature is used, the threshold level should be recorded along with the percentage of time the patient spends below that threshold.

A sample progress note is presented below:

Randy Greene

Visit 3. Patient reports that the headache is slightly improved (4 on 10-point scale). Has practiced relaxation at home 3 times since last visit. R and L wide cervical trapezius placement used. Relaxation-based therapy offered using autogenics heavy/warm to arms. Initial baseline R = 17, L = 12. Postbaseline R = 7.3, L = 5.3. Nice in-session response to autogenics therapy. Home-training exercises given with handout. Plan: check on transfer of initial baseline, deepen relaxation abilities.

DOCUMENTATION AS AN OUTCOME MEASURE

Surface EMG may be used as an outcome measure for other treatment modalities. To do this, sEMG baselines are collected in relevant postures and/or during functional movement patterns, prior to and following the alternate therapies (eg, mobilization). Such recordings may help to document the therapeutic effects of the alternative therapy and provide a basis for continuing or discontinuing a particular therapy.

RELATIONSHIP OF SURFACE ELECTROMYOGRAPHY TO OTHER MEASURES

Surface EMG information should be related to other forms of clinical information such as pain, manual muscle testing, range of motion, isolated joint control, and other indexes of function. If the patient is taking medications that might interact with the treatment, these should be noted. These medications include, but are not limited to, muscle relaxants, tranquilizers, some analgesics, central nervous system depressants, and antispasticity agents.

COMPREHENSIVE LIST OF ELEMENTS TO DOCUMENT

Below is a comprehensive list of all of the potential variables that could potentially affect sEMG recordings. Depending upon the setting, some variables may be more important to document than others. Attributes that are worthwhile to consider for medical-legal reasons are followed by *L*. Attributes considered germane to research protocols or procedures involving sEMG are followed by *R*. The research recommendations are adapted from those recommended by the International Society for Electromyography and Kinesthesiology.[2] Attributes considered essential for the clinical record are followed by *C*.

Recording Parameters

1. Target muscle (and use of anatomical markers if relevant) *(C,L,R)*
2. Recording electrode location, distance for anatomical markings, use of electrode locator templates or indelible markings for intersession reliability *(C,L,R)*
3. Electrode type, diameter, manufacturer, type of paste or gel used if relevant *(L,R)*
4. Interelectrode distance and orientation to muscle fibers *(C,L,R)*
5. Ground electrode placement location *(R)*
6. Instrumentation specifications: band-pass filter range *(C)*, site of preamplification (active electrode), notch filter, type of signal display (raw versus processed), integration times (time constants), common mode rejection ratio, input impedance, signal to noise ratio, time constant, type of signal processing (ie, RMS), and sampling rate for computerized systems *(L,R)*

Patient/Task Considerations

1. Subjective impressions associated with the clinical evaluations and procedures *(C,L)*
2. Informed consent for procedure and goals of training *(C,L,R)*
3. Associated physical exam findings *(C,L)*
4. Patient positioning and movement: task, trunk/limb support, open versus closed kinetic chain, control of single versus multiple joints, movement plane, etc *(C,L,R)*
5. Type of contraction: isometric, eccentric, concentric *(C,L,R)*
6. Joint angle *(R)*
7. Contraction intensity, load, and velocity *(R)*
8. Work: rest times, number of repetitions, exercise sets, task duration *(R)*
9. Relaxation strategy *(C,R)*
10. Threshold levels *(C,R)*

Surface Electromyography Characterization and Interpretation

1. Verification that sEMG placement records form the muscle of interest *(L,R)*
2. Verification that the clinician/scientist has attempted to document or eliminate cross-talk from neighboring muscles *(L,R)*
3. Baseline amplitude, maximum, minimum, standard deviation *(C,L,R)*
4. Peak magnitude or symmetry during a movement *(C,L,R)*
5. Average amplitude during a defined phase of cyclic movement *(C,L,R)*
6. Normalization methods *(C)* are becoming more common and are essential when the practitioner/scientist wants to compare sEMG levels across muscle groups. They are essential when one wants to quantify sEMG under dynamic conditions. They are just as important for the clinician as for the researcher. Many journals do not allow dynamic sEMG data to be presented unless it is normalized. When a

normalization procedure is used, it must be accompanied with conditions under which the maximum value was collected (ie, joint angle, intensity, positioning). Several types of normalization are described in Chapter 3. They are briefly described below. Types a and b are the most common, but types c through f are also very practical *(L,R)*

a. *Maximum voluntary isometric contraction*. Here the patient exerts the maximum muscular effort under isometric conditions. All sEMG values are calculated as a percentage of that value:

(sEMG activity ÷ maximum sEMG activity) × 100

This is highly reliable, but compliance and motivation of pain patients to exert a maximal effort is potentially problematic.

b. *Submaximal voluntary isometric contraction*. Here the patient is asked to exert a force against a dynamometer to a specified level. This sEMG level is then used to express all other values as a percentage of this:

(sEMG activity ÷ submaximal sEMG activity) × 100

This is a more realistic benchmark for pain-related disorders.

c. Surface EMG is defined as a *percentage of the peak magnitude* recorded during a defined dynamic movement.

d. Surface EMG is defined as a *percentage of the average magnitude* recorded during a defined dynamic movement.

e. Surface EMG values averaged over a defined movement sequence are expressed as a *percentage of the average* during another reference movement.

f. Surface EMG from homologous muscles are expressed as *a left-right percent difference*:

(Larger side − smaller side ÷ larger side) × 100

This may be done for resting tones or from peak contraction data. The peak conversion is commonly used in the work of Donaldson.[1]

7. *Frequency spectral analysis*. This has been used to monitor muscle fatigue. The initial frequency, the slope of the frequency during the exertive task, and the rate of recovery to the initial frequency are commonly measured *(R)*

ISSUES PERTAINING TO THIRD-PARTY REIMBURSEMENT

Surface EMG is generally considered to be a reimbursable procedure—simply one of the tools that the practitioner uses in his or her field. The secret to qualifying for third-party reimbursement is to use already existing codes for one's profession. For the physical medicine practitioner, the 97 series CPT code (the American Medical Association's *Current Procedural Terminology* code) is suggested. Some practitioners routinely use neuromuscular reeducation in conjunction with kinetic exercises. For mental health practitioners, the 98 series CPT code is suggested for "behavior therapy," interactive medical psychotherapy, or psychophysiologic therapy including biofeedback. Both physical medicine and psychology providers might consider using the 90901 CPT code for biofeedback. Unfortunately, this code is still somewhat controversial, even 20 years after its emergence.

Fortunately or unfortunately, depending upon one's point of view, there are no specific CPT codes that pertain to the diagnostic use of sEMG. Because of this ambiguity, there was a period of time in which many providers used the neurological section of the CPT code, billing the sEMG procedure as if it were the functional equivalent to a needle EMG study, charging a similar amount. Eventually, third-party carriers had these studies reviewed by their experts, all of whom were familiar with needle EMG procedures but knew very little about sEMG procedures. These reviewers stated, correctly, that sEMG procedures were not valid to study neurological conditions, and reimbursement for sEMG procedures were denied. Because of this confusion, many third-party carriers began to issue guidelines to deny all sEMG procedures. The clamor regarding this blurring of sEMG and needle EMG procedures led to responses from several professional organizations. In 1992, the Surface EMG Society of North America (SESNA) organized a multidisciplinary panel to produce a position paper, "Responsible Use of sEMG."[3] After studying the issues, it stated that sEMG procedures were valid for static and dynamic studies for musculoskeletal conditions, but for only 4 weeks following onset of injury. In 1992, a commission of 35 chiropractic physicians produced what is known as the Mercy Conference Guidelines.[4] It rated static assessment procedures as "experimental," while describing dynamic procedures as "promising." To some, this appeared to be a political move to stop the abuse of submissions for static assessments. In 1996, the American Association of Electrodiagnostic Medicine (AAEM) produced a position paper stating that there are no indications for the use of surface EMG in the diagnosis and treatment of disorder of nerve or muscle.[5] The AAEM position is correct: surface EMG is not intended to study muscle and nerve disease; this is to be done with needle EMG recordings. But, what AAEM is missing is the utility of sEMG for clinical or functional diagnoses, which is where sEMG is most valuable. Needle EMG studies for this purpose are considered to be overly invasive and a poor representative of gross and fine motor

activities. In fact, when a needle EMG assessment is done and the patient is asked to make a significant contraction, the term used for this phenomenon is *interference pattern*. This is because volume-conducted activity from surrounding motor units interferes with the needle electromyographer's ability to see the single motor unit—the primary area of interest. As Sihvonen et al noted,[6] sEMG recording better describes the flexion-relaxation phenomenon in the low back muscles than simultaneous needle EMG recordings. The needle EMG is designed to record from very specific muscle fibers and truly misses the larger picture that sEMG can see. The only case in which needle EMG performs better than sEMG in dynamic movement assessments is when the muscle of interest lies beneath other muscles. Here, the needle EMG could come closer to eliminating the volume conduction and cross-talk so commonly noted in sEMG. However, the needle recordings are also subject to volume-conducted activity or far-field potentials. So the political debate among different professional groups goes on.

Providers who wish to educate the insurance industry concerning the sensitivity, specificity, and clinical efficacy of sEMG should consider all of the references for the assessment and treatment chapters. A list of the most relevant ones appears in the Suggested Readings section. An asterisk (*) appears next to the most critical readings.

REFERENCES

1. Donaldson S, Donaldson M. Multi-channel EMG assessment and treatment techniques. In: Cram JR, ed. *Clinical EMG for Surface Recordings, II.* Nevada City, CA: Clinical Resources; 1990:143–174.

2. International Society for Electromyography and Kinesiology. Standards for reporting EMG data. *J Electromyogr Kinesiol.* 1996;6(1):III.

3. Surface EMG Society of North America. SESNA position paper: Responsible use of sEMG. *sEMG Potentials,* summer, 1992.

4. Haldeman S, Chapman-Smith D, Petersen D. *Guidelines for Chiropractic Quality Assurance and Practice*

Parameters: Proceedings of the Mercy Center Consensus Conference. Gaithersburg, MD: Aspen Publishers; 1992.

5. Haig AJ, Gelblum JB, Rechtein JJ, Gitter AJ. Technology assessment: the use of surface EMG in the diagnosis and treatment of nerve and muscle disorders. *Muscle Nerve.* 1996;19:392–395.

6. Sihvonen T, Partanin J, Osmo H, Soimakalio P. Electric behavior of low back muscles during lumbar pelvic rhythm in low back pain patients and healthy controls. *Arch Phys Med Rehab.* 1991;72:1080–1087.

SUGGESTED READINGS

Agency for Health Care Policy and Research. *Urinary Incontinence in Adults: Clinical Practice Guidelines.* Rockville, MD: Agency for Health Care Policy and Research; March, 1992. US Dept of Health and Human Services publication AHCPR 92-0038.

*Arena JG, Sherman R, Bruno G, Young T. Temporal stability of paraspinal electromyographic recordings in low back pain and non-pain patients. *Int J Psychophysiol.* 1990;9:31–37.

Basmajian JV, DeLuca C. *Muscles Alive.* 5th ed. Baltimore: Williams & Wilkins; 1985.

Bittman B, Cram JR. Surface EMG: An electrophysiological alternative in pain management. In: Weiner RS, ed. *Innovations in Pain Management: A Practical Guide for Clinicians.* St. Petersburg: Deutsche Press, 1993.

*Cram JR, Engstrom D. Patterns of neuromuscular activity in pain and non-pain patients. *Clin Biofeedback Health.* 1986;9:106–116.

*Cram JR, Steger JC. Muscle scanning and the diagnosis of chronic pain. *Biofeedback Selfregul.* 1983;8:229–241.

Dolce JJ, Raczynski JM. Neuromuscular activity and electromyography in painful backs: psychological and biomechanical models in assessment and treatment. *Psychol Bull.* 1985;97:502–520.

Fishbain DA, Goldberg M, Meagher BR, Steel R, Rosomoff H. Male and female chronic pain patients categorized by DSM-II psychiatric diagnostic criteria. *Pain.* 1986;26:181–197.

*Glazer HI, Rodke G, Swencionis C, Hertz R, Young A. Treatment of vulvar vestibulitis syndrome with electromyographic biofeedback of pelvic floor musculature. *J Reprod Med.* 1995;40:283–290.

*Kessler M, Cram JR, Traue H. EMG muscle scanning in pain patients and controls: a replication and extension. *Am J Pain Manage.* 1993;3:20–28.

*Klein AB, Snyder-Mackler L, Roy S, DeLuca C. Comparison of spinal mobility and isometric trunk extensor forces with electromyographic spectral analysis in identifying low back pain. *Phys Ther.* 1991;71(6):445–453.

Leach RA, Owens EF, Giesen JM. Correlates of myoelectric asymmetry detected in low back pain patient using hand held post style surface electromyography. *J Manipulative Physiol Ther.* 1993;16:140–149.

Mathiassen SE, Winkel J, Hagg GM. Normalization of surface EMG amplitude from the upper trapezius muscle in ergonomic studies: a review. *J Electromyogr Kinesiol.* 1995;5:197–226.

*Middaugh SJ, Kee WG, Nicholson JA. Muscle overuse and posture as factors in the development and maintenance of chronic musculoskeletal pain. In: Grzesiak RC, Ciccone DS, eds. *Psychological Vulnerability to Chronic Pain.* New York: Springer Publishing Co; 1994:55–89.

Peper E, Wilson V, Taylor W, et al. Repetitive strain injury. *Phys Ther Products.* September 1994:17–22.

Price JP, Clare MH, Ewerhardt RH. Studies in low backache with persistent spasm. *Arch Phys Med.* 1948;29:703–709.

Robinson ME, Cassisi JE, O'Connor PD, MacMillan M. Lumbar iEMG during isotonic exercise: chronic low back pain patients vs controls. *J Spinal Disord.* 1992;5:1.

*Roy SH, DeLuca CJ, Casavant DA. Lumbar muscle fatigue and chronic back pain. *Spine.* 1989;14:992–1001.

*Roy SH, DeLuca CJ, Snyder-Mackler L, et al. Fatigue, recovery and low back pain in elite rowers. *Med Sci Sports Exerc.* 1990;22:463–469.

Sherman R, Arena J. Biofeedback for assessment and treatment of low back pain. In: Basmajian JV, Wolf S, eds. *Rational Manual Therapies.* Baltimore: Williams & Wilkins; 1994:177–197.

Skubick D, Clasby R, Donaldson CCS, Marshall W. Carpal tunnel syndrome as an expression of muscular dysfunction in the neck. *J Occup Rehab.* 1993;3:31–43.

Soderberg GL, ed. *Selected Topics in Surface Electromyography for Use in the Occupational Setting: Expert Perspective.* Washington DC: National Institute for Occupational Safety and Health; 1992. US Dept of Health and Human Services publication NIOSH 91-100.

*Triano J, Schultz AB. Correlation of objective measurement of trunk motion and muscle function with low back disability ratings. *Spine.* 1987;12:561–565.

Veiersted KB, Westgaard RH. Work related risk factors for trapezius myalgia. *Int Arch Occup Environ Health.* 1990;62:31–41.

*Veiersted KB, Westgaard RH, Andersen P. Electromyographic evaluation of muscular work pattern as a predictor of trapezius myalgia. *Scand J Work Environ Health.* 1993;19:284–290.

Wolf S, Basmajian J. Assessment of paraspinal electromyographic activity in normal subjects and chronic back pain patients using a muscle biofeedback device. In: Asmussen E, Jorgensen K, eds. *International Series on Biomechanics; VI-B.* Baltimore: University Press; 1978.

Wolf S, Basmajian J, Russe C, Kutner M. Normative data on low back mobility and activity levels. *Am J Phys Med.* 1979;58:217–229.

Wolf S, LeCraw D, Barton L. Comparison of motor copy and targeted biofeedback training techniques for restitution of upper extremity function among patients with neurologic disorders. *Phys Ther.* 1988;69:719–735.

*Wolf S, Nacht M, Kelly J. EMG feedback training during dynamic movement for low back pain patients. *Behav Ther.* 1982;13:395–406.

Chapter Questions

1. Chart notes should include at least four basic elements. They are:
   a. name, age, Social Security number, and marital status
   b. subjective, objective, assessment, and planning information
   c. age, diagnosis, objective findings, and plan
   d. resting microvolt levels, peak micro-volt levels, recovery microvolt levels, and synergy pattern

2. How does the saying "can't see the forest for the trees" relate to electrodiagnosis?
   a. describes sEMG recordings
   b. describes needle EMG recordings
   c. none of the above

3. In functional kinesiology, needle EMG recordings are useful when:
   a. the practitioner wants to record from a deep muscle
   b. the practitioner wants a definitive quantification of gross motor activity
   c. both a and b
   d. none of the above

4. Surface EMG assessment procedures should be billed out as a neurological procedure.
   a. True
   b. False

CHAPTER 11

Surface Electromyography Past, Present, and Future

SURFACE ELECTROMYOGRAPHY AS AN EMERGING TECHNOLOGY

It is important to remember that surface electromyography (sEMG) is an emerging technology. Surface EMG is a very exciting instrument for assessing and treating conditions that may involve but go beyond strict, structural models. In addition to the issues of resting tone and functional recruitment patterns, the new information on "rest" and "noise" is particularly fascinating. The recent introduction of amplitude probability distributions[1-4] in understanding the etiology of tension myalgias in the workplace is particularly exciting. Perhaps it is not how we use our muscles during work that is important, but rather what we do with them between each effort. Taylor's single-case study[5] demonstrated that the interspersed rest epochs disappeared in a typist when she was placed under stress in the workplace. Adjusting the ergonomics of her work station to reduce the amount of effort needed to do her work would not eliminate the emotional component of her disorder. The recent work by White et al[6] on pelvic pain has also found "noise" to be a problem. These researchers found that the strongest and most consistent parameter to separate pelvic pain patients from their normal cohorts is the amount of postcontraction variability. The amount of noise in the sEMG signal indicated that slowness to return to baseline correctly identified 86% of the cases and the postcontraction variance correctly identified 93% of the cases. The sEMG practitioner constantly needs to remember and explore the three masters of muscle: posture, e-motions, and dynamic movement.

When the initial work by DeLuca on spectral analysis as a predictor of pain[7] was explored clinically by Roy et al[8] and Klein et al[9]; the limitations of working with amplitude-related values alone became quite clear. Amplitude-related variables (ie, peak root mean square, or RMS) could predict only 60% of the pain patients, while spectral sEMG data (ie, median frequency) indicated that recovery from fatigue following a sustained effort (80% maximum voluntary contraction, or MVC) predicted over 92% of the cases. Again, the sensitivity and specificity of sEMG information look quite promising. Perhaps, in the future, it will not be uncommon for the formal diagnosis of musculoskeletal pain (and related disorders) to entail sEMG monitoring.

The work by Bennett and Kornhauser[10] on the use of facial sEMG monitoring during general anesthesia is also quite interesting. Here sEMG is used to provide information on the consciousness and comfort of the patient while undergoing a major surgery. During general anesthesia, a neuromuscular blockade is administered to paralyze the patient, along with anesthesia to help the patient forget the trauma. Unfortunately, every year there are some 30,000 surgical patients (in the United States alone) who have an awareness experience during surgery; for whatever reason, the anesthesia is too light and the patient has a return of consciousness. But because of the chemically mediated paralysis, the patient cannot visually or verbally inform the surgeon or anesthesiologist of the dilemma. All the patient can do is lie there helplessly on the surgical table, feel the pain associated with the trauma of surgery, and hear the chatter of the operating room environment. For many, this leads to a posttraumatic stress disorder. However, monitoring the facial muscles for the grimace of pain can inform the anesthesiologist about the comfort and consciousness of the patient. Unlike the extremities, the exceptionally high level of innervation of the facial muscles, coupled with the power of the limbic system to drive the facial nuclei directly, allows the muscles of the face to penetrate the neuromuscular blockade and continue to provide trace amounts of information concerning nocioception. Although this recruitment is not strong enough to move the skin of the face, it can be detected by sEMG monitoring. As one can see, the importance of the emotional component of muscle cannot be overlooked.

Surface EMG instrumentation continues to evolve. One emerging aspect of this technology is the *double differential technique*.[11] Here, a linear electrode array is monitored (see Figure 11–1). The output from the first level of differential amplification (E_1, E_2, E_3) is then fed into a second set of differential amplifiers, which yields a smaller number of processed channels (S_1 and S_2). This second level of differential amplification also removes all elements of the sEMG signal common to the proximal and distal aspects of the electrodes. Researchers initially found this new technology to be useful in the study of conduction velocities of muscle fibers. In conduction velocity studies, the investigator wants to see the motor unit action potential (MUAP) travel from one electrode to the next, measuring the time it takes to travel the distance and thus deriving the velocity of the potential. The problem was that all four electrodes tended to see a large amount of common signal. Researchers believed that this was volume-conducted biologic potential common to all of the

electrodes. To eliminate the volume-conducted signal and to enable practitioners to see the movement of the MUAP down the muscle fiber, researchers developed the double differential technique. They discovered that this technique is useful for investigating and eliminating crosstalk among electrode pairs. As this new instrumentation and the phenomena it can detect are better understood, this technique will probably become more widespread.

Another interesting development in sEMG monitoring is the transfer of quantitative EEG techniques to the sEMG arena. Cram and Finley[12,13] used a dense two-dimensional electrode array (2-cm spacing in a four-by-six electrode array) and the LaPlacean transform to study the quadriceps muscle of the leg. The LaPlacean transform is a mathematical technique that sharpens a graphical display so that only the energy directly under the electrode is recorded. All volume-conducted information is mathematically eliminated (see Figure 11–2). The right quadriceps muscle was monitored during a step-up movement. In Figure 11–3, the leg is depicted with a window to see the muscle energy. The vastus medialis oblique and vastus lateralis can clearly be seen. The highlighted area above the vastus medialis oblique is thought to represent energy from the adductor muscles. The hip adductors may play a substantial role in patellofemoral pain syndromes.

THE USE OF SURFACE ELECTROMYOGRAPHY TO STUDY THE EFFECTS OF PRAYER

The last innovative application of sEMG involves using technology to study the metaphysics of the nonlocal effects of prayer.[14] This prayer study raises the question "What do sEMG instruments really measure?" Certainly, they measure motor unit action potentials; when we activate a muscle, the needle on the sEMG moves. But what about volume-conducted energy—the energy that the double differential technique so successfully eliminates? Where does that come from? What does it represent?

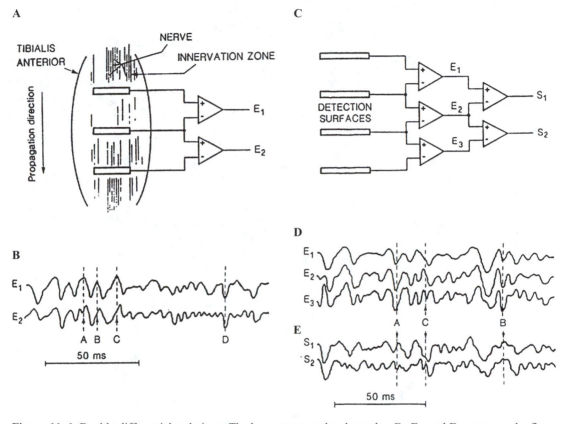

Figure 11–1 Double differential technique. The bars represent the electrodes; E_1, E_2, and E_3 represent the first level of differential amplification. S_1 and S_2 represent the second level of differential amplification. The sEMG output of (**A**) is displayed in (**B**). The sEMG output of (**C**) is shown in (**D**) and (**E**). *Source:* Adapted with permission from Broman et al, *IEEE Transaction on Biomedical Engineering,* Vol 32, pp 341–344, © 1985, IEEE.

The answers to these questions are truly a matter of speculation.

One theoretical framework that explains the flow of energy in the body is based on the concept of *nadis*.[15] In this more than 4000-year-old theory, the energy of the universe flows through an individual by traveling through metaphysical channels called *nadis*. According to this theory, there are more than 10,000 nadi channels in the body. There is a channel for each muscle group and organ, plus much more. Some of the channels are large, some are small. The three channels that flow around the spine are some of the largest: the *sushumna*, the *ida*, and the *pingala*. The sushumna travels directly up the center of the spine, while the ida and pingala crisscross back and forth as they travel up and down the spine. At the points along the spine where all three of these nadis meet, the *chakras* are found. According to this ancient theory, the chakras are sites in the body where the metaphysical energy is the greatest. Each of the seven chakras has its own purpose, its own characteristics.

In the prayer study,[14] the sEMG electrodes, 3 cm apart, were placed bilaterally (one electrode on the right side, one on the left side) at four of the chakra sites: the "third eye" (frontal), the "throat chakra" (C-4 paraspinals), the "heart chakra" (T-6 paraspinals), and the "lumbar chakra" (L-1/T-12 paraspinals). In modern

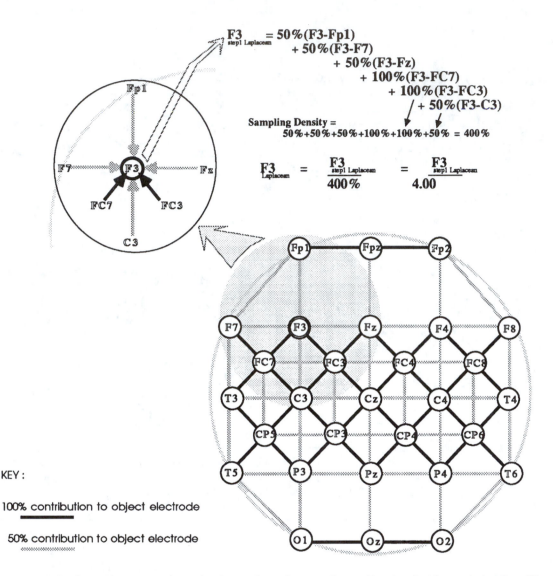

$$\mathbf{F3}_{\text{step1 Laplacean}} = 50\%(\text{F3-Fp1})$$
$$+ 50\%(\text{F3-F7})$$
$$+ 50\%(\text{F3-Fz})$$
$$+ 100\%(\text{F3-FC7})$$
$$+ 100\%(\text{F3-FC3})$$
$$+ 50\%(\text{F3-C3})$$

Sampling Density =
50%+50%+50%+100%+100%+50% = 400%

$$\mathbf{F3}_{\text{Laplacean}} = \frac{\mathbf{F3}_{\text{step1 Laplacean}}}{400\%} = \frac{\mathbf{F3}_{\text{step1 Laplacean}}}{4.00}$$

KEY :

100% contribution to object electrode

50% contribution to object electrode

Figure 11–2 The LaPlacean transformation for an electrode array. *Source:* Reprinted with permission from JR Cram et al, Topographic LaPlacean Source Derivation Analysis of the Quadriceps Muscle Group during Squatting, *Proceedings of the 8th International Congress of the International Society of Electrophysiological Kinesiology,* 1990.

Western terms, one could say that the electrodes were measuring the emotional displays of the face and the postural activity along the spine. In Eastern terms, one could say that the electrodes were measuring the qualities of the particular chakra. The prayer study was conducted using a randomized, double-blind, crossover design, which is the methodology utilized by drug companies to study and demonstrate the specific effects of medications. The 24 subjects did not know that they were involved in a study on prayer. They only knew that they were being asked to come and sit on a backless stool for 21 minutes twice, once in the morning and once in

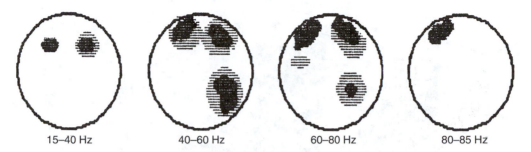

| 15–40 Hz | 40–60 Hz | 60–80 Hz | 80–85 Hz |

Figure 11–3 Topographic display of LaPlacean transformed sEMG of quadriceps muscle during a step-up procedure using a 24-channel electrode array. The top of each figure represents the knee, the bottom represents the hip. The left side is lateral and the right side is medial. The areas of lightness show little or no activity, while the areas of darkness show specific activation patterns. *Source:* Reprinted with permission from JR Cram et al, Topographic LaPlacean Source Derivation Analysis of the Quadriceps Muscle Group during Squatting, *Proceedings of the 8th International Congress of the International Society of Electrophysiological Kinesiology,* 1990.

the afternoon. Lunch was provided between sessions. Once the subject was connected to the electrodes, the experimenter left the room and called a prayer group (of two) to tell them that subject *X* was connected and ready to go, and the study was initiated. The first period of 7 minutes represented a baseline condition. The next 14-minute period entailed either prayer or a control condition. Once they received the call, the prayer group opened a sealed envelope with the subject number on it. If it contained a photograph of the subject, they initiated a heartfelt prayer of love. If it was a blank 3 × 5–inch card, they had tea instead. In either case, the experimenter did not know whether the subject was prayed for in the morning or afternoon, and thus could not intentionally or unintentionally influence the subject.

The results of the study are illustrated in Figure 11–4. When subjects sat and were not prayed for, the sEMG recordings at the heart and lumbar sites rose very slightly (approximately 10%). When the same subjects were prayed for (from a distance of 300 miles away), the energy at these sites fell by nearly 50%. In other words, the energy along the spine consistently relaxed as a function of nonlocal effects of prayer. The probability of this event happening purely by chance is 8 in 1 million.

So, what does all of this mean? It could mean that the Hindu theologians who wrote about the nadis knew something that people in the West know very little about. According to Hindu tradition, the heart chakra is the receiving center for prayer. And, interestingly enough, it was the heart chakra that showed the largest response in the prayer study. It is doubtful that the researchers would have had the same effects if they had measured muscle activity of the upper trapezius. After all, the neck and frontal regions did not change in any substantial way. However, the sEMG placements along the spine did monitor paraspinal muscle activity. The subjects were sitting, unsupported, on a stool for 21 minutes; when they were not prayed for, their muscles began to tire and they began to exert additional postural support energy to fight off the effects of fatigue. Yet, when these same subjects sat on the same stool and were prayed for, they did not resist the pull of gravity and relaxed along the spine.

Could there be a connection between consciousness and gravity? Again, in the Eastern tradition, one always learns to meditate sitting unsupported. Why is this? It could be that the energy needed in the spine to sit erect keeps the lamp of consciousness burning. In fact, anyone who has meditated for a period of time has experienced nodding off and being awakened by the

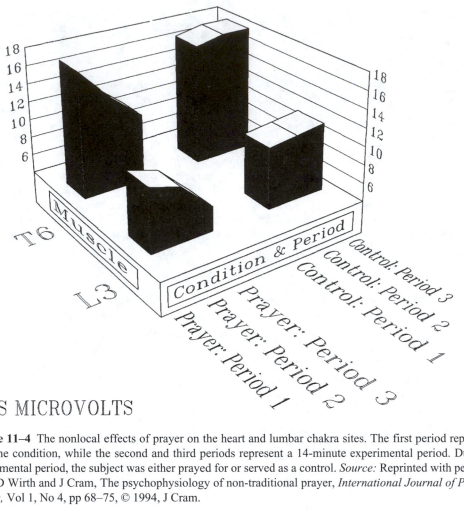

RMS MICROVOLTS

Figure 11–4 The nonlocal effects of prayer on the heart and lumbar chakra sites. The first period represents a baseline condition, while the second and third periods represent a 14-minute experimental period. During the experimental period, the subject was either prayed for or served as a control. *Source:* Reprinted with permission from D Wirth and J Cram, The psychophysiology of non-traditional prayer, *International Journal of Psychosomatics,* Vol 1, No 4, pp 68–75, © 1994, J Cram.

falling of the head or torso. These ancient teachers knew that energy in the spine was connected in some way to consciousness. But the Eastern yogis also noted that one should sit erect and keep the spine relaxed. In the prayer study, the two people who engaged in prayer used their consciousness and an open heart to send love to the subjects in this study. Perhaps their conscious love used the gravitational field to somehow connect with the subjects in the study. In any event, the prayer study shows the power of using these tools in innovative ways.

Researchers have just begun to tap into the domains of knowledge available to us when we study the *energy* of muscles rather than their *form.* In the future, we are certain to observe some exciting discoveries about how this energy moves us about.

REFERENCES

1. Jonsson B. Kinesiology: with special reference to electromyographic kinesiology. *Cont Clin Neurophysiol EEG Suppl.* 1978;34:417–428.

2. Jonsson BG, Persson J, Kilbom A. Disorders of the cervicobrachial region among female workers in the electronics industry: a two year follow up. *Int J Ind Ergon.* 1988;3:1–12.

3. Veiersted KB, Westgaard RH, Andersen P. Electromyographic evaluation of muscular work pattern as a predictor of trapezius myalgia. *Scand J Work Environ Health.* 1993;19:284–290.

4. Veiersted KB, Westgaard RH. Work related risk factors for trapezius myalgia. *Int Arch Occup Environ Health.* 1990;62:31–41.

5. Taylor W. Patterns of sEMG. Presented at the meeting of the Surface EMG Society of North America; 1993; Boston.

6. White G, Marek J, Glazer H. Towards establishing the diagnosis of vulvar vestibulitis. In press.

7. DeLuca C. Myoelectric manifestations of localized muscular fatigue in humans. *Crit Rev Biomed Eng.* 1984;11:251.

8. Roy SH, DeLuca CJ, Snyder-Mackler L, et al. Fatigue, recovery and low back pain in elite rowers. *Med Sci Sports Exerc.* 1990;22:463–469.

9. Klein A, Snyder Mackler L, Roy S, DeLuca C. Comparison of spinal mobility and isometric trunk extensor forces with electromyographic spectral analysis in identifying low back pain. *Phys Ther.* 1991;71(6):445–453.

10. Bennett H, Kornhauser S. Assessment of general anesthesia by facial muscle electromyography (FACE). *Am J Electromed.* 1995;6:94–97.

11. Broman H, Bilotto G, DeLuca CJ. A note on non-invasive estimation of muscle fiber conduction velocity. *IEEE Trans Biomed Eng.* 1985;32:341–344.

12. Cram JR, Finley WW, Lester ML, Rector DD. Topographic LaPlacean source derivation analysis of the quadriceps muscle group during squatting. In: *Proceedings of the 8th International Congress of the International Society of Electrophysiological Kinesiology.* Baltimore; 1990.

13. Finley WW, Lester ML, Cram JR, Rector DD. Topographic LaPlacean source derivation analysis of the quadriceps muscle group while standing on the right leg. In: *Proceedings of the 8th International Congress of the International Society of Electrophysiological Kinesiology.* Baltimore; 1990.

14. Wirth D, Cram J. The psychophysiology of non-traditional prayer. *Int J Psychosom.* 1994;1(4):68–75.

15. Rama S, Ballentine R, Hymes A. *The Science of Breath.* Honesdale, PA: Himalayan Institute; 1990.

CHAPTER 12

Conclusion

Surface electromyography (sEMG) has come quite a long way. It appeals to any professional who works with muscle. It is attractive because it is noninvasive. It is like an electronic stethoscope for muscles. Practitioners find it attractive because it examines muscle function rather than structure. Surface EMG has evolved from the days when it was conducted from within copper cages. While it began in the halls of scientific inquiry into muscle and muscle function, it has clearly found its way into clinical practice. Although this book has explored some of the scientific foundations of sEMG, its primary focus has been clinical.

This book is an introductory text. It only begins to scratch the surface of what we know about muscle energy and how it can be used clinically to assess and treat musculoskeletal disorders and pain. It presents an initial exploration of the anatomy and physiology of muscle. A vast amount of information is available on this topic—from introductory texts such as *Job's Body*, by Duane Juhan,[1] to advanced texts such as *Principles of Neural Science*, edited by Kandel, Schwartz, and Jessell.[2]

This book presents a brief introduction to the electrical concepts, the instrumentation, and the technology behind sEMG. For a more in-depth look at the basics, consider reading Peek's chapter on instrumentation in *Biofeedback: A Practitioner's Guide*, edited by Schwartz.[3] For a more sophisticated presentation, consider the first chapters of *Muscles Alive* (5th edition), by Basmajian and DeLuca.[4]

The electrode atlas in Part II of this book provides information concerning the placement of electrodes, along with the types of recruitment patterns one might see using such placements. In addition, it recommends clinical uses for the various placements and provides clinical information relevant to each site. Only 68 of the more than 600 muscles of the human body are explored, representing only a small portion (10%) of the total muscle energy of the human body. Fortunately, many of the muscles we currently can observe using sEMG are major muscles of the human body. Unfortunately, many offensive muscles (such as the levator scapulae) cannot be seen with today's sEMG instruments.

The assessment chapters emphasize normal resting tone and provide representative samples of the types of recruitment patterns seen on a very small subset of "normal" individuals. We encourage the practitioners to think about what type of recruitment pattern they would expect to see for a given muscle and then to test out those assumptions using sEMG. Through this type of inquiry, practitioners will expand their knowledge of how sEMG can aid in the understanding of muscle function and its applications to clinical problems.

Although the principles and issues pertaining to treatment are introduced in this book, only a few clinical examples are presented. For a more in-depth discussion of the use of sEMG in the treatment of musculoskeletal and pain-related disorders, see our companion book, *Clinical Applications in Surface Electromyography*.[5] In addition, the clinical protocol of Donaldson, Ettare, and Taylor is available in *Clinical EMG for Surface Recordings*, edited by Cram.[6]

To conclude, this book introduces the practitioner to the foundations and clinical uses of sEMG. It is our hope that practitioners have come to see that sEMG is a very powerful and exciting tool. However, along with its uses, come its abuses. We hope that practitioners take a conservative stance toward its use and in particular, toward the interpretations of clinical study results. Finally, the use of sEMG for treatment is very promising, but practitioners must be careful about the claims they make. Surface EMG is but a tool to enhance the already existing skills of the provider. If nothing else, it turbocharges providers' treatment efforts.

REFERENCES

1. Juhan D. *Job's Body.* Barrytown, NY: Station Hill Press; 1987.
2. Kandel E, Schwartz E, Jessell T. *Principles of Neural Science.* 3rd ed. Stamford, CT: Appleton & Lange; 1991.
3. Peek CJ. A primer of biofeedback instrumentation. In: Schwartz M, ed. *Biofeedback: A Practitioner's Guide.* New York: Guilford Press; 1987.
4. Basmajian J, DeLuca CJ. *Muscles Alive.* 5th ed. Baltimore: Williams & Wilkins; 1985.
5. Kasman G, Cram J, Wolf S. *Clinical Applications in Surface Electromyography.* Gaithersburg, MD: Aspen Publishers; 1997.
6. Cram J. *Clinical EMG for Surface Recordings: Volume 2.* Nevada City, CA: Clinical Resources; 1990.

PART II

Atlas for Electrode Placement

Jeffrey R. Cram and Glenn S. Kasman with Jonathan Holtz

CHAPTER 13

Electrode Atlas Overview

INTRODUCTION

The placement of the electrodes for surface electromyography (sEMG) recordings will, in large part, determine the quality of the recordings. Because the sEMG can "listen" only so deep and the sEMG signal is frequently contaminated by cross-talk from neighboring muscles, practitioners must decide whether they are interested in a specific or general recording and place the electrodes accordingly.

For a general recording, it is recommended that practitioners place the electrodes with a wide spacing. This will capture all of the muscle energy contributions between the two active electrodes, and more. For recording from a specific muscle group, the practitioner must know specifically where the muscle is located, the direction of its muscle fibers, and its depth. Palpation of the surface muscles is essential to ensure accurate placement. A general rule of thumb is that the depth and area of the sEMG recording are directly proportional to the interelectrode distance.[1] This is illustrated in Figure 13–1, where the darker fibers contribute more heavily than the lighter ones. This concept may be seen in cross-section in Figure 3–5. For both superficial and slightly deeper muscles, the practitioner must ask the patient to do the primary movement of the muscle, either through its active range of motion or in a resisted isometric fashion. In this way, the practitioner can verify that placement is correct. Finally, it is often useful to monitor si-multaneously the targeted muscle's synergist or antagonist so as to appreciate more fully the functional nature of the movement pattern.

INFORMATION CONTAINED IN ELECTRODE ATLAS

Type of Placement

Below are descriptions for general, specific, and quasi-specific electrode placements. Each description incorporates a variety of sources of information.

Some electrode placements monitor the muscular energy in a *general* region, while others are more *specific*. This atlas also includes a number of placements that are considered to be controversial; although sEMG recording from these controversial placements might appear to be specific, the muscles commonly lie beneath or adjacent to other muscles and are thus fraught with the possibility of cross-talk. These placements are called *quasi-specific*.

- *General:* This electrode placement strategy takes advantage of volume conduction and records from a general region rather than a specific muscle. For example, the frontalis (wide) placement is specifically designed to record from muscle activity of the upper and, perhaps, lower face (rather than specifically monitoring from the frontalis muscle).

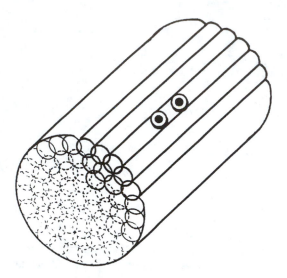

Figure 13–1 Relationship of interelectrode distance and depth of sEMG recordings.

• *Specific:* This electrode placement strategy attempts to detect the activity of a specific muscle group. Usually, these muscles are close to the surface and relatively easy to isolate. The position for placement and the spacing and orientation of the electrodes can play a significant role in the practitioner's success in recording from a specific muscle. The type of movement associated with a muscle recording may help isolate the muscle activity or contaminate it through volume conduction. For example, smaller movements that require less recruitment tend to necessitate few synergists and thus produce less volume conduction. As in muscle testing, correct positioning and instruction to the subject are necessary to ensure specificity in sEMG recordings.

• *Quasi-specific:* This electrode placement strategy uses the strategies of the specific placement, such as closely spaced electrodes oriented to record from specific muscles. However, specific recordings for certain muscles are difficult because of the proximity of neighboring muscles (particularly in the extremities) or the depth of the

muscle from the surface (as in the axial muscles). In both cases, it is difficult to identify clearly which muscle is contributing to the sEMG signal. Superficial muscles are typically easy to palpate and identify. However, they may be difficult to isolate using sEMG techniques if they are packed closely together. Cross-talk from neighboring muscles may contaminate your confidence in a specific recording. Examples of this include forearm recordings. Recordings from deep muscles are difficult, because the source sEMG must pass through the more superficial layers of muscles to reach the recording electrodes. It is impossible to state that the recording is primarily from the deeper muscle, because the sEMG recording could easily be contaminated by the more superficial layers of muscle. The proof of specificity of recording resides in demonstrating that the sEMG signal is activated during the movements ascribed to the muscle of interest and not during contraction of neighboring muscles.

Action or Purpose

For specific and quasi-specific sites, this section lists the primary function or action of the muscle. For general sites, it refers to the purpose of the sEMG recording.

Clinical Uses

This section highlights some of the conditions or procedures for which sEMG recordings at a particular site might be considered useful.

Muscle Insertions

This section describes the origins and insertions of the muscles of interest. This may be important in understanding the direction of the muscle fibers, because surface electrodes are commonly oriented in the direction of these fibers.

Innervation

In cases where specific and quasi-specific muscle sites are described, this section identifies the motor nerves associated with the muscle group.

Joint Considerations

When appropriate, the joints considered pertinent to and possibly affecting the sEMG recordings are highlighted.

Location

This section describes the actual placement of the electrodes in verbal terms. This verbal description augments the graphical description provided on the same page. *Experience with muscle testing and palpation helps the practitioner to place the electrode over the correct muscle group.* Information on muscle testing and palpation is available in *Muscles: Testing and Function* by Kendall, Kendall, and McCreary.[2] It is recommended that the practitioner palpate the described area during a muscle testing procedure to locate the exact position of the muscle belly and to assist in placing the electrode. Better quality sEMG recordings are obtained when the sEMG electrodes are placed parallel to the muscle fibers and slightly off the center of the belly of the muscle.

Behavioral Test

Whenever electrodes are placed over a muscle group, the practitioner should ask the patient to engage in a specific movement to determine whether the electrodes are over the muscle of interest. This section describes at least one of the main movements associated with the muscle. The sEMG tracing shown for the site usually reflects one or more of these movements.

Tracing Comment

These tracings illustrate the sEMG recording seen during one of the movements described in the "Behavioral Test" section above. Most of these tracings are presented in the raw sEMG format.* Whenever possible, this format was selected, because it provides the clearest view of the sEMG activity. In addition, a pregelled, recessed electrode at a fixed interelectrode distance (center to center) was used for many of the recordings to help obtain a clean signal and to provide a standard for later replication. These tracings are not intended to represent the "ideal" recruitment pattern, but rather what one would commonly see in the "normal" population. The tracings presented in this section are representative samples of sEMG tracings observed at a given site, on a given individual, using a given movement. The tracings are intended as a conceptual aid to electrode placement. They should not be taken as templates on which to base clinical decisions. No attempt has been made to evaluate systematically the variability of recruitment across a large population of normal subjects or patients. Simply put, these tracings demonstrate some of the expected recruitment patterns for the area of interest. Given the richness of human movement, it is important to note that these tracings do not represent comprehensive study of an area. Slight variations in electrode placement and movement patterns may produce different recruitment patterns.

Clinical Considerations

This section identifies some of the potential postural or positional elements that might affect the recordings. The sEMG activity may vary dramatically with the body in a different posture. This is due to the effects of gravity on the more axial muscles or changes in sEMG activity levels because of small changes in the elements of

---

*The sEMG recordings were done on a Norodyn 8000 sEMG instrument (raw) or J&J 1-330 M-501 sEMG instrument (processed). All recordings, unless otherwise specified, were conducted using the Norotrode 2.0 electrode. This electrode is a pregelled, recessed, or floating electrode with a 1.0-cm pellet and an interelectrode distance of 2.0 cm (center to center).

the kinetic chain. In addition, there may be a natural repositioning of the surface electrodes in relationship to the muscles beneath them during movement of an extremity. For example, placement of electrodes on the triceps muscle should be done with the arm in the position or plane in which the training will be taking place. This is because supination and pronation of the arm can alter the position of the electrodes in relation to the muscle belly.

In addition, the sEMG recording may be affected by dysfunctions in the joints and fascia. Comments regarding the impact of these restrictions are supplied, when appropriate. Finally, this section may list some of the common clinical uses for certain placements. Such descriptions are not intended to be exhaustive, nor are they intended to limit sEMG uses for a given muscle site.

Volume Conduction

This section identifies the common muscles that might contaminate the specificity of the recording through volume conduction.

Other Sites of Interest

This section identifies other sites that the practitioner may want to monitor concurrently with the muscle of interest. These additional sites may be synergists, agonists, or antagonists that participate with the muscle of interest in a given movement. Although this concept of relatedness is self-evident for kinesiologically oriented practitioners, there is no common term for it. Travell and Simons[3] have referred to this concept as a *myotatic unit*. The additional sites may be part of a larger mass action pattern, a kinetic chain, or simply some form of coordinated movement. This section helps the practitioner to see the "bigger picture" of muscle interaction patterns.

Referred Pain Considerations

Trigger points in a muscle group may affect features of the sEMG recording.[4,5] When appro-priate, the pain referral pattern for a trigger point located in the muscle group of interest is provided.[3]

Artifacts

This section identifies common artifacts associated with a given electrode placement.

Benchmark

This section provides a reference sEMG value for resting values. This information is provided for some sites but not others. The issues pertaining to dynamic sEMG recordings preclude meaningful benchmark values at this time. For example, it is unclear whether these values would be taken as an average of the entire tracing, the peak of the movement, the recovery back to baseline, the concentric component, the eccentric component, etc. In addition, the anthropomorphic variables may make absolute sEMG data less meaningful than normalized values. Normalized values may provide a more accurate picture of sEMG activity when one is comparing one muscle group to another. The percentage of asymmetry between the right and left homologous muscles of a particular group during a given movement may yield more meaningful information than absolute sEMG values.

The sEMG values associated with rest are considered meaningful. However, these values should be seen as guidelines rather than absolutes (see Chapter 6). Nearly all values have been converted to the J&J M-501 standard benchmark value. The benchmark values have been computed using the conversion factors listed in Table 3–1. To convert the benchmark value to a figure that is compatible with a particular instrument, simply multiply the benchmark value by the ratio associated with the particular sEMG instrument. For example, if the benchmark value is 5.0 microvolts and the practitioner is using a Davicon sEMG instrument, the practitioner would multiply the 5.0 by 1.67 to obtain a Davicon equivalent value (or 8.35 microvolts). If a particular instrument is not listed in Table 3–1, record root mean square

(RMS) values during rest from several muscle groups and compare the sEMG values to the benchmark value. If they consistently differ from the benchmark value by some factor (eg, if they are twice as high), then use that factor to convert the benchmark values to ones relevant to the sEMG system.

REFERENCE PLANES AND MOVEMENT DESCRIPTIONS

Certain terms are used to describe dynamic movements. Descriptions of some of the movements are provided below to help practitioners replicate these procedures during the studies of muscle function. For a more extensive review of descriptions of movement, see Gowitzke and Milner, *Scientific Basis of Human Movement,*[6] or Kendall, Kendall, and McCreary, *Muscles: Testing and Function.*[2]

There are three cardinal reference planes of movement. The *frontal plane* divides movement toward the front and the back of the body. The *sagittal plane* divides the movement into right and left planes. And the *horizontal* or *transverse plane* refers to the upper and lower portions of the body. These planes are shown in Figure 13–2.

Flexion, extension, rotation, and side bending are attributes used in movement of the head. These movements are clearly depicted in Figure 13–3. Flexion of the head brings the head forward, away from midline, chin to chest. The term *return* indicates a movement back to midline. Formal extension is movement backward, away from midline, letting the head fall back over the shoulders. Axial rotation of the head is associated with turning the head to look over the shoulder. Side bending involves bringing the ear toward the shoulder.

Movement of the jaw may also be described. In addition to opening and closing the jaw, it may be laterally deviated to the left or right and may be protruded outward from the cranium or retracted back toward the neck.

The study of shoulder functions is rather complex. Several forms and planes of movement are possible. *Shoulder abduction, adduction, flex-*

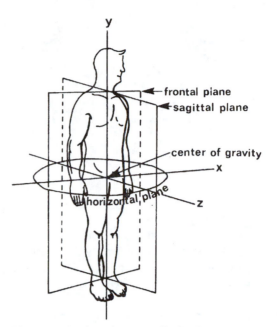

Figure 13–2 The primary cardinal reference planes. *Source:* Reprinted with permission from B Gowitzke and M Milner, *Scientific Basis of Human Movement,* p 9, © 1988, Williams & Wilkins.

ion, and extension are shown in Figure 13–4. Flexion and extension of the arm moves in the sagittal plane out in front of the chest (as if walking in one's sleep) and backward (as if to dive). Abduction moves the arm laterally out to the side, as if to form a *T* with the body. Many of the shoulder and arm movements presented in the atlas limit the abduction and flexion to 90 degrees, while others entail the full range of motion with the hands fully overhead. Adduction is associated with movement in toward the center of the body. *Scaption,* which is not shown in Figure 13–4, entails raising the arm out away from the body at an oblique 45-degree angle halfway between the frontal and sagittal planes or, in other words, halfway between flexion and abduction. *Internal and external rotation* of the shoulder is presented in Figure 13–5. Internal rotation rounds the shoulder in, while external rotation rounds the shoulder back. *Shoulder girdle elevation, depression, retraction,* and *protraction* reflect another dynamic range of motion for the shoulder. With elevation, one raises the

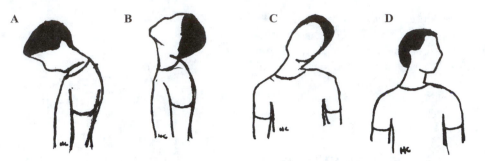

Figure 13–3 Cervical spine movements: (**A**) flexion, (**B**) extension, (**C**) lateral bending, and (**D**) rotation.

shoulder up around the ears; with depression, one pulls the shoulders down; with retraction, one pulls the shoulders back as if to stand in a military posture; with protraction, one moves the shoulders forward.

Movement of the upper extremities involves many aspects. *Elbow flexion* and *extension* are probably the easiest to define. The flexion component is presented in Figure 13–6. Here the biceps and brachialis shorten as the elbow bends. With elbow extension, the triceps shortens while the arm straightens. The forearm may also rotate. External rotation with the palm up is termed *supination*, while internal rotation with the palm down is termed *pronation*. These terms are graphically depicted in Figure 13–7. Wrist movements also need to be defined. Wrist extension (dorsiflexion) cocks the wrist up, wrist flexion (palmar flexion) curls the wrist down, radial abduction (deviation) moves the wrist toward the thumb side, and ulnar adduction (deviation) moves the wrist toward the little finger side. These are presented in Figure 13–8. Movement of the fingers and thumb may be isolated on sEMG recordings and are represented in Figures 13–9 and 13–10. Flexion and extension of the

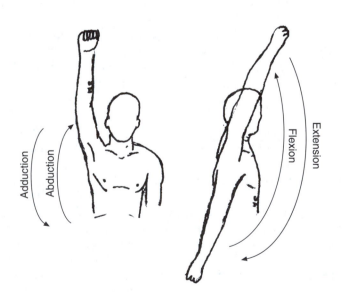

Figure 13–4 Primary movements of the shoulder.

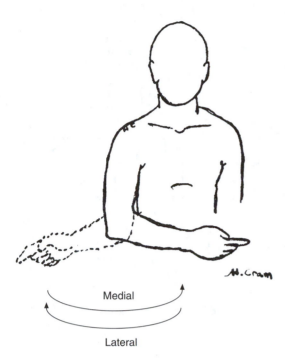

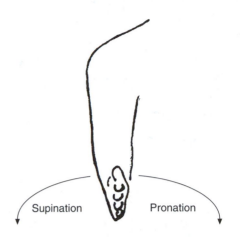

Figure 13–7 Pronation and supination at the radioulnar joint.

Figure 13–5 External (lateral) and internal (medial) rotation of the shoulder.

thumb allow one to hitchhike, while abduction and adduction of the thumb allow one to cut with scissors. Extending the fingers opens the hand, while flexing the fingers makes a fist.

Trunk movements have been studied primarily in terms of *flexion, extension, side bending, and rotation*. Flexion of the trunk brings one forward as if to touch the toes, while extension occurs when one leans back. The term, *return of the trunk* indicates a return to midline from a flexed position. Side bending occurs when the subject bends to the side while sliding the hand down the leg. Axial rotation of the trunk entails rotation of the chest relative to the pelvis. In some cases, the hips must be stabilized to facilitate and isolate rotation of the torso. Flexion and extension of the trunk are presented in Figure 13–11.

Hip and lower extremity movements are relatively straightforward. Figure 13–12 shows *hip flexion, extension, abduction, and adduction*. Hip flexion and extension occur when the leg moves forward and backward in the sagittal plane. One flexes the leg, moving it forward to take a step, and then extends the leg backward to push off to move the leg forward. Abduction moves the leg out to the side, while adduction moves the leg in toward midline. *Internal rotation* rotates the foot/knee in toward midline,

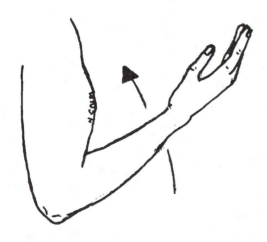

Figure 13–6 Elbow flexion.

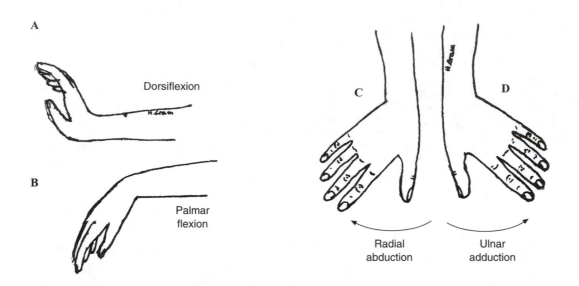

Figure 13–8 Function of muscles acting on the wrist. (**A**) Extension, (**B**) flexion, (**C**) radial abduction, (**D**) ulnar adduction.

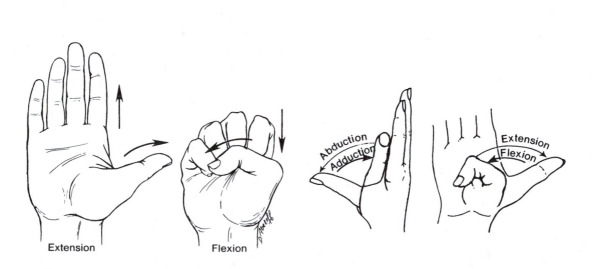

Figure 13–9 Finger flexion and extension of the thumb and fingers. *Source:* Reprinted with permission from J Basmajian, *Primary Anatomy*, p 159, © 1982, Williams & Wilkins.

Figure 13–10 Thumb abduction, adduction, flexion, and extension. *Source:* Reprinted with permission from J Basmajian, *Primary Anatomy*, p 95, © 1982, Williams & Wilkins.

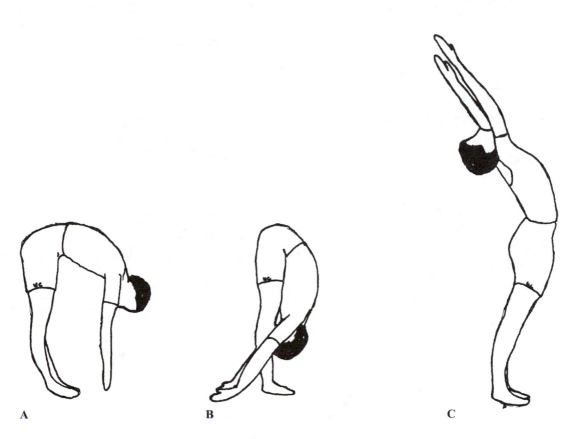

A   B   C

Figure 13–11 Movement of the vertebral column. (**A**) Flexion, (**B**) flexion combined with hip hyperflexion, and (**C**) extension.

while *external rotation* rotates the foot/knee out away from midline. *Knee flexion* occurs when hamstrings shorten and the knee bends, while *extension* occurs when the rectus femoris shortens and the leg straightens. *Plantar flexion* oc-

curs when the toe is pointed. *Dorsiflexion* occurs when the toes are pointed toward the knee. *Inversion and eversion* of the foot are illustrated in Figure 13–13. The foot is rolled inward to invert and rolled outward to evert it.

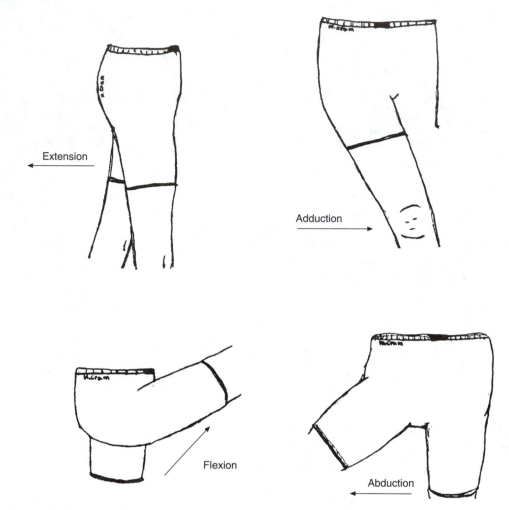

Figure 13–12 Muscle function and movement of the hip.

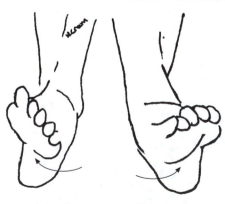

Figure 13–13 Inversion and eversion of the left foot.

REFERENCES

1. Lynn PA, Bettles ND, Hughes AD, Johnson SW. Influence of electrode geometry on bipolar recordings of the surface electromyogram. *Med Biol Eng Comput.* 1978;16:651–660.

2. Kendall FP, Kendall E, McCreary BA. *Muscles: Testing and Function.* 3rd ed. Baltimore: Williams & Wilkins; 1983.

3. Travell J, Simons D. *Myofascial Pain and Dysfunction: A Trigger Point Manual, I and II.* Baltimore: Williams & Wilkins; 1983.

4. Donaldson S, Skubick D, Donaldson M. *Electromyography, Trigger Points and Myofascial Syndromes.* Calgary, Alberta: Behavioral Health Consultants; 1991.

5. Donaldson S, Skubick D, Clasby B, Cram J. The evaluation of trigger-point activity using dynamic EMG techniques. *Am J Pain Manage.* 1994;4:118–122.

6. Gowitzke B, Milner M. *Scientific Basis of Human Movement.* 3rd ed. Baltimore: Williams & Wilkins; 1988.

CHAPTER 14

Electrode Placements

FRONTAL (WIDE) PLACEMENT

Type of Placement: General

Purpose: General recording of facial muscle activity; favors upper face

Clinical Uses: Psychophysiology, stress profiling, general relaxation

Location: Electrodes are placed on the forehead, with the ground electrode in the center and the two active electrodes one quarter inch above the eyebrow directly above the iris of the eyes (Figure 14–1A).

Behavioral Test: Ask the patient to raise the eyebrows, frown, clench teeth, and swallow. All of these movements will be seen by this wide placement.

Tracing Comment: In Figure 14–1B, the upper tracing shows surface electromyography (sEMG) from the wide frontal placement, while the lower tracing shows sEMG from the masseter muscle site. Following baseline, the patient is asked to raise the brow. Here, a clear separation between the frontal lead and the masseter may be seen. Next, the subject is asked to clench the teeth. Clenching of the jaw (masseteric activity) may be seen in frontal leads. This is an excellent example of volume conduction (processed: full-wave rectified recording).

Clinical Considerations: This site is considered a good barometer of general emotional state.[1,2] It is one of the original sites used in psychophysiological research,[3] particularly in assessing physiological responses to stress.[2] It is considered useful in the assessment of stress-related disorders such as anxiety, autonomic nervous system symptomology (eg, asthma, irritable bowel syndrome), headache, and temporal mandibular joint dysfunction.[4,5] This site has been used extensively to study and treat headache.[6] Biofeedback from this site is commonly used as an adjunct to general relaxation training.

Volume Conduction: Primarily frontalis, temporalis, corrugator, nasalis, and masseter

Other Sites of Interest: Temporal/mastoid, midcervical paraspinal, upper trapezius (wide), and forearm to assess and facilitate generalization

Artifacts: Swallowing, talking

Benchmark: Relaxed ($N = 46$): 2.5 µV (RMS) ($\pm$ 0.63)
Stressful Image ($N = 46$): 3.6 µV (RMS) ($\pm$ 0.78)
Recorded using Autogen 1700 set at 100-to-200–Hz filter.[7]

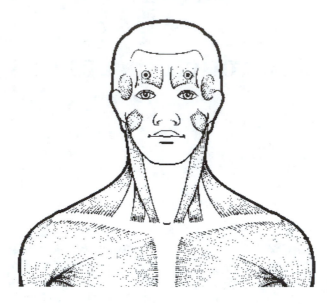

Figure 14–1A Electrode placement for frontal site. *Source:* Copyright © Clinical Resources, Inc.

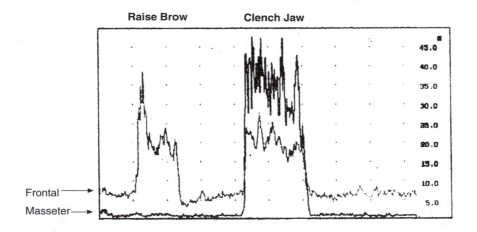

Figure 14–1B Frontal recordings during eyebrow flash and jaw clench. Note volume conduction to frontal leads during jaw clench. *Source:* Copyright © Clinical Resources, Inc.

TEMPORAL/MASTOID (WIDE) PLACEMENT

Type of Placement: General

Purpose: General recordings from the cephalic musculature. Accesses facial, cervical, and temporal muscle sets. Four sets of recordings may be taken from these electrodes.

Clinical Uses: Headache, tinnitus, other cephalgia

Location: Four electrodes are placed. An electrode is placed over the right and left anterior temporal muscles. Go lateral to the orbit of the eye, placing the electrodes approximately 3 cm above the zygomatic arch, just lateral to the eyebrow. The practitioner should palpate the muscle by placing the fingers in the temple area, just lateral to the eyebrow. Have the patient clench his or her teeth. The practitioner will feel the muscle bulge. Stay forward of the hairline. The other two electrodes are placed on the mastoid process, just below the hairline behind the ear (Figures 14–2A and 14–2B).

As a variation to the placement noted above, two electrodes can be placed at each of the four sites mentioned above. Two electrodes with a 2-cm spacing can be placed at the temporal sites so that one electrode is on the temporal location as noted above, and the second of the electrode pair is oriented obliquely toward the frontalis muscle. In addition, two electrodes with a 2-cm spacing can be placed at the mastoid site so that one of the electrode pairs is placed over the mastoid process as noted above, and the second pair is oriented obliquely toward the cervical paraspinals. In this way, four leads can be monitored simultaneously as is depicted in the tracing in Figure 14–2C.

Behavioral Test: Raise brow, frown, clench teeth, cervical flexion, extension and rotation of the head, wiggle ears

Tracing Comment: In Figure 14–2C, all four sets of recordings are shown simultaneously during eyebrow raise (F), head rotation (R), and ear wiggling (W). The top tracing is from the wide temporal leads, the second tracing is from the left temporal mastoid leads, the third tracing is from the right temporal mastoid leads, and the bottom tracing is from the wide mastoid leads. The mild asymmetry between the right and left temporal/mastoid recordings during ear wiggling is considered abnormal. To display all four recordings simultaneously may require a special cable or a variation of the electrode placement. These recordings were done using the variation of the electrode placement described above. In addition, it should be noted that recording the frontal and cervical leads separately (ie, at a later point in time) from right and left temporal/mastoid leads is acceptable (full-wave rectified recording).

Clinical Considerations: This placement was originally presented by Schwartz,[5] and was examined in the field by Hudzynski and Lawrence.[8] Its beauty lies in its ability to sample from the cephalic musculature, front and back and both sides, rather than relying on a single indicator such as the wide frontal placement. A comparison of the facial versus cervical activity is accomplished by monitoring the widely spaced temporal electrodes with one set of leads, and with the widely spaced cervical electrodes with the second set of leads. As an alternative or in addition to the frontal-cervical comparisons, the right and left cephalic muscles may be monitored by simultaneously recording from the temporalis and mastoid leads on the right and the left sides independently.

Volume Conduction: Frontalis-occipitalis, temporalis (anterior and posterior), corrugator, orbicularis oculi, masseter, capitis muscle groups, levator scapulae, sternocleidomastoid, and scalene

Other Sites of Interest: Upper trapezius (wide), forearm extensor bundle (wide) to promote generalization

Artifacts: Swallowing, breathing, talking

Benchmark: Left frontal cervical placement ($N = 25$): 3:32 µV (RMS) (± 1.22)

Right frontal cervical placement ($N = 25$): 3.09 µV (RMS) (± 1.12)

Recorded during quiet sitting using J&J M-57 set at 100-to-200–Hz filter.[8]

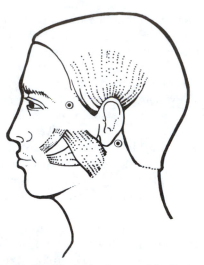

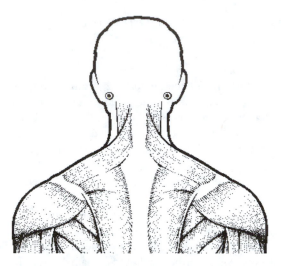

Figure 14–2A Electrode placement for the temporal/mastoid (wide) site. The temporal mastoid placements are shown from the side. *Source:* Copyright © Clinical Resources, Inc.

Figure 14–2B Electrode placement for the temporal/mastoid (wide) placement. The mastoid leads are shown from a posterior view. *Source:* Copyright © Clinical Resources, Inc.

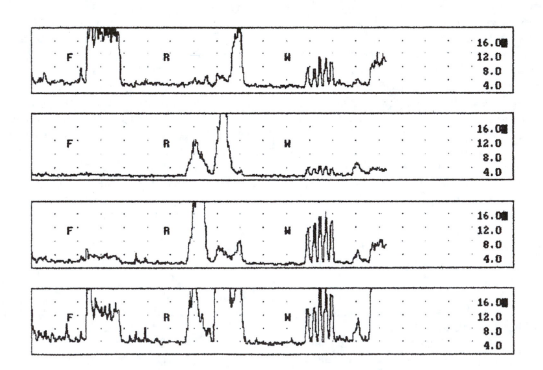

Figure 14–2C Surface EMG recordings using four leads from the temporal/mastoid electrodes. The top tracing is from the wide temporal leads, the second tracing is from the left temporalis/mastoid leads. The third tracing is from the right temporal/mastoid lead. The bottom tracing is from the wide mastoid leads. All four sets of recordings are shown simultaneously during (**F**) eyebrow raise, (**R**) head rotation, and (**W**) ear wiggling. *Source:* Copyright © Clinical Resources, Inc.

TEMPORAL/MASSETER (WIDE) PLACEMENT

Type of Placement: General

Purpose: General recording of mastication and facial muscles

Clinical Uses: Temporomandibular joint (TMJ) dysfunction and other oral facial pain disorders

Location: Right and left aspects are monitored separately. One electrode is placed on the anterior temporalis muscle, while the second electrode is placed on the masseter muscle. The anterior temporalis muscle is located in the temple region. Go lateral to the orbit of the eye, placing the electrodes approximately 3 cm above the zygomatic arch, just lateral to the eyebrow. Place fingers on the temple area and ask the patient to clench his/her teeth. Feel the muscle bulge and place electrode there. The masseter muscle group is located between the cheek bone and the corner of the jaw. Palpate the location by placing the fingers over that area; ask the patient to clench the teeth. Feel the muscle bulge. Place the electrode in the center of the muscle mass (Figure 14–3A).

Behavioral Test: Clench teeth, lateral excursion of the jaw, protraction and retraction of the jaw

Tracing Comment: In Figure 14–3B, recordings are from the right and left aspects of the temporal/masseter site. A brief rest is followed by clenching the teeth together. Note the symmetry of recruitment. The next four movements entail left lateral excursion, right lateral excursion, retraction, and protraction of the jaw. Note the asymmetrical recruitment during the asymmetrical movements of right and left lateral excursion. Also note the symmetrical recruitment during the symmetrical movement of protraction and retraction (processed: full-wave rectified recording).

Clinical Considerations: This placement records from both the upper and lower face, providing a very global view of functioning for the right and left aspects. Symmetry of electrode placement must be emphasized if one is concerned with asymmetrical patterns observed during movement. As a treatment site, it can provide the basis for a well-directed, general relaxation training protocol,[5] or it can be used for feedback for quiet movements of the jaw.[9]

Volume Conduction: Anterior and posterior temporalis, masseter, frontalis, corrugator, orbicularis oculi, orbicularis oris, buccinator, zygomaticus

Other Sites of Interest: Temporal mylohyoid, midcervical paraspinal, upper trapezius (wide) to assess and promote generalization

Artifacts: Swallowing, talking

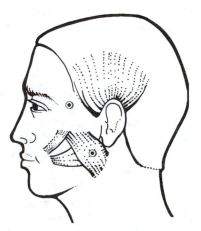

Figure 14–3A Electrode placement for temporal/masseter (wide) site. *Source:* Copyright © Clinical Resources, Inc.

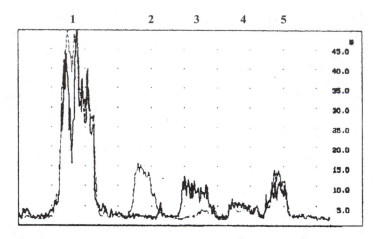

Figure 14–3B Surface EMG tracing for right and left temporal/masseter placement during (**1**) clench, lateral excursion of the jaw to the (**2**) left and then (**3**) right, followed by (**4**) protraction and (**5**) protrusion. *Source:* Copyright © Clinical Resources, Inc.

TEMPORAL/SUPRAHYOID (WIDE) PLACEMENT

Type of Placement: General

Purpose: To monitor general facial and perioral muscle activity

Clinical Uses: TMJ dysfunction, oral facial pain, and anxiety-related disorders

Location: An active electrode is placed on the anterior temporalis. Palpate the muscle belly by placing the fingers lateral to the notch in the eye and asking the patient to clench his/her teeth. Go lateral to the orbit of the eye, placing the electrode approximately 3 cm above the zygomatic arch, just lateral to the eyebrow. To locate the area of the mylohyoid/digastric muscles, palpate the area by placing the fingers under the patient's chin and asking the patient to open the jaw wide several times. Place the electrode over the muscle mass that is felt toward the anterior lateral border of the underside of the chin (Figure 14–4A).

Behavioral Test: Ask the patient to move the jaw through its range of motion (open, close/clench, lateral, protrusion, retraction), frown, raise the brow, smile. Any facial movement should be seen.

Tracing Comment: Figure 14–4B presents sEMG recordings from the right and left temporal/suprahyoid placement during teeth clench, mouth opening, and left and right lateral deviations. Symmetry is noted during symmetrical movements and separation of function during lateral deviations (full-wave rectified recording).

Clinical Considerations: This placement was introduced by Schneider and Wilson;[10] and Hudzynski and Lawrence[8] elaborated on a clinical protocol for its use. It provides a very general neuromuscular assessment of the perioral muscles for stress-related and movement components. As a treatment site, it can provide the basis for a well-directed, general relaxation-training protocol, or it may be used for feedback for quiet movements of the jaw.[9]

Volume Conduction: Frontalis, corrugator, anterior temporalis, orbicularis oculi, orbicularis oris, masseter, buccinator, mentalis, depressor, digastric, hyoid muscles, and tongue

Other Sites of Interest: Midcervical paraspinals, upper trapezius (wide) to assess and promote generalization

Artifacts: Swallowing, talking

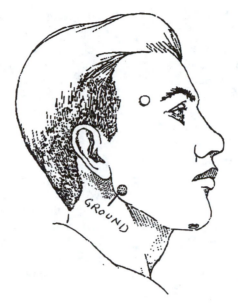

Figure 14–4A Electrode placement for temporal suprahyoid (wide) site. *Source:* Copyright © Clinical Resources, Inc.

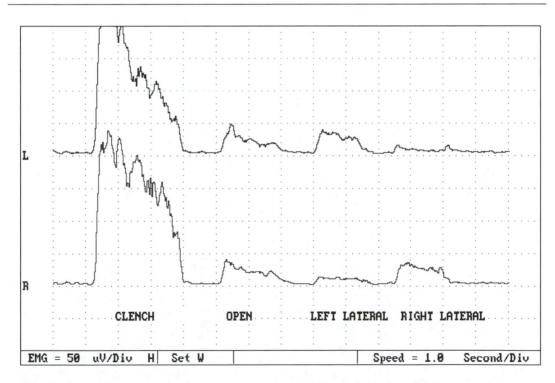

Figure 14–4B Surface EMG recordings from the right and left temporal/suprahyoid placement during teeth clench, mouth opening, and left and right lateral deviations. *Source:* Copyright © Clinical Resources, Inc.

SUPRAHYOID PLACEMENT

Type of Placement: Quasi-specific

Purpose: To record general muscle activity from the muscles that open the mouth, move the tongue, and elevate the larynx

Clinical Uses: Dysphagia, TMJ dysfunction

Muscle Insertions: The suprahyoid muscles (mylohyoids, digastrics, geniohyoids) originate on the mandible and insert on the hyoid bone. They primarily raise the hyoid bone in swallowing and/or opening the jaw.

Location: One set of electrodes is placed under the chin in the midline, running in the anterior-to-posterior direction. Palpate the area by placing the fingers under the chin; ask the patient to swallow a few times. Place the electrodes in the center of that mass (Figure 14–5A).

Behavioral Test: Swallowing, jaw opening

Tracing Comment: Figure 14–5B presents sEMG recordings from the right and left aspects of the suprahyoid site during swallowing, protruding of the tongue, and speaking (saying the alphabet). The amplitudes and derecruitment patterns are typical for the site (processed sEMG).

Figure 14–5C presents sEMG recording from the temporalis and suprahyoid sites during teeth clench, mouth opening, and left and right lateral deviations. Symmetry is noted during the symmetrical movements (eg, clench), and separation of function is noted during the lateral excursions. One can also see the role that the temporalis plays in clenching and the suprahyoids play in mouth opening (raw sEMG).

Also see tracings for temporalis/suprahyoid site (Figure 14–4B).

Clinical Considerations: This site is useful in the treatment of dysphagia.[11,12] An emphasis is placed on shaping and training the correct muscle recruitment pattern during swallowing.

Volume Conduction: Platysma, sternocleidomastoid

Other Sites of Interest: Masseter, buccinator, orbicularis oris during oral movements; temporal, midcervical paraspinal, upper trapezius (wide) to assess and treat generalized tension

Artifact: Talking

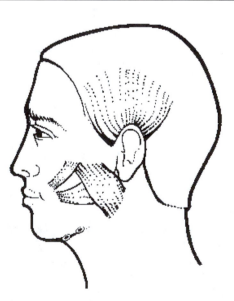

Figure 14–5A Placement of suprahyoid electrode. *Source:* Copyright © Clinical Resources, Inc.

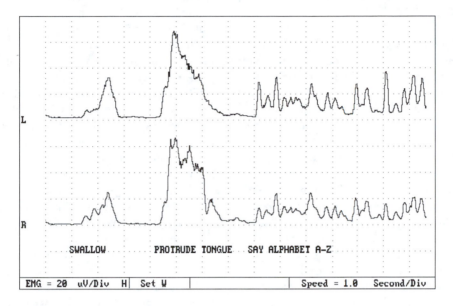

Figure 14–5B Surface EMG recordings from the right and left aspects of the suprahyoid site during swallowing, protruding of the tongue, and speaking (saying the alphabet). *Source:* Copyright © Clinical Resources, Inc.

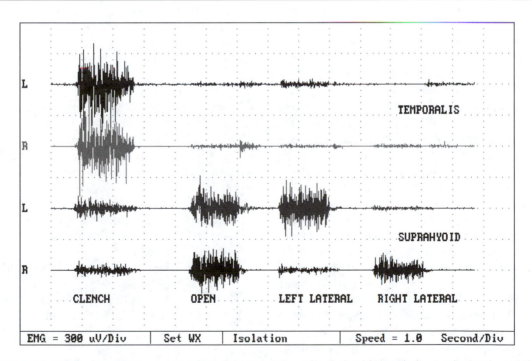

Figure 14–5C Surface EMG recording from the temporalis and suprahyoid sites during teeth clench, mouth opening, and left and right lateral deviations. *Source:* Copyright © Clinical Resources, Inc.

CERVICAL TRAPEZIUS (WIDE) PLACEMENT

Type of Placement: General

Purpose: To monitor general muscle activity from the upper back and neck, while assessing right and left side differences

Clinical Uses: Headaches, shoulder pain, upper quarter pain, repetitive strain injury (RSI), tension myalgias

Location: Two sets of electrodes are used—one for the right aspect and one for the left. For each side, one electrode is placed in the middle cervical area (approximately at C-4) and about 1 cm from midline over the muscle mass. Palpate to locate the muscle mass that parallels the spine. The second electrode is placed over the upper fibers of trapezius, along the ridge of the shoulder, approximately half the distance between the cervical vertebra at C-7 and the acromion. Palpate the muscle mass and place slightly lateral to that center point. See Figure 14–6A.

Behavioral Test: Shoulder elevation, retraction, protraction, cervical rotation, flexion, and lateral bending

Tracing Comment: Figure 14–6B provides a view of sEMG recorded from the cervical trapezius sites using both a 25-to-1000–Hz band-pass filter (wide) that shows the ECG artifact, and a 100-to-200–Hz filter (narrow). Notice how low and balanced the sEMG is for the 100-to-200–Hz filter setting. A noteworthy respiration artifact is present throughout. This is abnormal. When the 25-to-1000–Hz filter is used, the ECG artifact is quite striking on the left aspect for this subject. The respiration artifact continues to be clearly seen through the troughs of the recording. The amplitude attributed to the tracing would be determined by reading the value at the trough of the tracing. Because of the marked ECG artifact, using an integrated sEMG value would provide an inaccurate estimate of the sEMG amplitude for the left aspect (full-wave rectified recording).

Figure 14–6C presents sEMG recordings from cervical trapezius placement using the 100-to-200–Hz filter during head rotation to the right and left, followed by a shoulder girdle elevation (full-wave rectified recording).

Figure 14–6D presents right and left recordings from the placement sites using the 100-to-200–Hz filter during quiet sitting, standing, walking in place, standing a second time, and returning to the sitting posture.[13] Notice how quiet the sEMG recordings are except during the movements associated with the transition from one posture to another and during walking in place (full-wave rectified recording).

Also see tracings for cervical dorsal (Figures 14–18B, 14–18C) and dorsal lumbar (Figure 14–47B) placements for extensions of this wide placement strategy.

Clinical Considerations: Because this site monitors from the neck and upper back in general, it is particularly useful for assessing general levels of tension (resting levels).[14] This site is useful in teaching and reinforcing general relaxation skills. In addition, it is particularly useful as an indicator of how these muscles are affected by posture. Ettare and Ettare[13] have developed extensive clinical protocols for the use of this site in training patients to return to healthy levels of rest following changes in posture or movement.

Volume Conduction: Upper, middle, and lower trapezius; capitis muscle groups; levator scapulae; rhomboid; and scalene

Other Sites of Interest: Frontal (wide), temporalis (wide), forearm extensors (wide), wrist-to-wrist site to assess and promote generalization

Artifacts: ECG, breathing

Benchmark: Sitting quietly: 2.0 μV (RMS)
Standing, arms at sides: 2.0 μV (RMS)
Walking in place: 5.0 (± 1.0) μV (RMS)
Values from Ettare and Ettare[13] using J&J M-501 with 100-to-200–Hz filter.

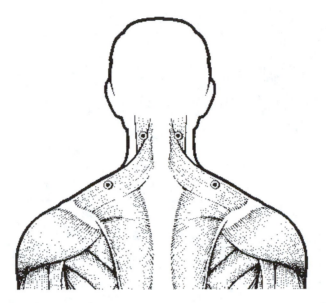

Figure 14–6A Electrode placement for cervical trapezius (wide) site. *Source:* Copyright © Clinical Resources, Inc.

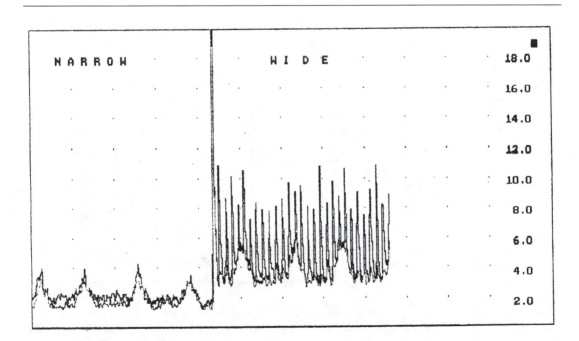

Figure 14–6B Surface EMG recordings from cervical trapezius at rest. The right aspect of the tracing was conducted using a 25-to-1000–Hz band-pass filter (wide) while the left aspect was conducted using a 100-to-200–Hz filter (narrow). Notice how the 100-to-200–Hz filter eliminates the ECG artifact, while the right aspect of the cervical trapezius leads shows a striking ECG artifact. Also note the respiratory artifact is present in both types of filtering. This is considered abnormal. *Source:* Copyright © Clinical Resources, Inc.

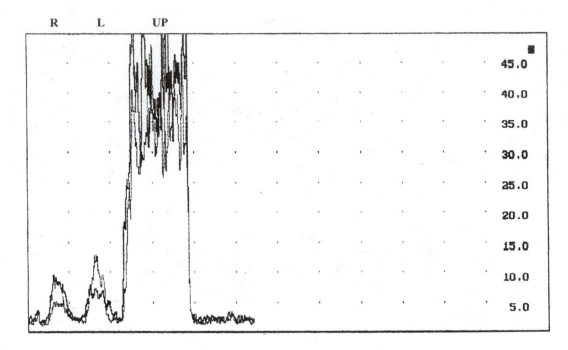

Figure 14–6C Surface EMG recordings from cervical trapezius placement using the 100-to-200–Hz filter during head rotation to the right and left, followed by a (**UP**) shoulder girdle elevation. There is separation of recruitment during rotation, and symmetry during elevation. *Source:* Copyright © Clinical Resources, Inc.

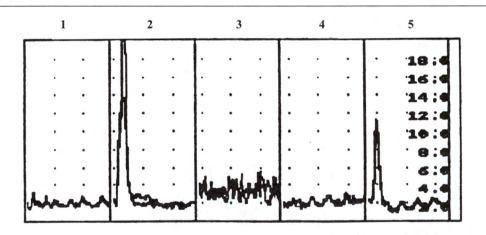

Figure 14–6D Surface EMG recording from the right and left cervical trapezius electrode placement during (**1**) sitting, (**2**) standing, (**3**) walking in place, (**4**) standing again, and (**5**) sitting. *Source:* Copyright © Clinical Resources, Inc.

UPPER TRAPEZIUS (WIDE) PLACEMENT

Type of Placement: General

Purpose: General recording of muscles of the upper back and neck

Clinical Uses: Headache, neck, shoulder pain, upper quarter pain, tension myalgias

Location: Electrodes are placed on the upper back, with the two active electrodes placed at the upper crest of the shoulder, halfway between the spine (C-7) and the acromion of the shoulder. Palpate the muscle at the crest and place over the area of largest mass (Figure 14–7A).

Behavioral Test: Ask the patient to raise the shoulders, rotate the head, and pull the shoulder blades together.

Tracing Comment: Figure 14–7B presents sEMG recordings from a wide upper trapezius placement during resting baseline, shoulder elevation (up), and retraction (back). The left aspect of the tracing, which was collected using a 25-to-1000–Hz band-pass filter, shows the ECG artifact. The right side of the tracing used a 100-to-200–Hz band-pass filter, which eliminated the ECG artifact. This may be seen during the rest periods between movements (full-wave rectified recording).

Clinical Considerations: This site is a good barometer of the shoulder elevation associated with an aroused emotional state.[3] It is useful in assessing and treating stress-related disorders, anxiety, asthma, hyperventilation syndromes, and headache.[5] It is also useful as part of an evaluation of neck and shoulder pain and RSI.[15]

Volume Conduction: Upper, middle, and lower trapezius; rhomboids; capitis muscle groups; levator scapulae; posterior deltoids

Other Sites of Interest: Frontal (wide), temporal (wide), forearm extensors (wide), wrist-to-wrist site to assess and promote generalization

Artifacts: ECG, breathing

Benchmark: At rest (sitting quietly): 3.3 (± 0.64) µV (RMS)
Stressful imagery: 3.8 (± 0.37) µV (RMS)
Recorded using Autogen 1700 with 100-to-200–Hz filter.

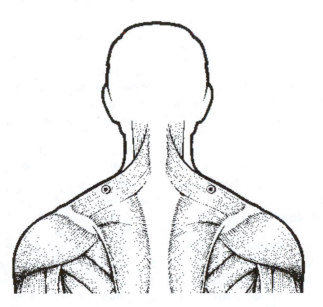

Figure 14–7A Electrode placement for upper trapezius (wide) site. *Source:* Copyright © Clinical Resources, Inc.

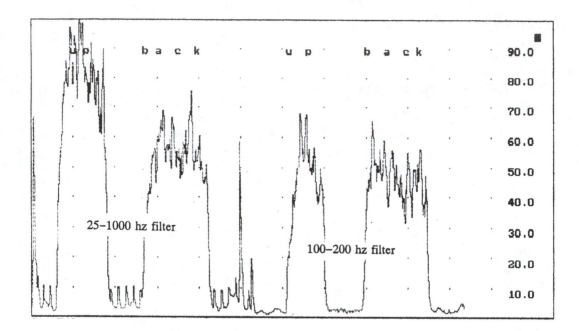

Figure 14–7B Surface recordings from upper trapezius leads using both a 25-to-1000–Hz filter (left side) and a 100-to-200–Hz filter (right side) during a shoulder elevation and retraction. Notice how the 100-to-200–Hz filter eliminates the ECG artifact during the resting baselines periods. *Source:* Copyright © Clinical Resources, Inc.

ANTERIOR TEMPORALIS PLACEMENT

Type of Placement: Specific

Action: Elevation of the mandible, retraction and lateral deviation of mandible, assistance in chewing

Clinical Uses: TMJ dysfunction and related disorders

Muscle Insertions: The anterior temporalis arises from the temporal fossa and inserts into the coronoid process of the mandible.

Innervation: Mandibular branch of the trigeminal nerve (fifth cranial nerve)

Location: To monitor the anterior portion of temporalis, palpate the temple region while the patient clenches his/her teeth. Two active electrodes, approximately 2 cm apart, are placed over the muscle mass so that they run parallel to the muscle fibers. The lowest electrode of the pair is placed just above the zygomatic arch or opposite the notch of the eye (Figure 14–8A).

Variations: The temporalis muscle also has posterior fibers, which are more consistently involved in retraction (retrusion) and lateral deviation of the mandible.[4,16] This placement is located on the lateral aspect of the head, behind the ear. Electrodes are placed on the bare skin, behind the flap of the ear.

Behavioral Test: Clench jaw, lateral deviation of the jaw, protraction and retraction of the jaw, swallowing

Tracing Comment: In Figure 14–8B, tracings of temporalis (top two tracings) and masseter (bottom two tracings) show synergistic functions during jaw clenching and chewing (raw sEMG).

Clinical Considerations: With normal dentition, gentle closure of the jaw is primarily associated with the anterior fibers of temporalis.[4] The temporalis muscle is responsible for keeping the mandible in the rest position while in the upright posture.[16] The patient may need to separate the teeth and intentionally relax the jaw musculature before quiet levels of recording are seen at this site with surface electrodes. Placing the tip of the tongue on the roof of the mouth just behind the front teeth can help quiet the perioral musculature. In addition, with patients who cannot intentionally relax the muscles at this site in the upright posture, the practitioner can attempt to do the procedure with the patient supine. Any training in the supine posture would then need to be generalized to the upright posture.

Volume Conduction: Posterior temporalis, frontalis, corrugator, orbicularis oculi, masseter

Other Sites of Interest: Masseter, posterior temporalis, suprahyoid sites to assess other potential muscles associated with movement; midcervical to assess for chewing in the neck

Referred Pain Considerations: Trigger points may refer pain to the temporal region, the eyebrow, and the upper teeth.[17]

Artifacts: Swallowing, talking

Benchmark: Sitting quietly ($N = 104$): 2.4 (± 2.1) µV (RMS)

Standing quietly ($N = 104$): 2.3 (± 2.1) µV (RMS)

Values taken using a J&J M-501 EMG set with a 100-to-200–Hz filter.[18]

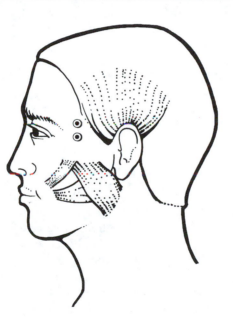

Figure 14–8A Electrode placement for anterior temporalis site. *Source:* Copyright © Clinical Resources, Inc.

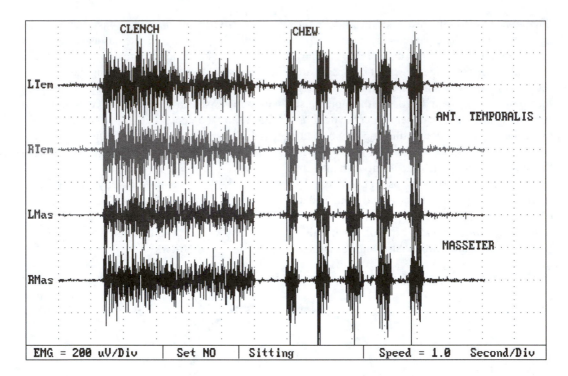

Figure 14–8B Surface EMG recordings from anterior temporalis and masseter during a clench and chewing. *Source:* Copyright © Clinical Resources, Inc.

MASSETER PLACEMENT

Type of Placement: Specific

Action: Elevation of the mandible; closure/grinding of jaw; mastication

Clinical Uses: TMJ dysfunction and oral-facial disorders

Muscle Insertions: The masseter muscle arises from the zygomatic arch (cheek bone) and inserts into the superior half of the lateral surface of the ramus of the mandible (corner of the jaw).

Innervation: The masseter is innervated by the masseteric aspect of the trigeminal nerve (fifth cranial nerve).

Location: Two active electrodes, approximately 2 cm apart, are placed along the direction of the fibers of the masseter muscle. Palpate the area while asking the patient to clench his/her teeth. Identify the muscle belly. Electrodes are

placed over the belly of the muscle. If symmetry of sEMG recording is an issue, the practitioner should be aware that slight differences in electrode placement and spacing may radically alter the sEMG recordings and conclusions regarding symmetry (Figure 14–9). Note that a forward head position may affect the resting value of the recordings.

Behavioral Test: Clench teeth, swallow, talk

Tracing Comment: In Figure 14–8B, temporalis (top two tracings) and masseter (bottom two tracings) show synergistic functions during jaw clenching and chewing (raw sEMG).

Clinical Considerations: Generally, masseter and temporalis are synergists and function concurrently. While the temporalis provides a basis for mandibular balance and postural control, the masseter is used during grinding and chewing.[19] During chewing, masseter responds before temporalis. Masseter, unlike temporalis, is not thought to be required to maintain the resting position of the mandible,[16] and it does not change its tonic levels as one moves from the sitting to supine postures.

Volume Conduction: Lateral pterygoid, buccinator, zygomaticus

Other Sites of Interest: Temporalis and suprahyoids to assess other potential muscles involved in movement of the mandible; mid-cervical paraspinals to assess for chewing in the neck

Referred Pain Considerations: Trigger points in the superficial layer of masseter may be projected to the eyebrow, maxilla, mandible, and upper or lower molar teeth.[17]

Artifacts: Swallowing, talking

Benchmark: Sitting quietly ($N = 104$): 1.7 ($\pm$ 1.3) μV (RMS)

Standing quietly ($N = 104$): 1.6 ($\pm$ 1.5) μV (RMS)

Values taken using a J&J M-501 with a 100-to-200–Hz filter.[18]

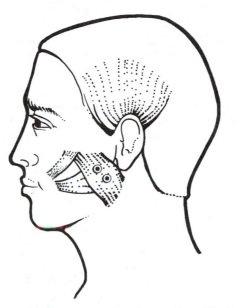

Figure 14–9 Electrode placement for the masseter site. *Source:* Copyright © Clinical Resources, Inc.

CHEEK (ZYGOMATICUS) PLACEMENT

Type of Placement: Quasi-specific

Action: Retraction and elevation of the lips, smiling

Clinical Uses: Psychophysiological studies, rehabilitation of facial muscles

Muscle Insertions: The zygomaticus arises from the zygomatic bone and the major aspect inserts into the corner of the mouth, while the minor aspect inserts into the upper portion of the lip.

Innervation: Facial nerve (seventh cranial nerve)

Location: Two active electrodes are placed so that they run parallel to the muscle fibers (cheek bone to corner of the mouth) and are placed at the midpoint (Figure 14–10A). A gross recording was obtained by using 1-cm electrodes placed 2 cm apart (Figure 14–10B). Recordings using 1-cm spacings did not improve the specificity of the recording dramatically (see also Figure 14–12B).

Behavioral Test: Smile

Tracing Comment: In Figure 14–10B, recordings with electrodes with 2-cm spacing are taken from orbicularis oculi, zygomaticus, and buccinator during a smile. Note the continual activation of orbicularis oculi throughout the tracing, indicating that the patient tends to squint, with an increased level during the smile itself. During the intentional smile, a very strong synergistic pattern occurs between zygomaticus and orbicularis oculi and buccinator. Note that a slightly different smiling expression could potentially bring out a different synergistic pattern. In addition, the smaller and more closely spaced electrodes seen in Figures 14–11B and 14–12B suggest that one cannot easily isolate the sEMG activity for zygomaticus, even with a more specific electrode placement (raw sEMG).

Clinical Considerations: The primary use of this site is in psychophysiological studies.[20] It has recently found its way into clinical use during anesthesia procedures.[21]

Volume Conduction: Masseter, buccinator, orbicularis oculi, and orbicularis oris

Other Sites of Interest: Orbicularis oculi, corrugator, frontal, and depressor anguli oris to study facial expressions

Referred Pain Considerations: Trigger points in zygomaticus major refers pain in an arch close to the side of the nose and reaching the forehead.[17]

Artifacts: Swallowing, talking

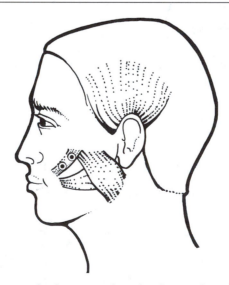

Figure 14–10A Electrode placement for the zygomaticus site. *Source:* Copyright © Clinical Resources, Inc.

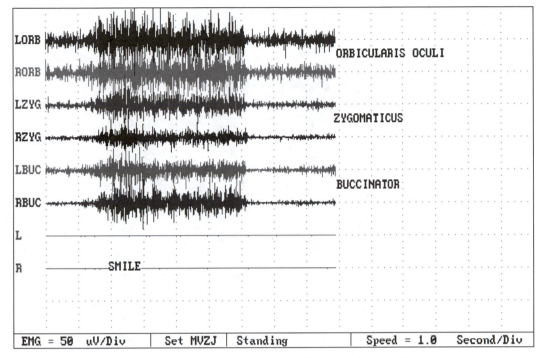

Figure 14–10B Surface EMG recordings from orbicularis oculi, zygomaticus, and buccinator using 1-cm electrodes 2 cm apart. The action is smiling. *Source:* Copyright © Clinical Resources, Inc.

ORBICULARIS OCULI PLACEMENT

Type of Placement: Specific

Action: Eye closure and squinting

Clinical Uses: Psychophysiological studies of emotions

Muscle Insertions: The orbital portion of this muscle wraps broadly around the orbit of the eye.

Innervation: Facial nerve (seventh cranial nerve)

Location: This muscle is most easily monitored by placing two closely spaced electrodes horizontally on the zygomatic bone just below the lower eyelid and toward the lateral aspect of the eye (Figure 14–11A). As can be seen in Figure 14–11B, the best recordings are obtained using miniature electrodes placed 1 cm apart. A grosser recording may be obtained by using 1-cm electrodes placed 2 cm apart (see Figure 14–12C). Compare the tracings seen in Figure 14–12C with those seen in Figure 14–11B.

Behavioral Test: Squint

Tracing Comment: Figure 14–11B presents sEMG recordings from zygomaticus and orbicularis oculi during smiling and squinting. In this individual, both muscles are active during smiling, but only the orbicularis oculi is active during squinting. Compared to Figure 14–12C, there is a slight improvement with narrowly spaced electrodes and the specificity of the sEMG recording (raw sEMG). See also the tracings for zygomaticus (Figure 14–10B) and buccinator (Figure 14–12C).

Clinical Considerations: The primary use of this site is in psychophysiological studies.[20] It has recently found its way into clinical use during anesthesia procedures.[21]

Volume Conduction: Masseter, temporalis, zygomaticus, corrugator

Other Sites of Interest: Corrugator, frontal, and zygomaticus to study emotional displays

Artifacts: Eye blinking, swallowing, talking

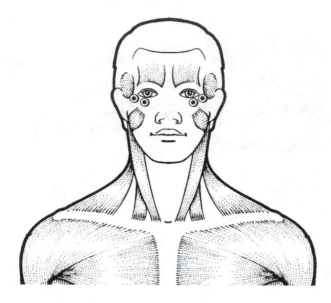

Figure 14–11A Surface EMG placement for the orbicularis oculi site. *Source:* Copyright © Clinical Resources, Inc.

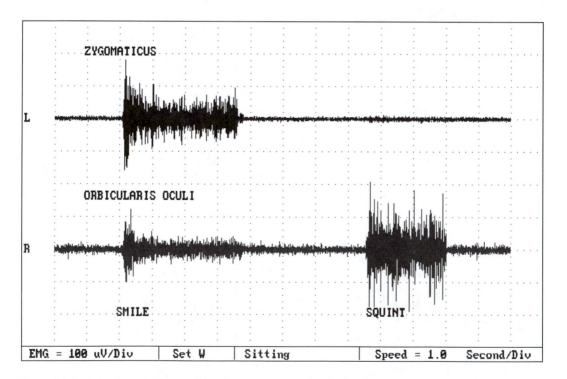

Figure 14–11B Surface EMG recordings from zygomaticus and orbicularis oculi during smiling and squinting using miniature electrodes and 1-cm spacing. *Source:* Copyright © Clinical Resources, Inc.

BUCCINATOR PLACEMENT

Type of Placement: Specific

Action: Retraction of cheek toward mandible; assists in chewing

Clinical Uses: Bell's palsy, dysphagia

Muscle Insertions: The buccinator arises from the mandible in the region of the first and second molars and extends to the corner of the mouth, blending with the orbicularis oris.

Innervation: Facial nerve (seventh cranial nerve)

Location: Two active electrodes are placed parallel to the muscle fibers. One electrode is placed just lateral to the corner of the mouth, with the second one just lateral to it (Figure 14–12A). As can be seen in a comparison of Figure 14–12B with Figure 14–12C, the best recordings are obtained using miniature electrodes placed 1 cm apart. A grosser recording may be obtained by using 1-cm electrodes placed 2 cm apart.

Behavioral Test: Press the cheeks against the sides of the teeth and pull corners of lips back as if to play a trumpet (buccinating).

Tracing Comment: Two tracings are shown with different levels of specificity. Figure 14–12B shows zygomaticus and buccinator using miniature electrodes set 1 cm apart, while Figure 14–12C shows zygomaticus, orbicularis oculi, and buccinator using larger and more widely spaced electrodes.

In Figure 14–12B, the buccinator recordings are clearly differentiated from zygomaticus recordings during buccinating but not during smiling (raw sEMG).

Figure 14–12C shows recordings from orbicularis oculi, zygomaticus, and buccinator during clenching, squinting, retracting the lips as if to play the trumpet (buccinating), and smiling. Note the volume conduction that appears on all channels during a jaw clench. The closer to the sEMG source, the larger the volume conduction. During the retraction of the lips, a strong burst of sEMG may be seen at the buccinator site. Collateral activity is also noted in zygomaticus (raw sEMG).

Clinical Considerations: This site may be useful in retraining the lips and cheek for dysphagia[11] and Bell's palsy patients.

Volume Conduction: Masseter, orbicularis oris, risorius, zygomaticus, depressor

Other Sites of Interest: Zygomaticus, depressor, orbicularis oris, and mentalis to study other muscles associated with lip and cheek movement

Artifacts: Swallowing, talking

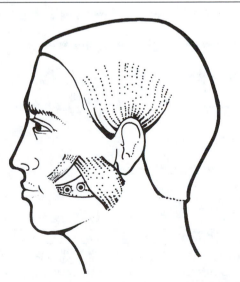

Figure 14–12A Electrode placement for buccinator site. *Source:* Copyright © Clinical Resources, Inc.

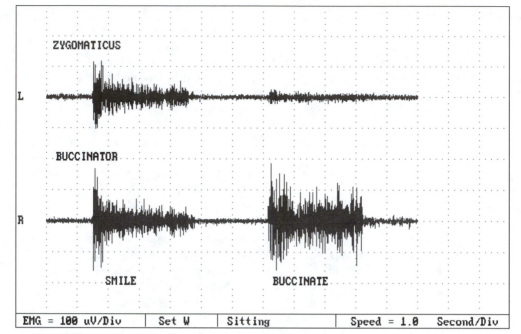

Figure 14–12B Surface EMG recordings from zygomaticus and buccinator using miniature electrodes and 1-cm spacing. The actions are smiling and buccinating. *Source:* Copyright © Clinical Resources, Inc.

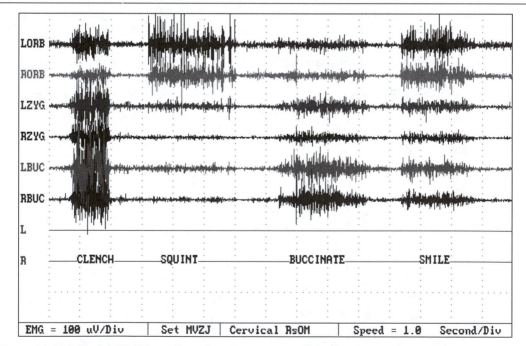

Figure 14–12C Surface EMG recordings from orbicularis oculi, zygomaticus, and buccinator using 1-cm electrodes at 2-cm spacings. The actions are clenching, squinting, buccinating, and smiling. *Source:* Copyright © Clinical Resources, Inc.

FRONTALIS (NARROW) PLACEMENT

Type of Placement: Specific

Action: Elevates the brow

Clinical Uses: Psychophysiological recordings of emotions (surprise, anger, sadness, fear)

Muscle Insertions: This muscle arises from the skin and subcutaneous tissue at the eyebrow and extends up over the crown of the head, joining the fibers of the occipitalis muscle.

Innervation: Facial nerve (seventh cranial nerve)

Location: Two active electrodes (2 cm apart) are placed vertically, half the distance between the eyebrow and the hairline, just lateral of midline and parallel to the muscle fibers of interest (Figure 14–13A). As can be seen in Figure 14–14B, the best recordings are obtained using miniature electrodes placed 1 cm apart. A grosser recording (see Figure 14–13B) may be obtained by using 1-cm electrodes placed 2 cm apart.

Variations: Due to the high innervation ratio of this muscle, the degree of lateral placement from midline may allow the practitioner to record different aspects of emotional displays.[22]

Behavioral Test: Raise the brow as in surprise.

Tracing Comment: Figure 14–13B shows recordings from two sets of electrodes, 2 cm apart, which have been placed over the frontalis. The most lateral electrodes were placed above the iris of the eye, and the medial electrodes were placed just lateral of midline. In addition, corrugator is monitored. Three emotional displays are studied: anger, surprise, and sadness. Note that the frontalis muscle is active during surprise and sadness, but only minimally active during anger. During sadness, there is a strong synergy pattern noted with corrugator. The practitioner should note that slight variations in the emotional expression could result in slightly different synergistic patterns. The specificity of the recordings is improved slightly with more narrowly spaced electrodes (see Figure 14–14B).

Clinical Considerations: Systematic study of the right and left aspects of the frontalis muscle may yield information concerning the emotionality of an individual. Sackeim and his colleagues[23] found that the left aspect of the frontalis is more active during emotional events. In addition, this site has recently been used by Bennett and Kornhauser[21] as part of an algorithm for assessing nocioception and consciousness during anesthesia.

Volume Conduction: Corrugator, temporalis, and masseter

Other Sites of Interest: Corrugator, orbicularis oculi, zygomaticus, depressor to study emotional displays; midcervical, upper trapezius, forearm extensor bundle (wide) to assess for general tension levels

Referred Pain Considerations: Trigger points in the belly of frontalis muscle projects pain diffusely over the local muscle belly.[17]

Artifacts: Swallowing, nonverbal communication

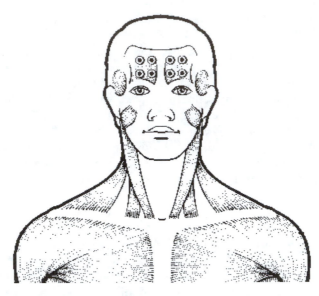

Figure 14–13A Electrode placement for frontalis (narrow) site. These electrodes are placed vertically so as to follow the direction of the muscle fibers. *Source:* Copyright © Clinical Resources, Inc.

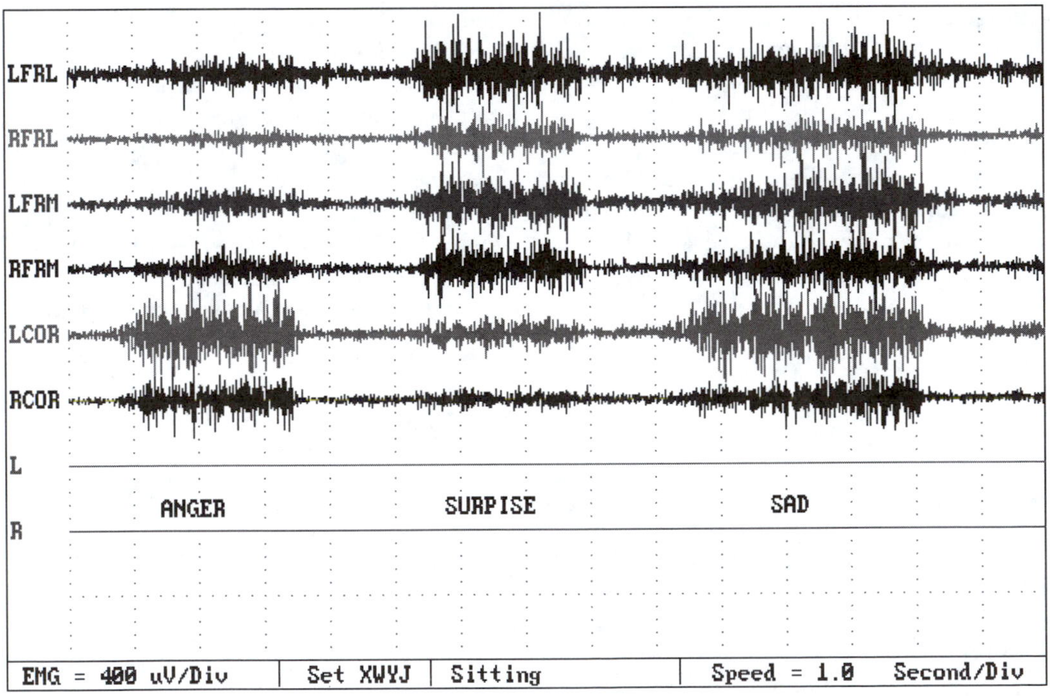

Figure 14–13B Surface EMG recordings using electrodes 2 cm apart placed on (FRL) lateral and (FRM) medial frontalis, along with (COR) corrugator. The subject is asked to display anger, surprise, and sadness. *Source:* Copyright © Clinical Resources, Inc.

CORRUGATOR PLACEMENT

Type of Placement: Specific

Action: Frowning at the brow

Clinical Uses: Psychophysiological studies of emotional displays

Muscle Insertions: This small muscle arises from the superciliary arch of the frontal bone (just above the nose) and inserts into the skin of the middle third of the supraorbital margin, at the eyebrow.

Innervation: Facial nerve (seventh cranial nerve)

Location: Two active electrodes are placed over the eyebrow just lateral of midline and at a slightly oblique angle (Figure 14–14A). As can be seen in Figure 14–14B, the best recordings are obtained using miniature electrodes placed 1 cm apart. Compare this to Figure 14–13B, in which a grosser recording is obtained by using 1-cm electrodes placed 2 cm apart.

Behavioral Test: Furrow the brow, frown

Tracing Comment: Figure 14–14B presents sEMG recordings using 1-cm spacings from corrugator and (medial) frontalis during the three facial expressions of anger, surprise, and sadness. Corrugator is more active during anger and sadness than surprise, while frontalis is most active during surprise and modestly active during sadness. Both corrugator and frontalis are active during expressions of sadness. By comparing Figure 14–13B with 14–14B, one can note that the more narrowly spaced electrodes (Figure 14–14B) provide a cleaner recording and separation of muscle function. Slight changes in any of the emotional expressions can result in changes in the synergistic patterns (raw sEMG).

Clinical Considerations: The corrugator is responsible for the furrowing of the brow, as in the display of anger. In addition, this site has recently been used by Bennett and Kornhauser[21] as part of an algorithm for assessing nocioception and consciousness during anesthesia.

Volume Conduction: Procerus, frontalis, orbicularis oculi

Other Sites of Interest: Frontalis, orbicularis oculi, zygomaticus, depressor to study emotional displays; masseter, temporalis, midcervical, and upper trapezius to assess generalized tension

Artifacts: Eye blink, nonverbal communication

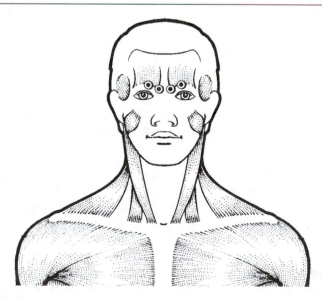

Figure 14–14A Surface EMG placement for corrugator site. *Source:* Copyright © Clinical Resources, Inc.

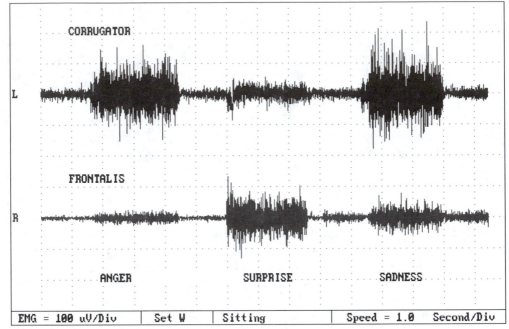

Figure 14–14B Surface EMG recordings from miniature electrodes, 1 cm apart, placed on the (medial) frontalis and corrugator muscles. The actions are anger, surprise, and sadness. *Source:* Copyright © Clinical Resources, Inc.

STERNOCLEIDOMASTOID (SCM) PLACEMENT

(Also known as sternomastoid)

Type of Placement: Specific

Action: Rotation of the head to the contralateral side, ipsilateral side bending, and forward flexion

Clinical Uses: Neck, shoulder, and headache pain

Muscle Insertions: This two-bellied muscle arises by one head from the sternum and the other head from the clavicle and inserts onto the mastoid process.

Innervation: The accessory nerve; via the cervical plexus, the ventral rami of the C-2 and C-3 spinal nerves

Joint Considerations: The SCM is attached to the anterior and superior surfaces of the sternum, and the superior border of the proximal third of the clavicle. The upper attachments include the mastoid process of the temporal bone and the lateral portion of the superior nuchal line of the occipital bone. Thus the joints directly related to

the muscle length include the S-C joint, the cervical joints as a group, and the O/A joint in particular.

Location: Palpate the large muscle belly on the anterior lateral aspect of the neck. Two active electrodes (2 cm apart) are placed half the distance between the mastoid process and the sternal notch, slightly posterior to the center of the muscle belly so that they run parallel to the muscle fibers. If the practitioner asks the patient to rotate the head to identify the muscle belly, electrodes should be placed once the patient has returned to the midline position (Figure 14–15A).

Behavioral Test: Rotate, side bend, or flex the head

Tracing Comment: In Figures 14–15B and 14–15D, the SCM, scalene, and C-4 paraspinals are monitored; in Figure 14–15C, the upper trapezius (narrow) placement has been added.

In Figure 14–15B, a comfortable, self-limited axial rotational pattern is studied. Note the cooperative functions between SCM and C-4 paraspinal during rotation. The left SCM activates first to provide movement during right rotation; the right C-4 paraspinal activates a little later. The opposite is true for left rotation. Also note how quiet the scalene muscles are during this movement, showing good isolation of the sEMG recordings for these sites in this individual (raw sEMG).

In Figure 14–15C, rotational patterns are studied again, but this time with the inclusion of the upper trapezius muscle. This tracing is similar to Figure 14–15B, in that the scalene remains relatively quiet (as does upper trapezius). If the end range of motion is pushed a little bit, there will be an increase in the activity of trapezius. This may be seen in Figure 14–17B (raw sEMG).

In Figure 14–15D, flexion of the head at the uppermost cervical segment is followed by return to midline. This is then followed by extension and return back to midline. Note how SCM and scalene work synergistically during flexion. The recruitment of the left SCM during the return to midline is mildly abnormal. The C-4 paraspinal site shows minimal recruitment during return to midline compared to extension of the head back over the shoulders. Here, a mild symmetry also is noted. Also note how the scalene site shows activity during this movement, while it did not during rotation (see Figure 14–15B). Examination of these two movement patterns allows for an assessment for synergistic movement patterns versus crosstalk. In this case, it appears that the scalene muscle participates in flexion but not rotation. The practitioner should note that the pattern of recruitment is radically altered when the flexion is conducted at the lowest possible cervical segment. The SCM muscle group would be less active, while the C-4 paraspinal site would be more active (raw sEMG).

Also note tracings for scalene (Figure 14–16B) and midcervical paraspinals (Figure 14–17B).

Clinical Considerations: Bilateral contraction of the SCM results in flexion of the lower and extension of the upper cervical spine.[24] Limitations in the ability of the upper cervical spine to flex will affect the ability of the lower cervical spine to extend. The converse is true for the impact of restricted extension in the lower cervical spine on the ability of the upper cervical spine to flex. Passive insufficiency (restricted excursion due to contracture or contraction) of the SCM can account for limited upper cervical spine flexion.[23]

The SCM muscles are phasic muscles that should show distinct patterns of activity associated with discrete motion. Their total amplitude is affected by the range of motion and the degree of excursion the muscle experiences in its motion. Postural forward head position is endemic to our sedentary society. Concomitant with this posture is the tendency for the SCM to shorten and thus alter the normal amount of excursion the muscle experiences in rotation and flexion/extension. Any additional increase in the gamma gain of a given SCM could have a significant effect upon the physiologically paired muscles, including sternalis, scalene, cervical paraspinal, upper trapezius, deep cervical flexors, clavicular portion of pectoralis, and platysma. Forward head posture with dysfunctional overlay in the SCM can be responsible for inhibited lower trapezius, cervical paraspinals, and other postural/functional problems.

The upper cervical spine has a unique morphology that allows for postural adaptations that return the eyes to the horizontal, regardless of the position of the neck and torso, via the righting reflex. Joint/muscle dysfunctions that limit the ability of the upper cervical spine to perform this function (eg, an O/A joint stuck in relative extension causing side flexion left and rotation right) should be compensated at C-1 or C-2, preferably, or in the upper thoracic spine and/or lower cervical spine. This will tend to shorten the ipsilateral and lengthen the contralateral SCM. Because the SCM is an accessory respiratory muscle, visceral and mechanical restrictions to respiration may cause increased SCM activity with inspiration. In craniomandibular dysfunctions, increased SCM activity can be related to a dysfunctional resting posture of the tongue[25] or cranial faults.[26]

Volume Conduction: Upper fibers of trapezius, scalene, cervicis, and capitis groups

Other Sites of Interest: Ipsilateral cervical paraspinals and upper trapezius during lateral bending and rotation, as well as scalene during deep inspiration

Referred Pain Considerations: Trigger points in the sternal division of the SCM refer pain to the vertex, to the occiput, across the cheek, and over the eye. Trigger points in the clavicular division commonly refer pain to the frontal region (frontal headaches) or the ear (earaches).[17]

Artifacts: ECG (This is augmented if electrodes are placed too far to the front.)

Benchmark: Sitting quietly at midline ($N = 104$): 1.3 (± 1.5) μV (RMS) Values taken using a J&J M-501 with a 100-to-200–Hz filter.[18]

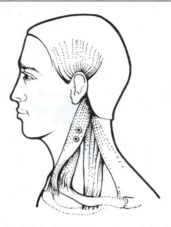

Figure 14–15A Electrode placement for SCM site. *Source:* Copyright © Clinical Resources, Inc.

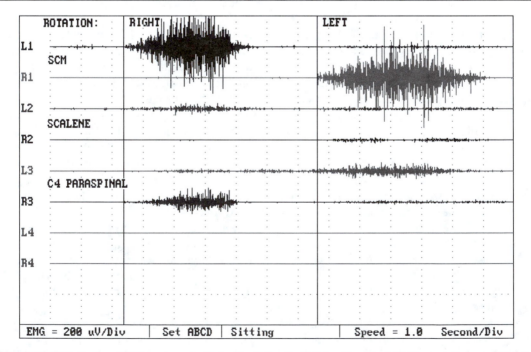

Figure 14–15B Surface EMG tracings during head rotation for SCM, midcervical (C-4) paraspinals, and scalene muscles. *Source:* Copyright © Clinical Resources, Inc.

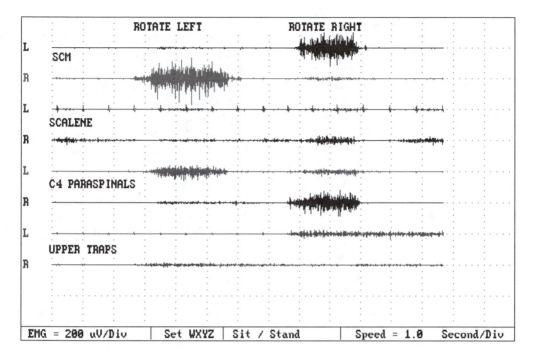

Figure 14–15C Surface EMG tracings during head rotation for SCM, scalene, midcervical (C-4) paraspinals, and upper trapezius. *Source:* Copyright © Clinical Resources, Inc.

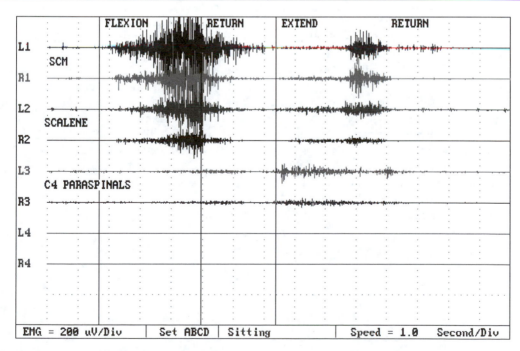

Figure 14–15D Surface EMG tracings during flexion and extension of the head for SCM, scalene, and midcervical paraspinals. *Source:* Copyright © Clinical Resources, Inc.

SCALENE (ANTERIOR) PLACEMENT

Type of Placement: Specific

Action: Lateral cervical flexor and stabilizer; assists in forward flexion; may play a role as an accessory muscle of respiration

Clinical Uses: Headache, repetitive strain injury

Muscle Insertions: Anterior scalene arises from the anterior tubercle of C-3, C-4, and C-5 vertebrae and inserts into the scalene tubercle of the first rib.

Innervation: The motor branch of the spinal nerves C-2 to C-7, depending upon location of attachment

Location: Palpate the SCM just lateral and above its attachment to the clavicle. Move posteriorly toward the outer superior edge of upper trapezius. Find the hollow triangle that lies just posterior to the SCM, just above the clavicle and anterior to the upper trapezius. Isolation of scalene is better when the electrodes are placed in the hollow by the clavicle than when placed higher up on the neck. Two active electrodes (2 cm apart) are placed on a slightly oblique angle just above the clavicle in the hollow triangle, so that they run parallel to the muscle fibers (Figure 14–16A).

Behavioral Test: Side bending of the neck, deep inspiration

Tracing Comment: In Figure 14–16B, SCM, midcervical paraspinals at C-4, scalene, and upper trapezius are monitored during a deep inspiration. Three out of the four muscle groups participate in this movement. Note the ECG artifact on the LSCA and LUTR sites (raw sEMG).

In Figure 14–16C, the SCM, scalene, C-4, paraspinals, and upper trapezius are monitored during lateral bending. The sternocleidomastoid and scalene are active, while the C-4 paraspinals and upper trapezius (narrow) are relatively quiet.

Figure 14–16D illustrates a synergy pattern between scalene and serratus anterior. During the first movement for flexion of the arms, serratus anterior activates while scalene remains relatively quiet. During the second movement of a sitting push-up, a clear synergy pattern between serratus anterior and scalene is noted. This is because the scalene group is being placed on stretch due to torsion on the rib cage by serratus anterior (raw sEMG).

Also note tracings for SCM (Figure 14–15D) and midcervical paraspinals (Figure 14–17B).

Clinical Considerations: The scalene muscles should be studied during deep inspiration as well as during movement. Scalene is seen as an ancillary muscle of respiration by some,[27] and a primary muscle of respiration by others.[28] A nice, symmetrical recruitment pattern should be observed or cultivated during treatment.

Volume Conduction: SCM, upper fibers of trapezius, and omohyoid

Other Sites of Interest: SCM during elevation of the chest and flexion of the head; upper trapezius during elevation of the shoulder; serratus anterior in the resisted flexion of the arm

Referred Pain Considerations: Trigger points in all three aspects of the scalene muscles can radiate pain into the pectoral region, laterally down to the front and back of the arm or into the thumb and index finger, and posteriorly to the upper vertebral border of the scapula.[17]

Artifacts: ECG and breathing

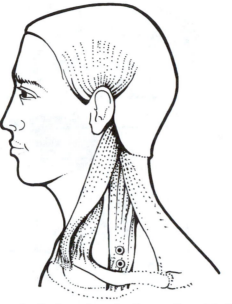

Figure 14–16A Placement of electrodes for the scalene site. *Source:* Copyright © Clinical Resources, Inc.

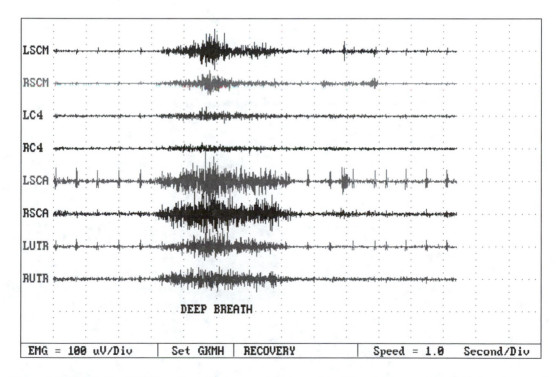

Figure 14–16B Surface EMG readings from sternocleidomastoid, midcervical paraspinals at C-4, scalene, and upper trapezius are presented during a deep inspiration. *Source:* Copyright © Clinical Resources, Inc.

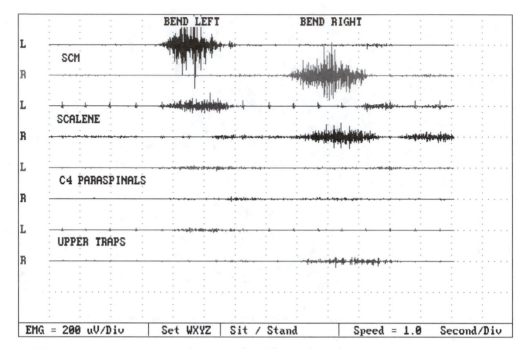

Figure 14–16C Surface EMG recordings from sternocleidomastoid, scalene, C-4 paraspinals, and upper trapezius are presented during lateral bending. *Source:* Copyright © Clinical Resources, Inc.

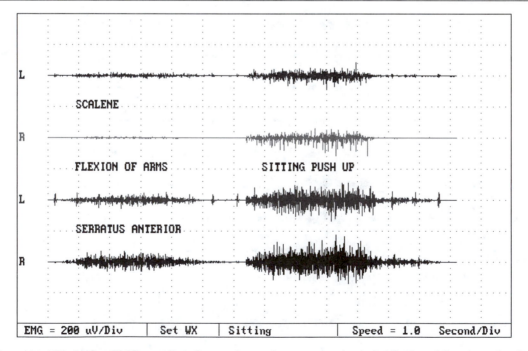

Figure 14–16D Surface EMG recordings from scalene and serratus anterior during flexion of the arms and push-up from chair (sitting). *Source:* Copyright © Clinical Resources, Inc.

MIDCERVICAL (C-4) PARASPINAL PLACEMENT

Type of Placement: Quasi-specific

Action: Stabilizes and extends the neck

Clinical Uses: Headache, neck pain, flexion/ extension injuries, and TMJ dysfunction

Muscle Insertions: This placement will record from the fibers of upper trapezius, along with the capitis and cervicis groups.

Innervation: Dorsal rami of the spinal nerves of the middle and lower cervical segments (C-3 to C-8). The dorsal ramus wraps around the articular pillar of the joint that makes up the posterior wall of the foramen. Arising off the dorsal ramus is the recurrent meningeal nerve; this retraces its path back into the spinal foramen and innervates the sensitive structures of the spinal segment as well as portions of the segments above and below, creating redundant innervation.[29]

Joint Considerations: When cervical segments are restricted due to postural habit, they are generally more symmetrical than those that are restricted due to trauma. In the middle and lower cervical spine, the motions of rotation and side flexion are conjoined. The resulting side flexion/rotation must be compensated for in the vertebral column, especially at the upper cervical spine.

Location: Palpate for the spinous processes of the cervical spine and the two muscle bellies that lie just lateral to it. Two active electrodes (approximately 2 cm apart) are placed so that they run parallel to the spine, approximately 2 cm from the midline, over the muscle belly at approximately C-4. Avoid the hairline (Figure 14–17A).

Behavioral Test: Cervical flexion and extension, lateral bending, and cervical rotation

Tracing Comment: In Figure 14–17B, the SCM, scalene, and C-4 paraspinals are monitored. In this tracing, rotational patterns are studied during rotation to the physiologic end of the range of motion. Note the cooperative functions between SCM and C-4 paraspinals during rotation. The left SCM activates to provide movement during right rotation, with the right C-4 paraspinals stabilizing. The opposite is true for left rotation. The scalene muscles are quiet during this movement, showing little cross-talk for the sEMG recordings for these three sites (raw sEMG).

Figure 14–17C monitors the same muscle sites during resisted rotation. The recruitment pattern for resisted rotation is very similar to the one collected during full range of motion (Figure 14–17B).

Also note tracings for SCM site (Figures 14–15B and 14–15C).

Clinical Considerations: The cervical paraspinals are made of groups of muscle; the most superficial is the splenius capitis, but these muscles include many others. These muscles have differing responsibilities regarding the motion of the head, neck, ribs, and thoracic spine. They can act in concert as cervical extensors. The practitioner should distinguish which layer of muscle and which direction of motion are most affected. As a whole, these muscles span many levels of the neck into the thoracic spine. They create functional links between distant regions of seemingly unrelated problems. A common example is the pulling and pain that many patients feel in the thoracic or lumbar region upon cervical flexion following a motor vehicle accident. This may be structural, as in restrictions in the free glide of the aponeurosis and fascia, or neurologically mediated, as in reflexive muscle contraction somewhere along the line of myofascium. Neurologically mediated restriction in multiple areas can also occur due to the redundant innervation within the spinal column. Palpation may reveal a motion segment responsible for the patient's symptoms, because unilateral pressure over one of the posterior vertebral joints of that segment reproduces the patient's symptoms, and perhaps some guarding muscle spasm is noted during palpation. However, passive motion testing may reveal restricted motion in the segment above or below.[24] The segment with restricted motion may actually be several segments away from the irritable segment.

Volume Conduction: Upper fibers of trapezius, deep cervical muscles, and levator scapulae

Other Sites of Interest: Upper trapezius and SCM during extension and rotation of the neck

Referred Pain Considerations: Trigger points in the splenius capitis muscle refer pain to the vertex of the head, while trigger points in the splenius cervicis refer pain intensely to the back of the orbit or downward toward the shoulder girdle and the angle of the neck.[17]

Artifacts: Respiration, electrode slippage during movement

Benchmark: Sitting quietly at midline ($N = 104$: 1.9 ($\pm$ 2.2) μV (RMS) Values taken using a J&J M-501 with a 100-to-200–Hz filter.[18]

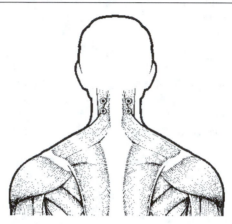

Figure 14–17A Electrode placement for midcervical paraspinals. *Source:* Copyright © Clinical Resources, Inc.

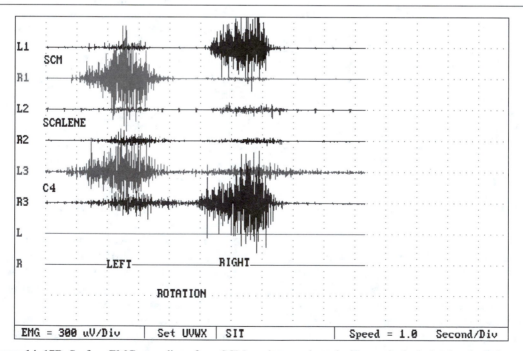

Figure 14–17B Surface EMG recordings from SCM, scalene, and cervical paraspinals during head rotation to full range of motion. *Source:* Copyright © Clinical Resources, Inc.

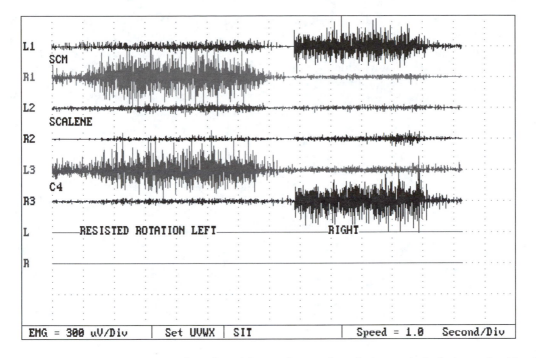

Figure 14–17C Surface EMG recordings from SCM, scalene, and cervical paraspinals during resisted head rotation. *Source:* Copyright © Clinical Resources, Inc.

CERVICAL DORSAL (WIDE) PLACEMENT

Type of Placement: General

Purpose: Monitor all cervical, shoulder, and thoracic movements

Clinical Uses: Headache, neck, shoulder, and arm pain

Location: The active electrodes are placed at the C-4 and T-10 levels approximately 2 cm out from the spine over the muscle mass of the paraspinals (Figure 14–18A).

Behavioral Test: Flex, extend, and rotate the head; elevate, retract, and protract the shoulders; abduct and flex the arms.

Tracing Comment: Figure 14–18B shows sEMG tracings from the cervical dorsal site during transitions between sitting and standing and forward flexion of the head. Note the general symmetry of the tracing, along with the activation that occurs during flexion of the head (processed sEMG).

Figure 14–18C shows sEMG activity from cervical dorsal leads during repeated sitting, walking, and sitting activities. The tracings are from a patient who has been trained to use minimal muscular effort in this region[13] (processed sEMG).

Also note tracings for cervical trapezius placements (Figures 14–6B, 14–6C, 14–6D).

Clinical Considerations: This site is particularly influenced by posture, with higher sEMG values commonly seen as patients go from sitting to standing. Patients may be taught, however, to rapidly quiet this region following movement.[13] This task involves intentionality (ie, becoming aware that the muscles remain active following a postural change) and postural adjustments of the rib cage (sternal lift) and head position (better alignment of the head over the shoulders).

Volume Conduction: Cervical and thoracic paraspinals; upper, middle, and lower trapezius; levator scapulae; rhomboids; and scaleni

Other Sites of Interest: SCM and scalene to assess other muscles that contribute to cervical motion; dorsal lumbar (wide) to consider movement of the spine as a whole. More specific monitoring sites should be considered if these more generalized treatments are ineffective.

Artifacts: ECG and breathing
Benchmark: Sitting: 2.0 µV (RMS)
             Standing: 2.0 µV (RMS)
             Values based upon the observation of Ettare and Ettare.[13]

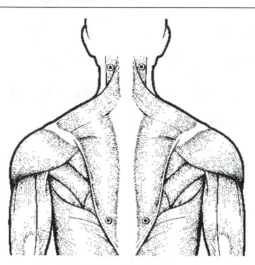

Figure 14–18A Electrode placement for cervical dorsal (wide) site. *Source:* Copyright © Clinical Resources, Inc.

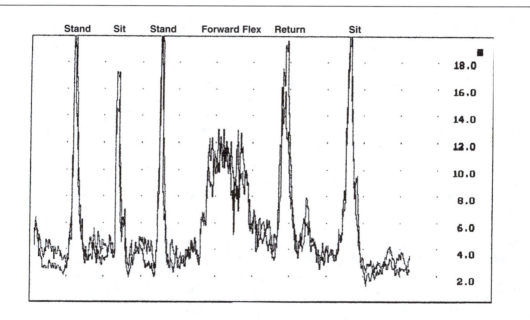

Figure 14–18B Surface EMG activity from cervical dorsal leads during sitting-standing transitions and forward flexion of the head. *Source:* Copyright © Clinical Resources, Inc.

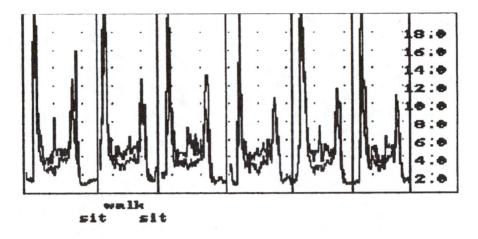

Figure 14–18C Surface EMG activity from cervical dorsal leads during repeated sitting, walking, and sitting activities. *Source:* Copyright © Clinical Resources, Inc.

UPPER TRAPEZIUS (NARROW) PLACEMENT

Type of Placement: Specific

Action: Adduction, upward rotation, and elevation of the scapula; side bending of head

Clinical Uses: Headaches, shoulder pain, upper quarter pain, repetitive strain injury, tension myalgia

Muscle Insertions: The upper fibers of trapezius arise from the superior nuchal line, the external occipital protuberance, and the ligamentum nuchae. They insert into the lateral third of the clavicle and the spine of the scapula.

Innervation: C-3, C-4 myotome via sensory nerves of the ventral rami of the C-3 and C-4 spinal nerves

Joint Considerations: O/A; C-6 through T-3 spinous process; acromioclavicular and sternoclavicular joints

Location: Place two active electrodes (2 cm apart) so that they run parallel to the muscle fibers (origins and insertions) of upper trapezius, along the ridge of the shoulder, slightly lateral to and one half the distance between the cervical spine at C-7 and the acromion. Palpate the muscle mass and place over the muscle belly (Figure 14–19A). *Variations:* Due to the broad nature of the trapezius muscle, the farther the electrode placement is moved down from the crest of the shoulder, the more the sEMG recording will register the actions associated with scapular adduction.

Behavioral Test: Shoulder elevation/shrug, lateral bending of the head

Tracing Comment: Figure 14–19B shows upper and lower trapezius recruitment during shoulder girdle elevation (shrug). The upper trapezius shows a large recruitment pattern as the shoulder girdle is raised (raw sEMG).

Figure 14–19C shows upper trapezius, supraspinatus, infraspinatus, posterior deltoids, and latissimus dorsi during the movements of shoulder girdle elevation, external rotation, and extension of the arm. Shoulder girdle elevation brought about the largest recruitment pattern for the upper trapezius tracing. The infraspinatus was most active during external rotation. The posterior deltoid and latissimus dorsi were more active during extension of the arm. The electrodes placed above the supraspinatus fossa (upper trapezius and supraspinatus) did not differentiate during any of the movements (raw sEMG).

See also the tracings for lower trapezius (Figures 14–21B, 14–21C, 14–21D, 14–21E) and suprascapular/supraspinatus site (Figures 14–23C, 14–23D).

Clinical Considerations: Sitting unsupported may yield higher values than when the back is supported. Arms in the lap may yield lower values than when arms are at the sides. Standing values are commonly higher than sitting values.[18] Acting unilaterally, the upper trapezius bends the neck and head toward the same side.[16] In synergy with other muscles, it assists in the abduction and flexion of the arm. Bilateral activation may be seen during resisted extension of the head.

Upper trapezius could be affected by dysfunction in segments C-3 through T-2 because of its insertions on the ligamentum nuchae. Forward head posture and associated changes in position of scapula, ribs, O/A joints, and other cervical structures may also cause upper trapezius dysfunction. Irritable contralateral scalene, possibly due to underlying cervical joint structures, may create hypertonicity in the upper trapezius. Myofascial restrictions in latissimus dorsi, deltoids, and biceps may affect upper trapezius recordings. Finally, elevations in the upper trapezius have been noted in multidirectional instabilities of the shoulder.

Cook et al monitored the sEMG activity of shoulder muscle during the throwing of a ball in pitchers and non-pitchers.[30]

Volume Conduction: Middle fibers of trapezius, levator scapulae, supraspinatus

Other Sites of Interest: Lower trapezius, middle trapezius, serratus anterior, supraspinatus, biceps, deltoid, infraspinatus, teres major, and pectoralis major during movements of the upper extremities

Referred Pain Considerations: Trigger points in the upper trapezius characteristically refer pain along the posterolateral aspect of the neck behind the ear and up into the temple.[17]

Artifacts: ECG, breathing

Benchmark: Sitting quietly at midline (N = 104): 2.2 (± 2.6) μV (RMS)

Standing quietly at midline (N = 104): 3.1 (±3.1) μV (RMS)

Values taken using a J&J M-501 with a 100-to-200–Hz filter.[18]

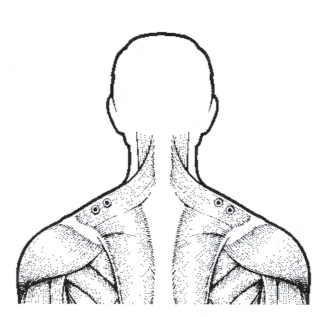

Figure 14–19A Electrode placement for upper trapezius site. *Source:* Copyright © Clinical Resources, Inc.

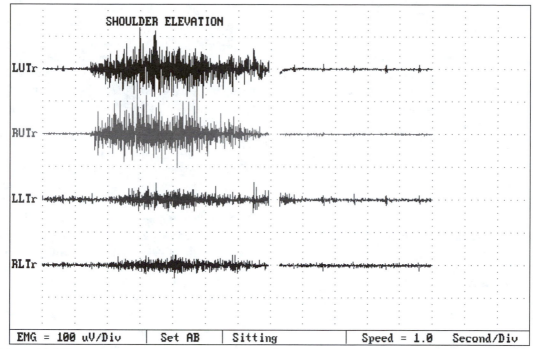

Figure 14–19B Surface EMG activity from upper and lower trapezius during shoulder girdle elevation. *Source:* Copyright © Clinical Resources, Inc.

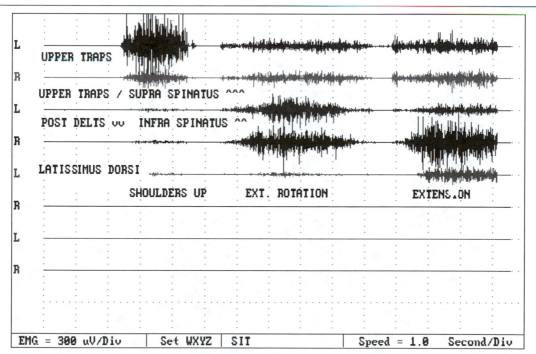

Figure 14–19C Surface EMG activity from upper trapezius, supraspinatus, infraspinatus, posterior deltoids, and latissimus dorsi during shoulder girdle elevation, external rotation, and extension of the arm. *Source:* Copyright © Clinical Resources, Inc.

INTERSCAPULAR (MIDDLE TRAPEZIUS) PLACEMENT

Type of Placement: Quasi-specific

Action: Scapular stabilization; adduction, retraction, and upward rotation of the scapula during flexion and abduction of the arms, especially near its full range of motion

Clinical Uses: Shoulder rehabilitation

Muscle Insertions: These fibers arise from the spinal processes of C-6 to T-3 and insert on the acromion and superior lip of the spine of the scapula.

Innervation: Spinal portion of the accessory nerve (11th cranial nerve), and the ventral ramus C-2, C-3, and C-4.

Location: To place the electrodes, locate the medial border of the spine of the scapula (root). The electrodes are placed horizontally, 2 cm apart, next to the root (Figure 4–20A).

Behavioral Test: Retract the scapula and abduct the arms through the full range of motion.

Tracing Comment: Figure 14–20B shows recordings from the interscapular site during shoulder retraction. While middle trapezius fibers are thought to contribute to this recording, it is difficult to separate out this muscle's sEMG contribution from the sEMG contributions of rhomboid (raw sEMG). Also see tracings for lower trapezius (Figure 14–21B).

Clinical Considerations: The middle fibers of trapezius are known to adduct and retract the scapula.[31] They are thought to play a larger role in abduction of the arm near its full range.[32]

Volume Conduction: Upper trapezius, levator scapulae, rhomboids, erector spinae

Other Sites of Interest: Upper trapezius, lower trapezius, serratus anterior, supraspinatus, biceps, deltoid, infraspinatus, teres major, and pectoralis major during movements of the upper extremities and shoulder girdle

Referred Pain Considerations: Trigger points in this region tend to refer pain toward the vertebrae and the interscapular region in general.[17]

Artifacts: ECG, breathing

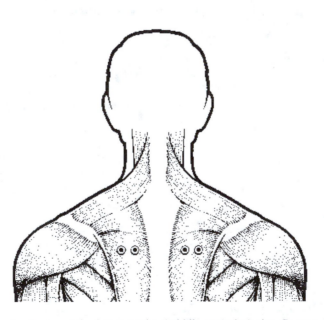

Figure 14–20A Electrode placement for interscapular (middle trapezius) site. *Source:* Copyright © Clinical Resources, Inc.

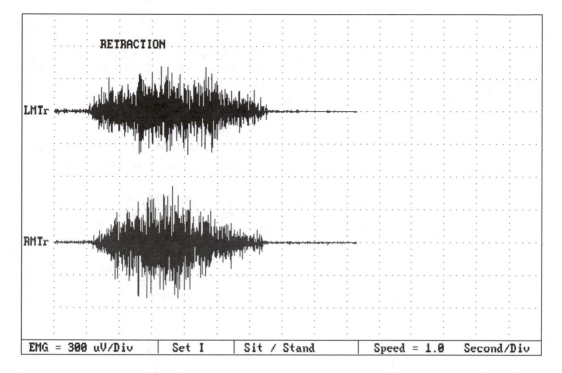

Figure 14–20B Surface EMG recordings from the middle trapezius site during scapular retraction. *Source:* Copyright © Clinical Resources, Inc.

LOWER INTERSCAPULAR (LOWER TRAPEZIUS) PLACEMENT

Type of Placement: Quasi-specific

Action: Scapular stabilization; upward rotation, retraction, and depression of the scapula during abduction, flexion, and scaption of the arms

Clinical Uses: Shoulder, neck, and upper quarter pain; repetitive strain injury

Muscle Insertions: The fibers arise from the 3rd to the 12th thoracic vertebrae (T-3 through T-12) and insert onto the scapular spine.

Innervation: Spinal portion of the accessory nerve (11th cranial nerve), and the ventral ramus C-2, C-3, and C-4

Location: Palpate the interscapular region. Have the patient retract and depress the scapula and then flex the arm to at least 90 degrees. Palpate the inferior medial border of the scapula for the muscle mass that emerges. Place the electrodes on an oblique angle, approximately 5 cm down from the scapular spine. The two active electrodes (2 cm apart) are placed next to the medial edge of the scapula at a 55-degree oblique angle (Figure 14–21A).

Behavioral Test: Abduction of arms; retraction of the shoulder back and down at a 45-degree angle

Tracing Comment: Four tracings are shown for a variety of muscle groups and movements to provide the practitioner with an appreciation of the complexity of recruitment patterns and synergy at this site.

Figure 14–21B shows a normal tracing of abduction through 90 degrees, followed by an isolated movement of retraction and depression of the scapula. Both upper and lower trapezius muscles are roughly equally active during the abduction. In this example, during the return phase, the lower trapezius continues in its recruitment pattern slightly longer than the upper trapezius. The key attribute of a normal synergy pattern during this movement is symmetry between the right and left and the upper and lower trapezius. Isolation of the lower trapezius is also presented and is characterized by active retraction and depression of the scapula.

Figure 14–21C represents an abnormal recruitment pattern during abduction to 90 degrees. The lower trapezius is dominant, which suggests excessive scapular depression. Normally, during the last third of the active recruitment, the lower trapezius has a slightly greater activation associated with the return phase of the movement. As a rough rule of thumb, when abduction is done to 90 degrees, the upper trapezius to lower trapezius ratio should be approximately less than 1.0. An abnormal synergy is noted when activation of upper fibers of trapezius exceeds activation of lower fibers at 90 degrees.[33]

Figure 14–21D shows sEMG recordings from upper trapezius, middle trapezius, lower trapezius, and serratus anterior. The first half of the tracing represents abduction to 180 degrees for the right arm. A separate, isolated flexion of the right arm to 180 degrees follows. The lower trapezius activates more briskly during abduction, while the upper trapezius and serratus anterior activate more briskly during flexion of the arm.

Figure 14–21E shows upper trapezius, middle trapezius, lower trapezius, and serratus anterior during three isolated movements of abduction, scaption, and flexion for the right upper extremity only. The recruitment pattern in this example is slightly different from that in Figure 14–21D. All three of the trapezius recording sites play a role in controlling the scapula. The role of the upper trapezius gradually diminishes as one moves from abduction through scaption to flexion of the arm, as does the middle trapezius. The lower trapezius appears to be constant across all three movements, while the recordings at the serratus anterior site increase across the three movements (raw sEMG).

Also see the tracings for the suprascapular/supraspinatus site (Figures 14–23C and 14–23D).

Clinical Considerations: The lower trapezius interacts with upper trapezius through the process of reciprocal inhibition.[33] Whenever the upper trapezius is found to be hyperactive, it is worthwhile to monitor the lower trapezius simultaneously; it is commonly found to be inhibited. When uptraining the lower trapezius, it is useful to explore how the position of the sternum affects the muscle recruitment patterns. Allowing the person to engage in a sternal lift prior to attempted isolation of the lower trapezius may enhance the probability of successful isolation of recruitment.

Volume Conduction: Middle trapezius, rhomboids, and erector spinae

Other Sites of Interest: Upper trapezius, middle trapezius, serratus anterior, supraspinatus, biceps, deltoid, infraspinatus, teres major, and pectoralis major during movements of the upper extremities and shoulder girdle

Referred Pain Considerations: Trigger points in this muscle group refer pain sharply to the upper cervical region of the paraspinal muscles.[17]

Artifacts: ECG, breathing

Benchmark: Sitting quietly at midline ($N = 104$): 2.3 (± 2.3) µV (RMS)
Standing quietly at midline: 2.5 (± 2.5) µV (RMS)
Values taken using a J&J M-501 with a 100-to-200–Hz filter.[18]

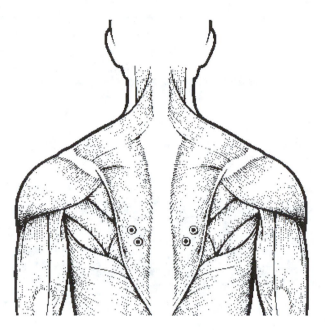

Figure 14–21A Electrode placement for lower interscapular (lower trapezius) site. *Source:* Copyright © Clinical Resources, Inc.

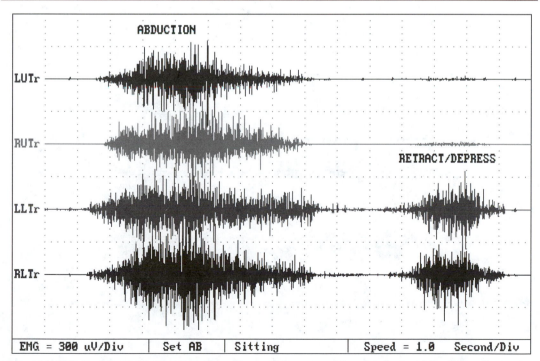

Figure 14–21B Surface EMG recordings from upper and lower trapezius sites during abduction and retraction. Note the balance of recruitment between upper and lower trapezius during abduction, while only the lower trapezius muscles are active during retraction. *Source:* Copyright © Clinical Resources, Inc.

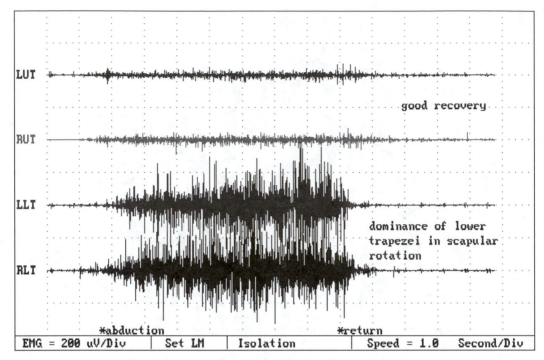

Figure 14–21C Abnormal surface EMG recordings from upper and lower trapezius sites during abduction. Note how lower trapezius appears to be dominant. *Source:* Copyright © Clinical Resources, Inc.

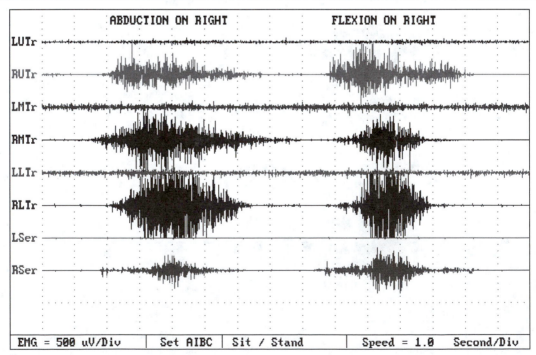

Figure 14–21D Surface EMG recordings from (UTr) upper, (MTr) middle, and (LTr) lower trapezius sites, along with (Ser) serratus anterior during abduction and flexion for the right side only. *Source:* Copyright © Clinical Resources, Inc.

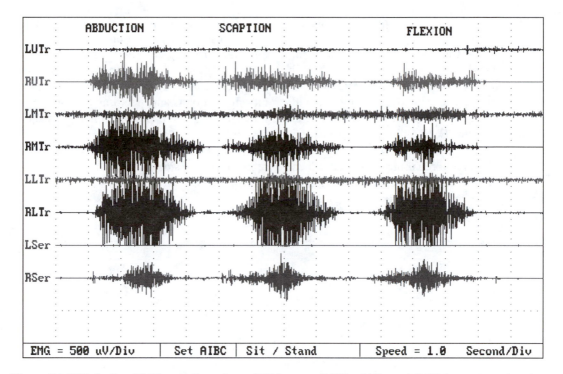

Figure 14–21E Surface EMG recordings from (UTr) upper, (MTr) middle, and (LTr) lower trapezius sites, along with (Ser) serratus anterior during abduction, scaption, and flexion. *Source:* Copyright © Clinical Resources, Inc.

SERRATUS ANTERIOR (LOWER FIBERS) PLACEMENT

Type of Placement: Specific

Action: Upward rotation, depression, and abduction of the scapula during abduction and flexion of the arm; protraction of scapula during pushing activities

Clinical Uses: Upper quarter, neck, and headache pain, (ie, with upper trapezius placements in overuse syndromes)

Muscle Insertions: The fibers of this multibellied muscle usually arise by nine slips from the first to ninth ribs. The lowest portion of this muscle inserts on the costal surface of the inferior angle of the scapula.

Innervation: The anterior rami of the C-5 through C-8 spinal nerves

Location: Have the patient flex the arm against resistance. Palpate this contraction in an area just anterior to the border of the latissimus dorsi muscle at the level of the inferior tip of the scapula. Place two active electrodes horizontally (2 cm apart) just below the axillary area, at the level of the inferior tip of the scapula, and just medial of the latissimus dorsi. It is important that the electrodes are anterior to the latissimus dorsi muscle (Figure 14–22A).

Behavioral Test: Forward flexion of the arms, protraction of the shoulders, push-ups

Tracing Comment: Figure 14–22B shows recordings from serratus anterior during a series of push-up maneuvers: wall push-up, knee push-up, and floor push-up. Note the increasing level of recruitment associated with the increasing efforts. Also note a mildly abnormal asymmetry between the right and left aspects (raw sEMG).

Figure 14–22C shows sEMG recordings from upper trapezius, lower trapezius, pectoralis (clavicular head), and serratus anterior during flexion of the arms. The pectoralis group shows the greatest activation pattern. The serratus anterior also recruits during this movement for this subject, while the upper and lower trapezius do not (raw sEMG).

Also see the tracings for scalene placement (Figure 14–16D).

Clinical Considerations: The EMG activity of this muscle during neutral rest position should be quiet.[16] Protraction of the scapula has been noted along with sEMG activity during forward pushing movements.[32,34] The portion of the serratus anterior monitored using the site described in this section is most active during flexion of the arm, and slightly less active during abduction.[16]

Volume Conduction: Latissimus dorsi, intercostal muscles, costal portion of pectoralis

Other Sites of Interest: Upper trapezius, middle trapezius, lower trapezius, supraspinatus, biceps, deltoid, infraspinatus, teres major, latissimus dorsi, and pectoralis major during movements of the upper extremities and shoulder girdle

Referred Pain Considerations: Trigger points refer pain to the side and back of the chest.[17]

Artifacts: ECG, respiration

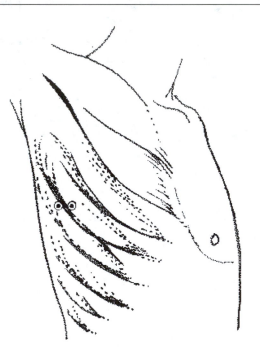

Figure 14–22A Electrode placement for serratus anterior site. *Source:* Copyright © Clinical Resources, Inc.

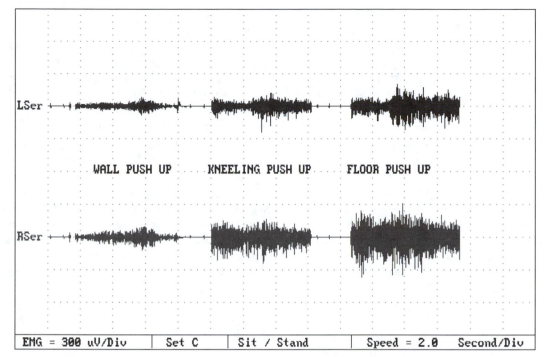

Figure 14–22B Surface EMG recordings from serratus anterior during wall push-up, kneeling push-up, and floor push-up. *Source:* Copyright © Clinical Resources, Inc.

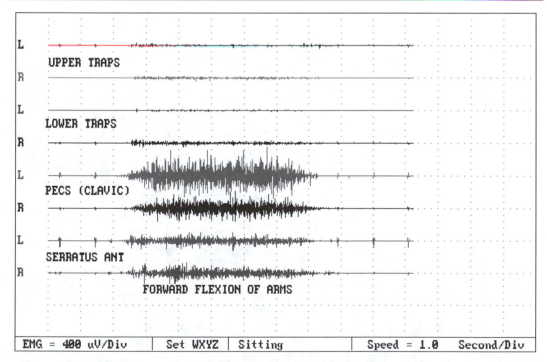

Figure 14–22C Surface EMG recordings from upper trapezius, lower trapezius, pectoralis (clavicular head), and serratus anterior during flexion of the arms. *Source:* Copyright © Clinical Resources, Inc.

SUPRASCAPULAR FOSSA (UPPER TRAPEZIUS/SUPRASPINATUS) PLACEMENT

Type of Placement: Quasi-specific

Action: Abduction of the arm; controls the head of the humerus in the glenoid fossa

Clinical Uses: Shoulder rehabilitation

Muscle Insertions: The fibers of supraspinatus lie beneath middle and upper fibers of trapezius. They arise from the supraspinatus fossa and insert on the greater tubercle of the humerus.

Location: Palpate the spine of the scapula, locating its lateral distal aspect. The electrodes are placed there 2 cm apart, directly above the spine of the scapula, over the suprascapular fossa (Figure 14–23A).

Behavioral Test: Abduction of the arm

Tracing Comment: Figure 14–23B shows recordings taken from the right side only of the upper trapezius, supraspinatus, infraspinatus, and middle deltoid during shoulder elevation (shrug) and abduction with the thumb in the down and then up positions. Shoulder elevation is associated with contractions at the upper trapezius and supraspinatus site but does not involve the middle deltoid. The recruitment pattern noted during abduction indicates that deltoid fires first during the initiation of the movement. The contraction of the upper trapezius is thought to facilitate a stable length-tension relationship for the deltoid. Note that the thumb up and thumb down portions of the tracing are very similar for all sites for this subject (raw sEMG).

In Figures 14–23C and 14–23D, two studies were conducted on the right side of another subject during abduction with the thumb up, palm down, and thumb down. The upper trapezius (narrow), suprascapular/supraspinatus, middle deltoid, infraspinatus, lower interscapular (lower trapezius), and latissimus dorsi placement sites were monitored. In Figure 14–23C, the subject was standing with a slight flexion to the upper back during the movement patterns of abduction, while in Figure 14–23D, these movements were conducted during a sternal lift, raising the rib cage and upper torso into a more upright posture. By comparing the recruitment patterns for a given muscle under the two different postural loads, one can see that during the sternal lift (Figure 14–23D), the suprascapular/supraspinatus site shows a stronger distinction between the thumb up and thumb down movement, with a more robust recruitment pattern during the thumb down abduction. The thumb down movement is predicted to augment recruitment of the supraspinatus. Such augmentation, however, may not be seen unless the rib cage is in the proper position. In addition, the sternal lift brings about a stronger recruitment pattern for the lower trapezius during all three abduction movements. Using the rules regarding relationships for upper and lower trapezius presented in Chapter 7, the level of recruitment during abduction should be approximately the same for both the upper and lower trapezius sites. In Figure 14–23C, when abduction is conducted with a slightly flexed upper back, the lower trapezius recruitment pattern appears slightly abnormal because it is so much smaller than the upper trapezius pattern. In Figure 14–23D, however, the sternal lift augments the recruitment of the lower trapezius, thus making the abduction movement look more normalized (raw sEMG).

Clinical Considerations: The supraspinatus muscle is extremely difficult to monitor electromyographically using surface electrodes because the middle and upper trapezius muscles overlie it. To record from supraspinatus, indwelling electrodes are needed. For the most part, recordings from this site correlate remarkably well with those of middle and upper trapezius. However, under isolated circumstances, using particular movements and with the correct posture (such as the ones seen in Figures 14–23C and 14–23D), recruitment from the supraspinatus can be inferred.

Volume Conduction: Major problems of cross-talk arise from the middle and upper fibers of trapezius. It is impossible to isolate EMG activity from the supraspinatus (relative to the upper trapezius) with surface electrodes. These muscles are layered next to each other and function synergistically. Movements that attempt to separate out differential muscle function fail to show differential recruitment patterns from upper trapezius at this site.

Other Sites of Interest: Upper trapezius, middle trapezius, lower trapezius, serratus anterior, biceps, deltoid, infraspinatus, teres major, and pectoralis major during movements of the upper extremities and shoulder girdle

Referred Pain Considerations: Trigger points at this site refer pain to the middle deltoid region and may include the lateral epicondyle region.[17]

Artifacts: ECG

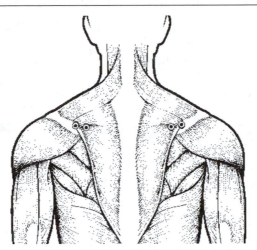

Figure 14–23A Electrode placement for upper suprascapular fossa (trapezius/supraspinatus) site. *Source:* Copyright © Clinical Resources, Inc.

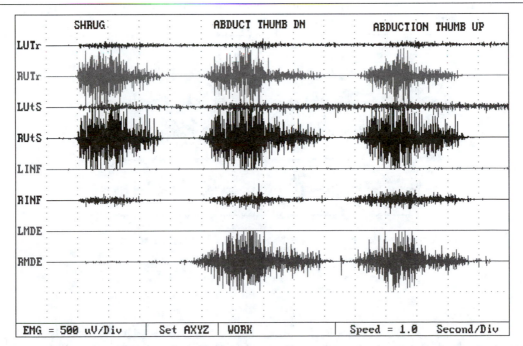

Figure 14–23B Surface EMG recordings from upper trapezius, suprascapular (upper trapezius/supraspinatus), infraspinatus, and middle deltoid site during a shoulder shrug, abduction of the arm with the thumb down, and abduction with the thumb up. *Source:* Copyright © Clinical Resources, Inc.

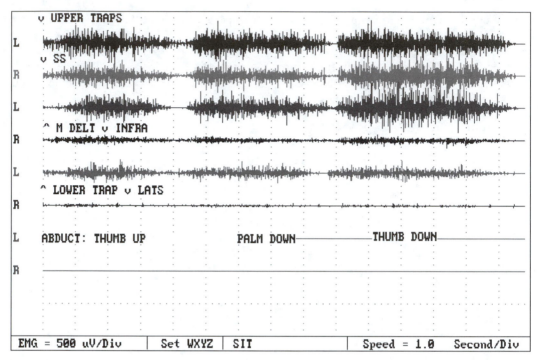

Figure 14–23C Surface EMG recordings from the upper trapezius (narrow), suprascapular/supraspinatus, middle deltoid, infraspinatus, lower interscapular (lower trapezius), and latissimus dorsi placement sites during abduction with thumb up, palm down, and thumb down and with a slightly flexed upper back. *Source:* Copyright © Clinical Resources, Inc.

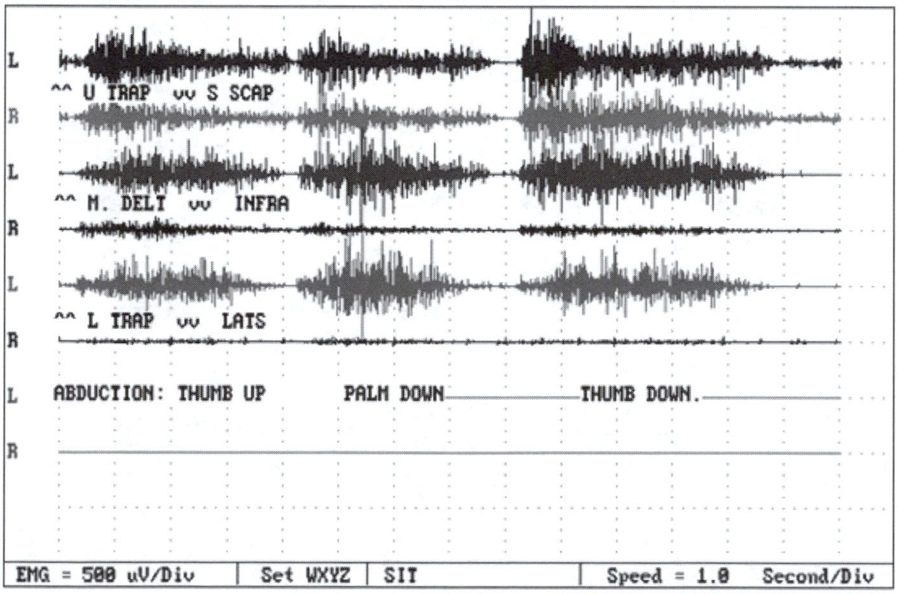

Figure 14–23D Surface EMG recordings from the upper trapezius (narrow), suprascapular/supraspinatus, middle deltoid, infraspinatus, lower interscapular (lower trapezius), and latissimus dorsi placement sites during abduction with thumb up, palm down, and thumb down following a sternal lift. *Source:* Copyright © Clinical Resources, Inc.

INFRASPINATUS PLACEMENT

Type of Placement: Specific

Action: Lateral rotation of the shoulder joint, along with stabilization of the head of the humerus in the glenoid cavity

Clinical Uses: Treatment of stroke patients to facilitate use of upper extremity; treatment of shoulder instability and orthopedic impingement syndromes

Muscle Insertions: The fibers arise from the infraspinatus fossa, below the spine of the scapula, and insert on the greater tubercle of the humerus.

Innervation: The superior cord of the brachial plexus, from the spinal nerves of segments C-4, C-5, and C-6

Joint Considerations: The joints of the cervical spine related to the muscle (C-4, C-5, and C-6) may affect the sEMG resting or recruitment patterns, along with the glenohumeral joint (particularly the anterior glide stability and the inferior glide capacity) and the acromioclavicular (AC) joint.

Location: Palpate the spine of the scapula. Two closely spaced electrodes (2 cm apart) are placed parallel to and approximately 4 cm below the spine of the scapula, on the lateral aspect, over the infrascapular fossa of the scapula. Avoid placement over posterior deltoid (Figure 14–24A).

Behavioral Test: Elbow bent to 90 degrees with lateral (external) rotation of the bent arm out to the side; abduction of the arm

Tracing Comment: Figure 14–24B shows sEMG tracings from infraspinatus and posterior deltoid during lateral rotation with the right arm flexed at the elbow, and external rotation and extension of the right arm with the elbow extended. During lateral rotation, the activity at the infraspinatus site is greater, while during lateral rotation with extension of the shoulder, the sEMG activity of the posterior deltoid site is greater (raw sEMG).

Also see tracing from upper trapezius (Figure 14–19C) and triceps (Figure 14–34B).

Clinical Considerations: Forward head posture and thoracic kyphosis, with the downward pull of the rib cage, may allow the internal rotators of the shoulder (both scapular and glenohumeral) to shorten, altering the normal length-tension relationship for the infraspinatus.

During abduction, the supraspinatus requires external rotation of the humeral head to clear the greater tubercle from impinging against the coracoacromial ligament. With slight dysfunction (tightness of the supraspinatus muscle, slight anterior capsule laxity, excessive tightness of the internal rotators, spurring of the AC joint, etc), the infraspinatus overworks and develops triggers.

In full overhead elevation, as in throwing, the lower trapezius is in a functional line with the infraspinatus and posterior deltoids. Inhibition of the lower trapezius alters the ability of the scapula stabilizers to protect the length-tension advantage of the deltoids. With the deltoids working at a disadvantage and the lower trapezius dysfunctional, the infraspinatus is asked to overwork.

Volume Conduction: Posterior deltoid, teres major, and teres minor

Other Sites of Interest: Upper trapezius, middle trapezius, lower trapezius, serratus anterior, supraspinatus, biceps, deltoid, teres major, and pectoralis major during movements of the upper extremities and shoulder girdle

Referred Pain Considerations: Trigger points at this site refer pain to the anterior deltoid region and the shoulder joint.[17]

Artifacts: ECG

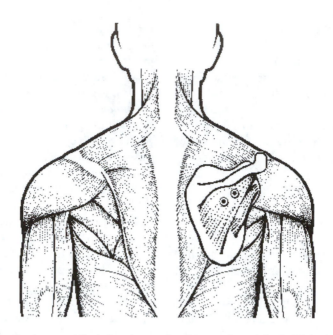

Figure 14–24A Electrode placement for infraspinatus site. *Source:* Copyright © Clinical Resources, Inc.

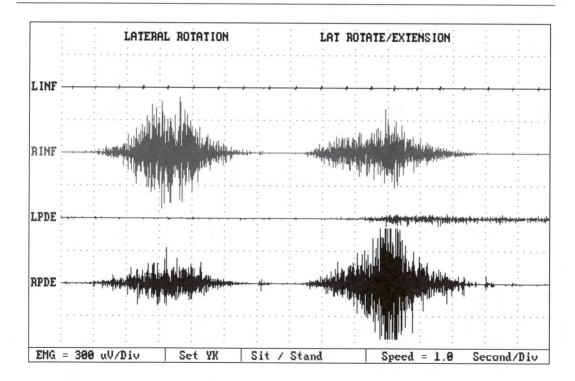

Figure 14–24B Surface EMG recordings from infraspinatus and posterior deltoid during lateral rotation of the arm and lateral rotation and extension of the shoulder. *Source:* Copyright © Clinical Resources, Inc.

ANTERIOR DELTOID PLACEMENT

Type of Placement: Specific

Action: Forward flexion, medial rotation, and abduction of the arm

Clinical Uses: Shoulder rehabilitation

Muscle Insertions: This muscle arises from the lateral third of the clavicle and inserts on the deltoid tuberosity of the humerus.

Innervation: Via the axillary nerve from the posterior cord of the brachial plexus (These carry fibers from the spinal nerves of segments C-5 and C-6.)

Joint Considerations: Deltoid muscle dysfunctions can arise from neurogenic causes from the cervical spine (C-5 primarily, but also C-6, C-7, C-8, and T-1). Joint motion dysfunctions that would affect the tension of the posterior cord of the plexus (namely, the costovertebral articulations of the first rib, the sternocostal junctions, and the scapulothoracic positioning as seen via the acromioclavicular joints, the sternoclavicular joints, and the posture of the scapula) could also affect sEMG recordings.

Location: Palpate the clavicle. Two active electrodes, 2 cm apart, are placed on the anterior aspect of the arm, approximately 4 cm below the clavicle, so that they run parallel to the muscle fibers (Figure 14–25A).

Behavioral Test: Forward flexion, abduction, and horizontal adduction of the arm

Tracing Comment: Figure 14–25B shows sEMG recordings from anterior, middle, and posterior deltoid monitored during flexion, abduction, and extension of the right side only. The largest recruitment of anterior deltoid is seen during flexion of the arm. It also contributes during abduction (raw sEMG).

Also see tracing from triceps (Figure 14–34B) and pectoralis major (Figure 14–28B).

Clinical Considerations: Simultaneous activation of the anterior, middle, and posterior deltoids abduct the arm.[16] The anterior portion flexes the arm,[16] and also plays a role in the horizontal flexion of the arm across the chest.[32] Movement of the hand to the face requires adequate function of anterior deltoids and serratus anterior muscles.[31]

The position of the humeral head in the glenohumeral joint, and that of the scapula on the chest wall, are important to the function of the deltoids. Behavioral nuances of movement strategy in the initiation of elevation of the upper extremity are also important. It is necessary to attempt to control and standardize these factors for successful testing at this site.

Myofascial factors that would tend to activate the neural pathway of the deltoids and dysfunction include: scalene, latissimus dorsi, teres minor, and the muscles of the arm and forearm supplied by the radial nerve. Factors from the contralateral side that activate the neural tree also must be considered. Inhibition of the lower trapezius with hyperactivity of the upper trapezius could affect the functions of elevation, reaching, and weight bearing through the upper extremity. Elevation of the arm into abduction is normally a result of the force couple of the scapular rotators (upper trapezius, lower trapezius, serratus anterior) and the force couple of the supraspinatus and deltoids. Imbalance in the shoulder elevator group could be related to imbalance between elements of the elevators and the supraspinatus/deltoid force couple.

Volume Conduction: Medial deltoid, biceps, and pectoralis major

Other Sites of Interest: Clavicular aspect of pectoralis, long head of biceps, serratus anterior, upper and lower trapezius, suprascapular fossa site, and middle and posterior deltoid during movements of the upper extremities

Referred Pain Considerations: Trigger points at this site refer pain locally.[17]

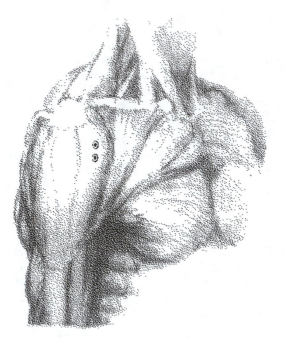

Figure 14–25A Electrode placement for anterior deltoid site. *Source:* Copyright © Clinical Resources, Inc.

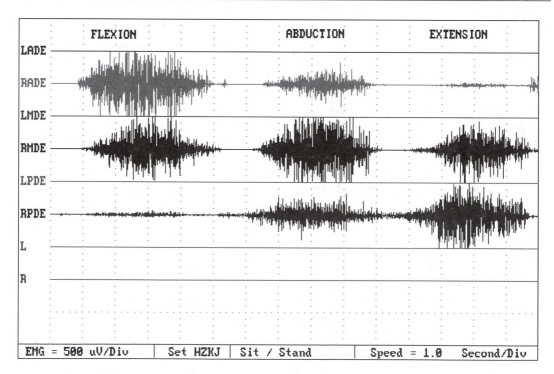

Figure 14–25B Surface EMG recordings from anterior, middle, and posterior deltoid during flexion, abduction, and extension. *Source:* Copyright © Clinical Resources, Inc.

MIDDLE DELTOID PLACEMENT

Type of Placement: Specific

Action: Abduction of the arm

Clinical Uses: Shoulder rehabilitation

Muscle Insertions: This muscle arises from the acromion and inserts on the deltoid tuberosity of the humerus.

Innervation: The axillary nerve, spinal segments C-5 and C-6

Location: The active electrodes are placed on the lateral aspect of the upper arm, 2 cm apart, and approximately 3 cm below the acromion, over the muscle mass so that the electrodes run parallel to the muscle fibers (Figure 14–26).

Behavioral Test: Abduction of the arm

Tracing Comment: Figure 14–25B for anterior deltoid shows how the middle deltoid is active during all three phases of movement: flex-ion, abduction, and extension. Also see Figure 14–23B (suprascapular fossa), where timing issues relative to other synergists are highlighted.

Clinical Considerations: Simultaneous activation of the anterior, middle, and posterior deltoids abducts the arm.[16] Abduction is the primary function of the middle deltoid, and this muscle is also active during flexion and extension of the arm.

Volume Conduction: Anterior and posterior deltoids, biceps, and triceps

Other Sites of Interest: Suprascapular fossa site; anterior and posterior deltoids; upper, lower, and middle trapezius; pectoralis; teres major; and latissimus dorsi during movements of the upper extremities

Referred Pain Considerations: Trigger points at this site refer pain locally.[17]

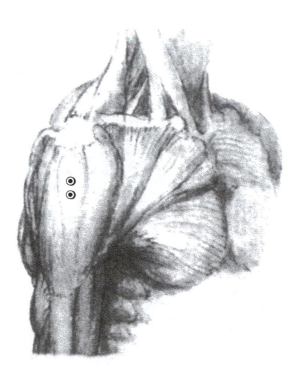

Figure 14–26 Electrode placement for the middle deltoid site. *Source:* Copyright © Clinical Resources, Inc.

POSTERIOR DELTOID PLACEMENT

Type of Placement: Specific

Action: Extension, lateral (external) rotation, and abduction of the arm

Clinical Uses: Shoulder rehabilitation

Muscle Insertions: This muscle arises from the lower border of the spine of the scapula and inserts on the deltoid tuberosity of the humerus.

Innervation: The axillary nerve, spinal segments C-5 and C-6

Joint Considerations: Deltoid muscle dysfunctions can arise from neurogenic causes from the cervical spine (C-5 primarily, but also C-6, C-7, C-8, and T-1). Joint motion dysfunctions that affect the tension of the posterior cord of the plexus (namely, the costovertebral articulations of the first rib, the sternocostal junctions, and the scapulothoracic positioning as seen via the acromioclavicular joints, the sternoclavicular joints, and the posture of the scapula) could also affect sEMG recordings.

Location: Palpate the spine of the scapula. Two active electrodes are placed 2 cm apart and approximately 2 cm below the lateral border of the spine of the scapula and angled on an oblique angle toward the arm so that they run parallel to the muscle fibers (Figure 14–27).

Behavioral Test: Extension, abduction, and lateral rotation of the arm

Tracing Comment: Figure 14–25B (anterior deltoid) shows that for posterior deltoid the largest recruitment occurs during extension, but that it also contributes to abduction. Figures 14–19C (upper trapezius) and 14–24B (infraspinatus) indicate that the posterior deltoid is active during lateral rotation of the arm and extension of the shoulder.

Clinical Considerations: Simultaneous activation of the anterior, middle, and posterior deltoids abduct the arm.[16] The posterior deltoid, however, is primarily active in extension of the arm.

The posterior deltoid seems to be hypoactive more often than the anterior deltoid, possibly because it gets fatigued and stretched; there is currently no scientific evidence to support this theory. There is documentation that the internal rotators are naturally stronger than the external rotators.[35]

Compared to the anterior and middle compartments, there is almost always more atrophy and less sEMG of the posterior deltoid. Clinically, this might be due to the increased length of the posterior deltoid with anterior translated head of the humerus associated with forward shoulders. In patients with multidirectional shoulder instability, the posterior deltoid is the most important muscle to train. In these patients, the deltoid should be trained isometrically to restore its ability to approximate the glenoid into the fossa to prevent excessive caudal glide.[36]

Volume Conduction: Middle deltoid, infraspinatus, teres major, and triceps

Other Sites of Interest: Long head of triceps, latissimus dorsi, teres major, middle and anterior deltoid, and upper and lower trapezius during movements of the upper extremities

Referred Pain Considerations: Trigger points at this site refer pain locally.[17]

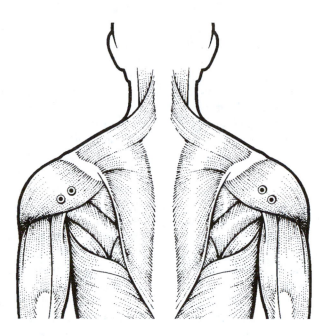

Figure 14–27 Electrode placement for the posterior deltoid site. *Source:* Copyright © Clinical Resources, Inc.

PECTORALIS MAJOR (CLAVICULAR AND STERNAL) PLACEMENT

Type of Placement: Specific

Action: Medial (internal) rotation and flexion of the shoulder; horizontal adduction of the arm; depression of the shoulder (sternal aspect)

Clinical Uses: Shoulder and arm rehabilitation

Muscle Insertions: The clavicular aspect arises from the medial third of the clavicle. The sternal aspect arises from the sternal membrane and the cartilage of the second to sixth ribs. Both insert on the greater tubercle of the humerus.

Innervation: This area is innervated by the medial and lateral pectoralis nerves. The clavicular aspect is innervated mainly via the C-5 and C-6 spinal nerves; the sternal aspect is innervated mainly via the C-6 and C-7 spinal nerves.

Joint Considerations: In addition to the spinal joints that might affect the nerve roots (C-5 through T-1), other joints that should be cleared of problems include the sternoclavicular (and thus the AC) joint, the sternomanubrial junction, the costocartilaginous and costosternal junctions, and the second through sixth ribs.

Location: For clavicular placement, palpate the clavicle. Two active electrodes (2 cm apart) are placed on the chest wall at an oblique angle toward the clavicle, approximately 2 cm below the clavicle, just medial to the axillary fold (Figure 14–28A).

For sternal placement, locate the anterior axillary fold (armpit). Palpate just medial to the fold while the patient medially rotates the arm against resistance. Place two active electrodes (2 cm apart) horizontally on the chest wall over the muscle mass that arises (approximately 2 cm out from the axillary fold) (Figure 14–28A).

Behavioral Test: Flexion of the arm, abduction of the arm above 90 degrees, medial rotation, and horizontal adduction of arm

Tracing Comment: Figure 14–28B shows sEMG recordings from the clavicular and sternal pectoralis sites, along with anterior deltoids and posterior deltoids. The motions of right arm flexion, chair push-up, and right palm to left ear (medial rotation and adduction) are represented.

Note the primary role of anterior deltoid and the clavicular aspect of pectoralis during forward flexion. During a chair push-up, all muscle groups are used for movement and stabilization. When the right palm is moved toward the left ear, both the clavicular and sternal aspects are active, with the sternal aspect coming into play toward the end of the movement pattern. Anterior deltoid also contributes to this movement (raw sEMG).

Also see tracings for serratus anterior (Figure 14–22C).

Clinical Considerations: Chronically protruded shoulders can lead to shortening of the internal rotators of the shoulder, which include the pectoralis major. Thoracic kyphosis leads to shortening of the pectoralis.

The brachial plexus, with its diverse connections, is complex. The suprascapular nerve leaves the anterior division of the superior trunk and goes cranially and posteriorly; a short distance more distally, the lateral pectoral nerve goes in the opposite direction. The pectoralis major has many fascial connections to the neck, abdomen, lateral trunk, and upper extremity. The clavicular portion can be seen as an extension of the clavicular portion of the sternocleido-mastoid, particularly if the upper extremity is in slight depression/extension and the face is rotated away.

The distal insertion of the clavicular portion is immediately adjacent to the fibers of the anterior deltoid muscle. These muscles are strong synergists and are often dysfunctional in shoulder conditions. The sternal portion's tendinous insertion can blend into the shoulder capsule. The lower portion of the pectoralis major arises off the aponeurosis of the external obliques. This may be a connection in addition to the latissimus dorsi for the many myofascial patients who complain of shoulder and pelvic pain.

Pectoralis is an accessory respirator, particularly if the upper extremities are weight bearing. Care should be taken to assess breathing habits and correct dysfunctional patterns.

Volume Conduction: Anterior deltoid, sternal or clavicular aspect of pectoralis major, pectoralis minor

Other Sites of Interest: Deltoids, upper trapezius, lower trapezius, serratus anterior, teres major, the long head of the triceps during movements of the upper extremities; SCM, scalene with extreme respiration

Artifacts: ECG

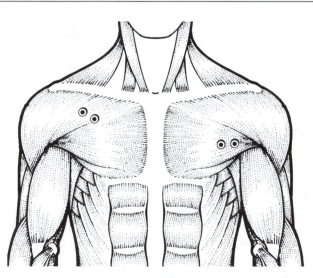

Figure 14–28A Electrode placement for the pectoralis major clavicular (right side) and sternal (left side) sites. *Source:* Copyright © Clinical Resources, Inc.

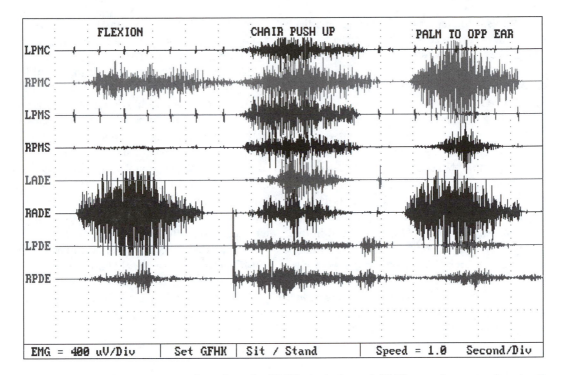

Figure 14–28B Surface EMG recordings from the (PMC) clavicular and (PMS) sternal aspects of pectoralis major, along with (ADE) anterior and (PDE) posterior deltoid during flexion of the arm, chair push-up, and movement of the right palm to left ear during horizontal adduction. *Source:* Copyright © Clinical Resources, Inc.

WRIST-TO-WRIST (WIDE) PLACEMENT

Type of Placement: General

Purpose: General index of tension in the upper extremity, shoulders, neck, and torso

Clinical Uses: Commonly used in relaxation-based treatments for upper extremity, neck, chest wall, and headache pain

Location: The active electrodes are placed on a more distal part of the arm. The wrist or back of the hands are convenient locations. The ground electrode is placed next to one of the active electrodes (Figure 14–29A).

Behavioral Test: Systematically ask the patient to tense and relax the muscles of the arm, shoulder, and torso (forearm flexors, extensors, biceps, shoulder elevation, shoulder retraction). The farther away the contracting muscles are from the active electrodes, the lower the recorded sEMG level should be.

Tracing Comment: In Figure 14–29B, (top to bottom) the wrist-to-wrist placement, upper trapezius (wide) placement, and upper trapezius (narrow) placement on the right side were monitored simultaneously. The left half of the tracing was recorded using a narrow 100-to-200–Hz band-pass filter, while the right half was conducted using a wide 25-to-1000–Hz band-pass filter. ECG artifact is present during the second half of the tracing for the two upper panels, but not for the lower panel (narrow upper trapezius placement). ECG artifact is more problematic when the two recording electrodes cross the midline and are placed farther apart. Surface EMG recordings from the left side of the upper back, even when using narrow placements, are typically more contaminated with ECG artifact compared to right-sided placements. In addition, the wider 25-to-1000–Hz filter passes more of the sEMG spectrum along for amplification and thus shows a higher level of RMS microvolts. This is most clearly seen in the lower panel. Although the tracing does not show the heart rate artifact once the filters are changed to 25-to-1000–Hz range, it does show an increase in the sEMG levels (processed sEMG).

Figure 14–29C presents recordings from (top to bottom) the wrist-to-wrist placement, the cervical trapezius (wide) placement for the right side only, and the upper trapezius (narrow) placement for the left side only. The 100-to-200–Hz band-pass filter is used, which is usually recommended for the wrist-to-wrist placement. Three sets of activation patterns are seen in the tracing. The first set represents right and then left wrist extension. The second represents right and then left elbow flexion. The third represents right and then left shoulder girdle elevation. Note how the wrist-to-wrist leads pick up volume-conducted sEMG activity from the forearm extensors during wrist extension, from the bi-ceps during elbow flexion, and to a lesser extent from the upper trapezius during shoulder girdle elevation (processed sEMG).

Clinical Considerations: Head, shoulder, arm, hand, and finger position can alter the resting levels. One can readily demonstrate how this placement records from all of the muscles in both upper extremities and upper torso by asking the patient to systematically tense and release each major muscle group in the left upper extremity, left shoulder, right shoulder, and right lower extremity. If the sEMG system allows a choice of filters, the narrow 100-to-200–Hz band-pass filter eliminates the ECG artifact.

Volume Conduction: This placement detects sEMG activity from all of the muscles of the arm, shoulder, and upper back.

Other Sites of Interest: Frontalis (wide) and ankle-to-ankle (wide) to assess and promote generalization

Artifacts: ECG, breathing

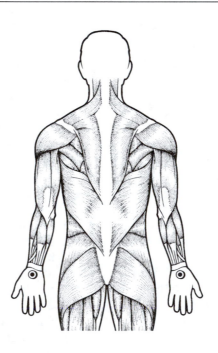

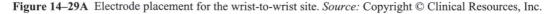

Figure 14–29A Electrode placement for the wrist-to-wrist site. *Source:* Copyright © Clinical Resources, Inc.

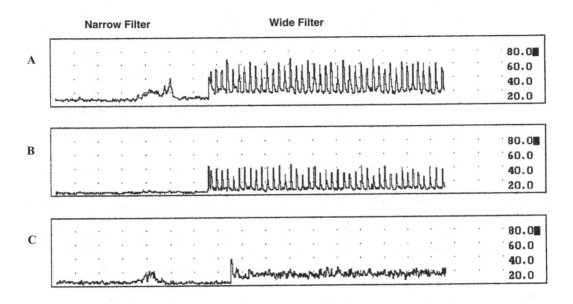

Figure 14–29B Surface EMG recordings from (**A**) the wrist-to-wrist placement, (**B**) upper trapezius (wide) placement, and (**C**) upper trapezius (narrow) placement on the right side were monitored simultaneously. The first half of the tracing was recorded using 100-to-200–Hz band-pass filter; the second half was conducted using a 25-to-1000–Hz band-pass filter. *Source:* Copyright © Clinical Resources, Inc.

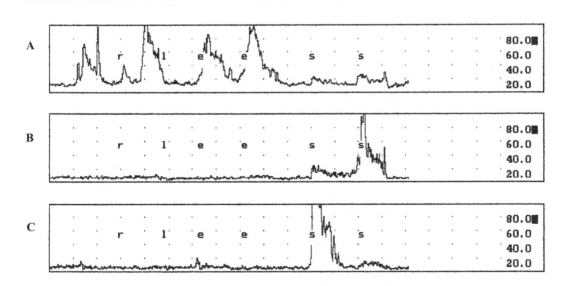

Figure 14–29C Surface EMG recordings from (**A**) the wrist-to-wrist placement, (**B**) the cervical trapezius (wide) placement for the right side only, and (**C**) the upper trapezius (narrow) placement for the left side only are shown using the 100-to-200–Hz band-pass filter. Three sets of activation patterns are seen in the tracing. The first set (*r* and *l*) represents right and then left wrist extension. The second (*e* and *e*) represents right and then left elbow flexion. The third (*s* and *s*) represents right and then left shoulder girdle elevation. *Source:* Copyright © Clinical Resources, Inc.

FOREARM FLEXOR/EXTENSOR (WIDE) PLACEMENT

Type of Placement: General

Purpose: To monitor the general level of muscle tension in the forearm bundles

Clinical Uses: To study general tension of the body, and the forearm in particular; to assess and treat arm-related pains such as repetitive strain injury; for use in industrial medicine and ergonomics

Location: One active electrode is placed over the wrist extensor bundle (top of the arm) and the other is placed over the flexor bundle (bottom of the arm). The extensor site is found on the dorsal aspect of the arm, approximately 5 cm distal from the elbow. The practitioner should place the fingers on that surface and ask the patient to extend his/her wrist. Place electrode in the center of the muscle mass that emerges. The flexor site is located on the ventral aspect of the arm, approximately 5 cm distal from the elbow. Ask the patient to flex his/her wrist. Place the electrode in the center of the muscle mass that emerges (Figure 14–30A).

Behavioral Test: Flexion, extension, pronation, and supination of the wrist and hand

Tracing Comment: In Figure 14–30B, sEMG recordings from the wide flexor extensor site are presented along with recordings from wide placements for flexor and extensor. Activation patterns during wrist extension, flexion, and cocontraction (making a fist) are presented. This wide placement shows recruitment for all movements, while the wide extensor and wide flexor sites show specificity of function and recruitment only during their movement (processed sEMG).

Clinical Considerations: The sEMG values may change radically as a function of the arm/wrist being supported. Sitting with arms in the lap provides different values than standing with arms at the sides. Degree of pronation/supination or ulnar deviation can also alter resting levels.

This site is commonly used to monitor the upper extremity in cases of repetitive strain injury or carpal tunnel syndrome. Lundervold[37] studied a large number of normal subjects and patients with occupational myalgias using needle EMG recordings and noted that patients showed increased and prolonged recruitment patterns during typing compared to normal subjects. He noted that activity in the asymptomatic arm could cause recruitment in the symptomatic arm while at rest and that forearm muscle activity could be readily induced by physical or emotional stress. Skubick et al[38] noted that, in patients with carpal tunnel syndrome, the forearm flexors and extensors tend to become active during cervical rotation. He attributed this to a return of the tonic neck reflex in these symptomatic individuals. In addition, it has been noted that there is an increase in the sEMG levels of distal segments when there is scapular instability. Singh and Karpovich[39] also provide information concerning isotonic and isometric contractions in the flexors and extensors.

Volume Conduction: All of the muscles of the forearm; to a lesser extent, muscles of the upper arm

Other Sites of Interest: Biceps, triceps, deltoids, upper trapezius, midcervical paraspinals, SCM

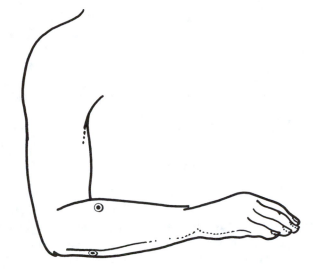

Figure 14–30A Electrode placement for forearm flexor/extensor (wide) site. *Source:* Copyright © Clinical Resources, Inc.

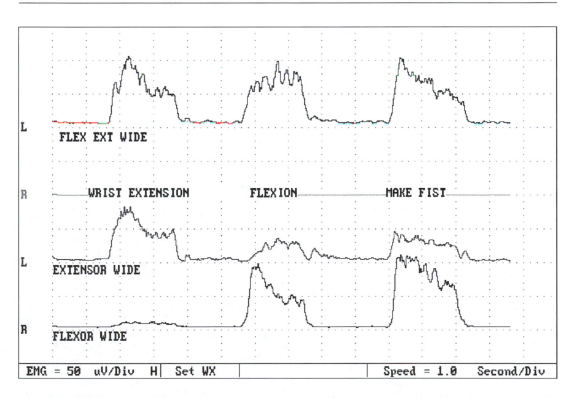

Figure 14–30B Surface EMG recordings from the forearm extensor/flexor site, along with recordings from wide placements of the flexor and extensor sites during the movements of wrist extension, flexion, and cocontraction (making a fist). *Source:* Copyright © Clinical Resources, Inc.

FOREARM EXTENSOR BUNDLE (WIDE) PLACEMENT

Type of Placement: Quasi-specific

Purpose: To measure the muscle bundle associated with wrist extension (primarily extensor digitorum)

Clinical Uses: Rehabilitation of the wrist and hand, assessment and treatment of repetitive strain injury, industrial medicine, ergonomics

Location: The extensor site is found on the dorsal aspect of the arm, approximately 5 cm distal from the elbow. The practitioner should place the fingers on that surface and ask the patient to extend his/her wrist. Place the electrodes 3 to 4 cm apart in the center of the muscle mass that emerges, with the electrodes oriented in the direction of the muscle fibers. The wide placement will ensure volume-conducted pickup from the extensor carpi radialis and extensor carpi ulnaris, as well as the extensor digitorum (Figure 14–31A).

Behavioral Test: Extension of the wrist

Tracing Comment: In Figure 14–31B, sEMG recordings for both the wide forearm extensor site (upper) and the wide forearm flexor site are presented during left and right wrist flexion. The extensor groups recruit vigorously during wrist extension (raw sEMG).

In Figure 14–31C, the flexor and extensor sites for the left arm are monitored. The subject first makes a fist, coactivating both the extensor and flexor groups. This action is followed by wrist extension and then wrist flexion in the neutral position.

Also see tracings from wrist flexors (Figure 14–32B).

Clinical Considerations: Resting values may be affected by arm, wrist, and finger positions, along with the degree of pronation and supination.

This site is commonly used to monitor the upper extremity in cases of repetitive strain injury or carpal tunnel syndrome. Lundervold[37] studied a large number of normal subjects and patients with occupational myalgias, using needle EMG recordings, and he noted that patients showed increased and prolonged recruitment patterns in extensor carpi radialis during typing compared to normal subjects. He noted that activity in the asymptomatic arm could cause recruitment in the symptomatic arm while at rest and that forearm muscle activity could be readily induced by physical or emotional stress. Skubick et al[38] noted that, in patients with carpal tunnel syndrome, the forearm flexors and extensors tend to become active during cervical rotation. He attributed this to a return of the tonic neck reflex in these symptomatic individuals. In addition, it has been noted that there is an increase in the sEMG levels of distal segments when there is scapular instability. Singh and Karpovich[39] also provide information concerning isotonic and isometric contractions in the flexors and extensors.

Volume Conduction: Extensor digitorum, brachioradialis, extensor carpi radialis (longus and brevis), and pronator teres

Other Sites of Interest: Forearm flexor (wide) placement, biceps, triceps, deltoids, upper trapezius, midcervical paraspinals, SCM

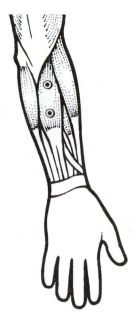

Figure 14–31A Electrode placement for the forearm extensor (wide) site. *Source:* Copyright © Clinical Resources, Inc.

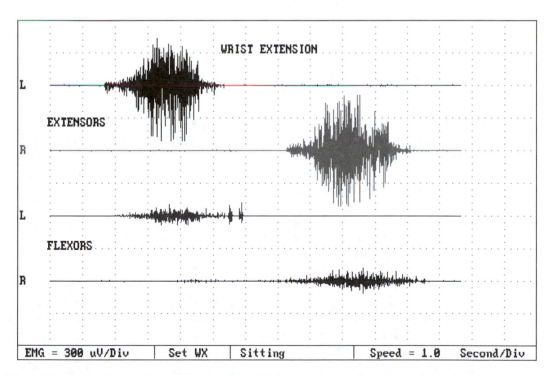

Figure 14–31B Surface EMG recording from the wide forearm extensor (upper) and flexor (lower) sites during wrist extension. *Source:* Copyright © Clinical Resources, Inc.

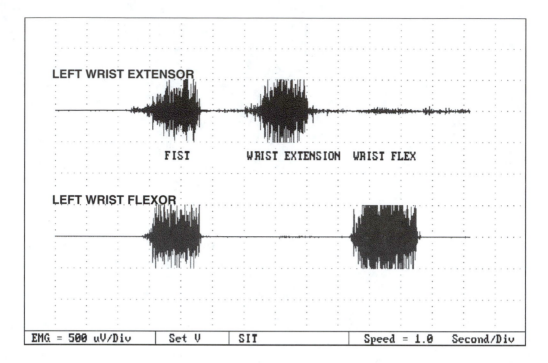

Figure 14–31C Surface EMG recordings from the forearm extensor and flexor (wide) sites during making a fist, wrist extension, and wrist flexion. *Source:* Copyright © Clinical Resources, Inc.

FOREARM FLEXOR BUNDLE (WIDE) PLACEMENT

Type of Placement: Quasi-specific

Purpose: To monitor the muscles associated with wrist flexion

Clinical Uses: To assess and treat arm pain and repetitive strain injury; used in industrial medicine and ergonomics

Location: The flexor site is located on the ventral aspect of the arm, approximately 5 cm distal from the elbow. Hold the patient's dorsal side of the arm. Ask the patient to flex his/her wrist and palpate the muscle mass that emerges. Place two active electrodes 3 to 4 cm apart over the belly of the muscle in the direction of the muscle fibers (Figure 14–32A).

Behavioral Test: Flexion of the wrist

Tracing Comment: In Figure 14–32B, both the flexor and extensor bundles are monitored simultaneously during flexion of the left and right wrists (raw sEMG).

Also see tracings from wrist extensors (Figure 14–31B).

Clinical Considerations: Position and support of the hand, fingers, and arm may affect sEMG values. The resting tone is greatly affected by arm, finger, and wrist position. Degree of supination or pronation during flexion may affect the readings, depending upon electrode placement.

This site is commonly used to monitor the upper extremity in cases of repetitive strain injury or carpal tunnel syndrome. Lundervold[37] studied a large number of normal subjects and patients with occupational myalgias, using needle EMG recordings, and he noted that patients showed increased and prolonged recruitment patterns during typing compared to normal subjects. He noted that activity in the asymptomatic arm could cause recruitment in the symptomatic arm while at rest and that forearm muscle activity could be readily induced by physical or emotional stress. Skubick et al[38] noted that, in patients with carpal tunnel syndrome, the forearm flexors and extensors tend to become active during cervical rotation. He attributed this to a return of the tonic neck reflex in these symptomatic individuals. Singh and Karpovich[39] also provide information concerning isotonic and isometric contractions in the flexors and extensors.

Volume Conduction: Flexor digitorum (superficialis and profundus), flexor carpi (ulnaris and radialis), and flexor pollicis longus

Other Sites of Interest: Forearm extensor (wide) placement, biceps, triceps, deltoids, upper trapezius, midcervical paraspinals, SCM

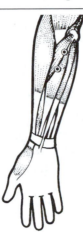

Figure 14–32A Electrode placement for forearm flexor bundle (wide) site. *Source:* Copyright © Clinical Resources, Inc.

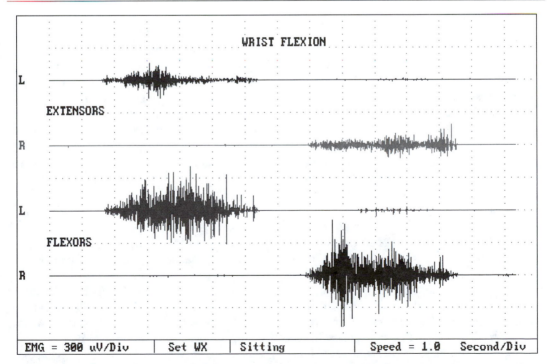

Figure 14–32B Surface EMG recordings from forearm extensor (wide) placement and forearm flexor (wide) placement during left and right wrist flexion. *Source:* Copyright © Clinical Resources, Inc.

BICEPS-BRACHIUM PLACEMENT

Type of Placement: Specific

Action: Forearm flexion, supination, and shoulder flexion

Clinical Uses: Rehabilitation

Muscle Insertions: The biceps is a two-bellied muscle. The long head arises from the superior margin of the supraglenoid tubercle of the scapula and passes over the head of the humerus. The short head arises from the coracoid process of the scapula. Both insert into the tuberosity of the radius.

Innervation: The musculocutaneous nerve via the lateral cord and spinal nerves C-5 and C-6

Location: Ask the patient to flex his/her forearm in the supinated position. Palpate the muscle mass in the dorsal aspect of the upper arm that emerges. Place two active electrodes (2 cm apart) parallel to the muscle fibers and in the center of the mass (Figure 14–33A, left arm).

Variations: Due to the compartmentalization of this muscle, placing the active electrodes more laterally will emphasize detection of shoulder flexion (in addition to forearm flexion), and placing the electrodes more medially will emphasize detection of adduction and internal rotation. If electrodes are placed too distally with the lateral placement, there will be volume conduction from brachialis (Figure 14–33A, right arm).

Behavioral Test: Flex the forearm. Resisted flexion augments the signal.

Tracing Comment: The tracings for biceps also include recordings from other related muscles such as triceps, deltoids, brachioradialis, and pronator teres. Refer to tracings for these sites, as well.

For biceps/triceps isolation, see Figure 14–33B, in which three sites for placement of electrodes on the biceps and triceps are used. The top three tracings show the lateral, intermediate, and medial aspects of the biceps. The lower three tracings show the lateral, intermediate, and medial aspects of the triceps. Two movements are depicted: resisted elbow flexion in the supinated position and resisted elbow extension. Here, there is clear isolation of biceps during flexion and fairly clear isolation of triceps during extension. There is minor cross-talk to the lateral and medial biceps (raw sEMG).

For biceps during supination, see Figure 14–33C, in which the intermediate biceps and pronator teres are studied during supination and pronation. During supination, biceps is active while pronator is quiet. However, during pronation, the pronator teres is active while the biceps is quiet (raw sEMG).

For biceps during elbow flexion, see Figure 14–33D, in which brachioradialis (top) and biceps (bottom) are studied during elbow flexion in three positions. During elbow flexion with supination (palm up), both muscles recruit briskly. In the neutral position (thumb up), the muscles display the same pattern, only more reduced. During flexion with pronation (palm down), the biceps is no longer involved and brachioradialis does all of the work of flexion (raw sEMG).

In Figure 14–33E, elbow and shoulder flexion are shown while monitoring biceps (intermediate), anterior deltoids, long head of triceps, lateral triceps, posterior deltoids, and latissimus dorsi. During elbow flexion, the biceps show a very strong recruitment pattern. During shoulder flexion, the anterior deltoid recruits robustly, with some recruitment seen in biceps.

Clinical Considerations: Positioning of the arm can dramatically alter the resting tone and recruitment patterns. Consider how the arm is supported while in the seated position. As seen in Figure 14–33D, the degree of supination/pronation is important. Length-tension relationships that are altered by the amount of flexion at the elbow can dramatically alter biceps recruitment patterns.

Recruitment of biceps during elbow flexion is enhanced during supination and diminished during pronation.[16,40]

Volume Conduction: Brachialis, deltoids, triceps, forearm, extensors

Other Sites of Interest: Brachioradialis during flexion of the forearm; brachioradialis, anterior deltoid, suprascapular fossa site (supraspinatus) during abduction of the arm; triceps

Referred Pain Considerations: Trigger points in this muscle refer pain mainly upward, to the anterior deltoid region.[17]

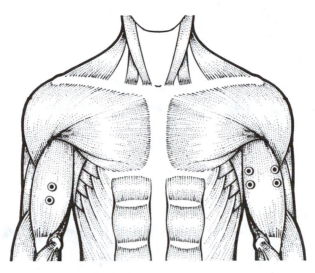

Figure 14–33A Electrode placement for the biceps-brachium site. *Source:* Copyright © Clinical Resources, Inc.

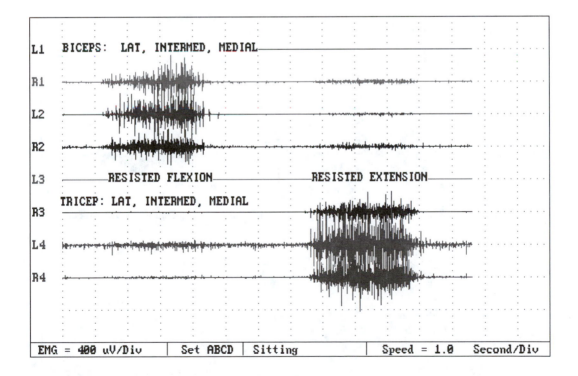

Figure 14–33B Surface EMG recordings from biceps and triceps are presented. The top three tracings show the (**R1**) lateral, (**L2**) intermediate, and (**R2**) medial aspects of biceps. The lower three tracings show the (**R3**) lateral, (**L4**) intermediate, and (**R4**) medial aspects of the triceps. Resisted elbow flexion and extension are presented. *Source:* Copyright © Clinical Resources, Inc.

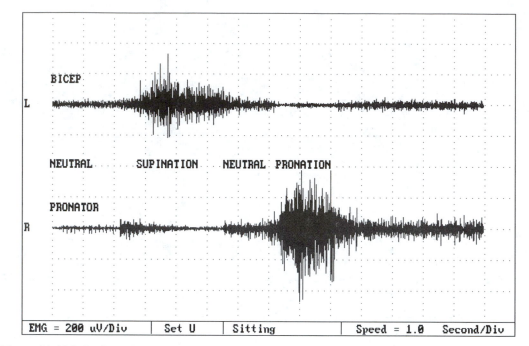

Figure 14–33C Surface EMG recordings from biceps and pronator teres are presented during supination and pronation. *Source:* Copyright © Clinical Resources, Inc.

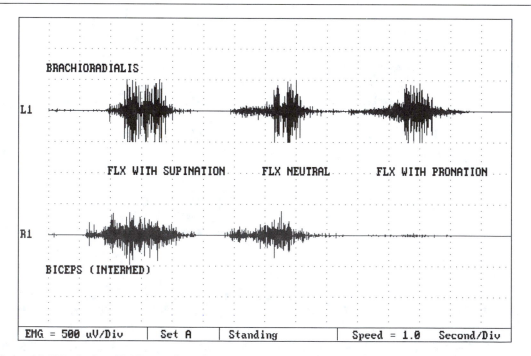

Figure 14–33D Surface EMG recordings from brachioradialis and biceps are shown during elbow flexion in supinated and pronated positions. Note the absence of biceps recruitment during pronated elbow flexion. *Source:* Copyright © Clinical Resources, Inc.

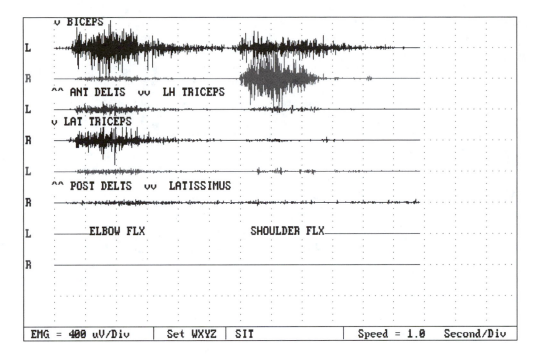

Figure 14–33E Surface EMG monitoring of biceps (intermediate), anterior deltoids, long head of triceps, lateral triceps, posterior deltoids, and latissimus dorsi during elbow and shoulder flexion. *Source:* Copyright © Clinical Resources, Inc.

TRICEPS PLACEMENT

Type of Placement: Specific

Action: Extension of elbow and adduction and extension of the shoulder

Clinical Uses: Rehabilitation

Muscle Insertions: The long head of this three-bellied muscle arises from infraglenoid lip of the scapula; the medial and lateral heads of this muscle arise from the medial and lateral aspects of the radial groove of the humerus, respectively; and all three fuse and insert on the olecranon process of the ulna via a common tendon.

Innervation: Branches of the radial nerve via the posterior cord and the spinal nerves C-7 and C-8

Location: To monitor from the long head of the triceps, two active electrodes (2 cm apart) are placed parallel to the muscle fibers, 2 cm medial from midline of the arm, approximately 50% of the distance between the acromion and the olecranon or elbow. Caution should be exercised

not to place electrode too distally. Because electrode position on the skin relative to muscles below may change as a function of arm/palm position, palpate and place the electrodes in the arm position to be studied. To place electrode on the lateral aspect of the triceps muscle, palpate the lateral aspect of the triceps region during an isometric contraction. As with the long head placement, two active electrodes (2 cm apart) are placed parallel to the muscle fibers, approximately 2 cm lateral from midline of the arm, approximately 50% of the distance between the acromion and the olecranon or elbow (Figure 14–34A).

Behavioral Test: Extension of the forearm (resistance of this movement augments the sEMG signal)

Tracing Comment: In Figure 14–34B, sEMG recordings from the right posterior deltoid, medial triceps, lateral triceps, and infraspinatus are shown during isometric extension with the elbow at 90 degrees with three angles of shoulder flexion and again with the elbow at 0 degrees and resisted extension of the shoulder and arm. The posterior deltoid appears to be deactivated when the shoulder is at 160 degrees of flexion, and becomes more active as the shoulder reaches 90 degrees of flexion. Both aspects of triceps are active during all four movements. The level of recruitment is stronger when the arm is straight than when it is bent and, particularly, when the shoulder and elbow are extended. The infraspinatus is active primarily during the shoulder and arm extension (raw sEMG).

Figure 14–34C presents sEMG recordings from the right posterior deltoid, general triceps, and infraspinatus during resisted elbow flexion at 90 degrees, with the shoulder flexed to 90 degrees. This level of shoulder flexion allows the recruitment of triceps to be seen (raw sEMG).

See biceps tracings for additional tracings of triceps (Figure 14–33B).

Clinical Considerations: Surface EMG values may differ when patient is sitting with arm supported from when patient is standing. Arm position may affect the recordings and should be noted.

Although the medial head of triceps is the main "workhorse" for elbow extension,[16,41] the long head of the triceps is strongly involved in adduction.[31]

Volume Conduction: Biceps, posterior and medial deltoids

Other Sites of Interest: Forearm extensors; latissimus dorsi and teres major during adduction and extension of the shoulder

Referred Pain Considerations: Trigger points in this muscle project primarily up and down the posterior aspect of the arm and to the lateral epicondyle with potential spillover into the fourth and fifth digits.[17]

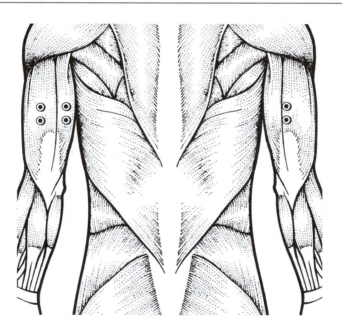

Figure 14–34A Electrode placement for long head and lateral triceps sites. *Source:* Copyright © Clinical Resources, Inc.

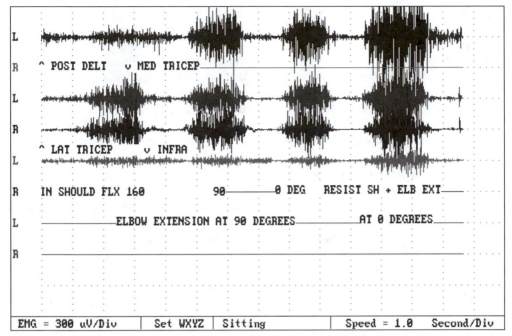

Figure 14–34B Surface EMG recordings from the right posterior deltoid, medial triceps, lateral triceps, and infraspinatus are shown during isometric extension with the elbow at 90 degrees with three angles of shoulder flexion and again with the elbow at 0 degrees and resisted extension of the shoulder and arm. *Source:* Copyright © Clinical Resources, Inc.

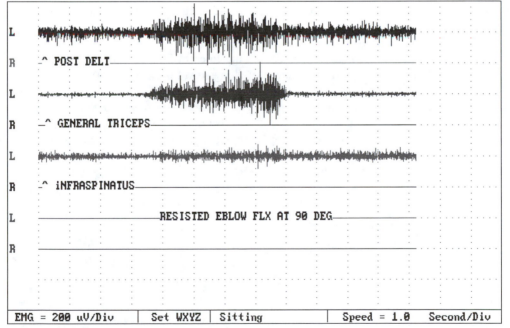

Figure 14–34C Surface EMG recordings from the right posterior deltoid, general triceps, and infraspinatus are shown during resisted elbow flexion at 90 degrees, with the shoulder flexed to 90 degrees. *Source:* Copyright © Clinical Resources, Inc.

BRACHIORADIALIS PLACEMENT

Type of Placement: Quasi-specific
Action: Elbow flexion
Clinical Uses: Rehabilitation
Muscle Insertions: This muscle arises from the lateral supracondylar ridge of the humerus and the related intermuscular septum and inserts into the tendinous attachments of the styloid process of the wrist.
Innervation: The radial nerve from the posterior cord and spinal nerves C-5 and C-6
Location: Palpate the muscle mass just distal to the elbow while resisting elbow flexion with the wrist in the neutral position (thumb up). Two active electrodes, 2 cm apart, are placed approximately 4 cm distally from the lateral epicondyle of the elbow on the medial fleshy mass that covers that area, so that they run parallel to the muscle fibers (Figure 14–35A).
Behavioral Test: Flex the forearm.
Tracing Comment: In Figure 14–35B, three muscle sites are monitored: extensor carpi ulnaris, extensor carpi radialis, and brachioradialis. Four isolated movements are shown with the elbow at 90 degrees, thumb up. During resisted elbow flexion with the wrist relaxed, brachioradialis shows the strongest activation pattern with suspected cross-talk at the extensor carpi ulnaris and extensor carpi radialis sites. During wrist extension with the rest of the arm well supported and relaxed, the extensor carpi ulnaris and extensor carpi radialis sites show strong burst patterns. Activation in the brachioradialis site during this movement probably reflects minor cross-talk. During resisted radial deviation, the extensor carpi radialis shows its strong recruitment pattern, with minor cross-talk or compensatory stabilization activity noted at the extensor carpi ulnaris and brachioradialis sites. During ulnar deviation, the extensor carpi ulnaris shows its strongest recruitment pattern, with minor cross-talk or stabilization activity noted at the extensor carpi radialis site. There is little or no cross-talk or activation noted at the brachioradialis site during this movement (raw sEMG).

Also see tracings for biceps (Figure 14–33D), flexor carpi radialis (Figure 14–40B), and flexor carpi ulnaris (Figure 14–41B).

Clinical Considerations: The position of the wrist can affect the level of recruitment as is seen in Figure 14–33D. The degree of elbow flexion can affect the amplitude and time of recruitment due to length-tension relationships. The activity of this muscle is augmented during quick elbow flexion movements, when a weight is to be lifted, and when the arm is in the neutral position.[16]

Volume Conduction: Volume conduction is a major problem. Signals from extensor carpi radialis (longus and brevis) and brachioradialis are common.

Other Sites of Interest: Biceps brachium during forearm flexion, and extensor carpi radialis (longus and brevis) during wrist extension and grasping

Referred Pain Considerations: Trigger points in this muscle refer pain primarily to the lateral epicondyle, as well as down the length of the muscle to the web of the hand.[17]

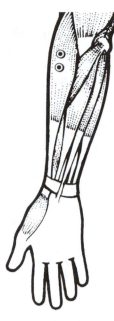

Figure 14–35A Electrode placement for the brachioradialis site. *Source:* Copyright © Clinical Resources, Inc.

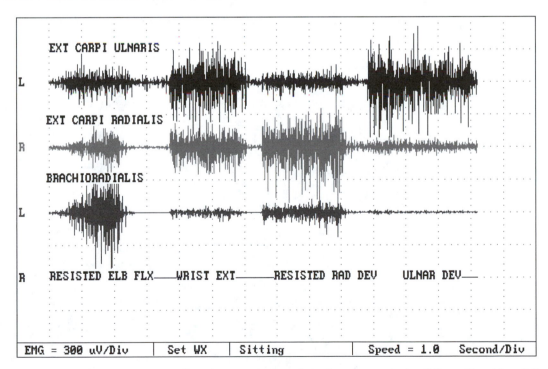

Figure 14–35B Surface EMG recordings from extensor carpi ulnaris, extensor carpi radialis, and brachioradialis during resisted elbow flexion, wrist extension, resisted radial deviation, and ulnar deviation. *Source:* Copyright © Clinical Resources, Inc.

VENTRAL FOREARM (PRONATOR TERES) PLACEMENT

Type of Placement: Quasi-specific

Action: Pronation of the arm

Clinical Uses: Rehabilitation

Muscle Insertions: The pronator teres arises from the humeral head of the epicondyle and the ulnar head of the coronoid process, and inserts into the middle of the lateral surface of the radius.

Innervation: The median nerve through spinal nerves C-6 and C-7

Location: Support the arm in the palm-up (supinated) position. Palpate in the soft valley in the middle of the ventral aspect of the forearm just below the elbow. Ask the patient to pronate (palm up to palm down) the arm and feel for the muscle mass. Place two active electrodes (2 cm apart) on an oblique angle so that they run parallel to the muscle fibers (Figure 14–36A).

Behavioral Test: Pronate the arm.

Tracing Comment: In Figure 14–36B, recordings are made from the flexor carpi radialis and pronator teres placement. The elbow is bent at 90 degrees with the wrist in a neutral position (thumb up). Two isolated movements are shown. During wrist flexion in the neutral position, the flexor carpi radialis shows a clear burst pattern. Minor cross-talk is suspected at the pronator site. Resisted pronation was accomplished by securing the patient's wrist, then asking the patient to rotate the arm toward the palm-down position while keeping the fingers relaxed. Note the poor separation of these two recording sites, suggesting cross-talk between recording sites (raw sEMG).

Also see tracings for biceps (Figure 14–33B).

Clinical Considerations: Support of the arm may affect the initial resting tone of the muscle. The beginning wrist position would, of course, affect the observed recruitment pattern. The degree of elbow flexion does not appear to affect the activity in this muscle.[16]

Volume Conduction: Expect considerable cross-talk from flexor carpi radialis, palmaris longus, and brachioradialis.

Other Sites of Interest: Brachioradialis

Referred Pain Considerations: Trigger points in this muscle commonly refer pain to the base of the thumb.[17]

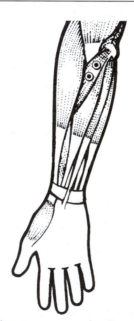

Figure 14–36A Electrode placement for the pronator teres site. *Source:* Copyright © Clinical Resources, Inc.

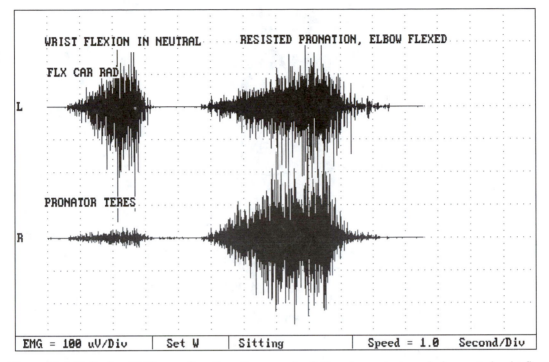

Figure 14–36B Surface EMG recordings from flexor carpi radialis and pronator teres during neutral wrist flexion and resisted pronation. *Source:* Copyright © Clinical Resources, Inc.

EXTENSOR CARPI ULNARIS PLACEMENT

Type of Placement: Quasi-specific

Action: Wrist extension, ulnar deviation

Clinical Uses: Hand rehabilitation, industrial ergonomics

Muscle Insertions: This muscle arises from the common extensor tendon from the lateral epicondyle of the humerus and the aponeurosis from the border of the ulna, and inserts on the pisiform bone in the hand and the fifth metacarpal.

Innervation: The radial nerve from spinal nerves C-6, C-7, and C-8

Location: Support the patient's arm in the palm-down position. Palpate the ulnar (little finger) side of the arm a few cm below the elbow. Have the patient do an ulnar deviation of the wrist, and palpate for the active muscle mass. Place two active electrodes 2 cm apart in the direction of the muscle fibers (Figure 14–37A).

Behavioral Test: Ulnar deviation of the wrist

Tracing Comment: In Figure 14–37B, extensor carpi radialis and extensor carpi ulnaris sites are monitored while the wrist is supported in the neutral position (thumb up), and the hand is out over the edge of the table. Radial deviation is resisted to augment and isolate the recruitment pattern. Note the burst of activity at extensor carpi radialis site. Next, an unresisted ulnar deviation is conducted. Clear isolation of the extensor carpi ulnaris is present. Finally, an unresisted wrist extension is examined with both sites showing a synergy pattern (raw sEMG).

Also see brachioradialis tracings (Figure 14–35B).

Clinical Considerations: The degree of support of the arm affects the resting tone. Wrist position alters initial resting amplitudes and recruitment patterns.

Volume Conductor: Extensor carpi radialis, brachioradialis, and extensor digitorum

Other Sites of Interest: Extensor carpi radialis, brachioradialis, flexor carpi ulnaris

Referred Pain Considerations: Trigger points in this muscle refer pain to the dorsal side of the wrist.[17]

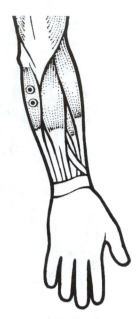

Figure 14–37A Electrode placement for extensor carpi ulnaris. *Source:* Copyright © Clinical Resources, Inc.

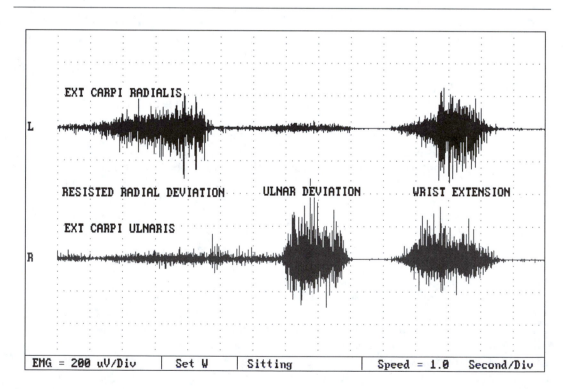

Figure 14–37B Surface EMG recordings from extensor carpi radialis and extensor carpi ulnaris sites during resisted radial deviation, unresisted ulnar deviation, and wrist extension. *Source:* Copyright © Clinical Resources, Inc.

EXTENSOR CARPI RADIALIS (LONGUS AND BREVIS) PLACEMENT

Type of Placement: Quasi-specific

Action: Wrist extension, abduction, radial deviation

Clinical Uses: Hand rehabilitation, industrial ergonomics

Muscle Insertions: The brevis component arises from the common head of the lateral epicondyle of the humerus and related ligaments and inserts into the base of the third metacarpal. The longus component arises from the margin of the humerus and related septum and inserts into the base of the second metacarpal.

Innervation: The radial nerve via the spinal nerves at C-6 and C-7

Location: Ask the patient to flex the wrist and palpate the muscle mass approximately 5 cm distal from the lateral epicondyle of the elbow, on dorsal side of the arm just lateral to brachioradialis. Place two active electrodes 2 cm apart over the muscle mass that emerges, with the electrodes running in the direction of the muscle fibers (Figure 14–38A).

Behavioral Test: Wrist extension and radial deviation

Tracing Comment: In Figure 14–38B, sEMG recordings from the extensor carpi radialis, extensor indicis proprius, and abductor pollicis sites are presented while the wrist was supported in the neutral position (thumb up). Three movements were studied in isolation. (1) During wrist extension with the fingers remaining relaxed, the extensor carpi radialis shows clear isolation. (2) During extension of first finger with the wrist in the neutral position, a clear burst pattern is seen at the extensor indicis proprius site not involving abductor pollicis. Some activity is also noted in extensor carpi radialis. It is uncertain as to whether this is a synergy pattern or cross-talk. (3) During thumb and finger extension (spreading the palm), a clear burst pattern is seen from the abductor pollicis site, along with strong activity from extensor indicis proprius. Extensor carpi radialis shows some minor activity (raw sEMG).

Also see tracings for brachioradialis (Figure 14–35B), extensor carpi ulnaris (Figure 14–37B), and extensor digitorum (Figure 14–39B).

Clinical Considerations: The way in which the wrist is supported may affect sEMG values associated with resting tone. Because finger extension activity is noted at this site (Figure 14–38B), finger position may also affect recording levels. This site is known to play a role in the power grip.[42]

Volume Conduction: Brachioradialis and extensor digitorum

Other Sites of Interest: Extensor carpi ulnaris and finger extensors during extension; flexor carpi radialis during ulnar deviation; flexor carpi ulnaris during flexion

Referred Pain Considerations: Trigger points in these muscles refer pain primarily to the lateral epicondyle, lightly over the dorsum of the arm, and dorsal aspect of the web of the thumb.[17]

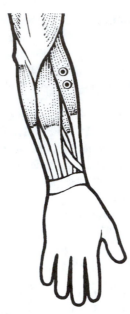

Figure 14–38A Electrode placement for the extensor carpi radialis (longus and brevis) site. *Source:* Copyright © Clinical Resources, Inc.

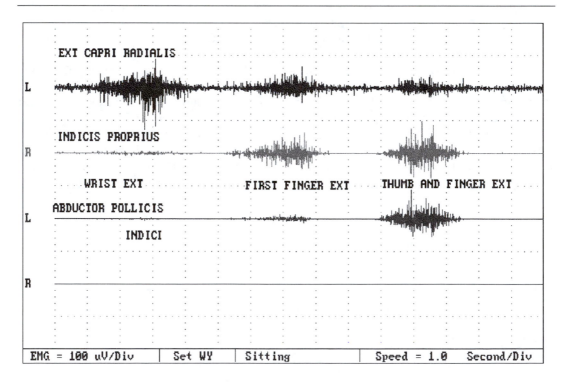

Figure 14–38B Surface EMG recordings from extensor carpi radialis, extensor indicis proprius, and abductor pollicis during wrist extension, first-finger extension, and thumb and finger extension. *Source:* Copyright © Clinical Resources, Inc.

EXTENSOR DIGITORUM PLACEMENT

Type of Placement: Quasi-specific

Action: Finger extension

Clinical Uses: Hand rehabilitation

Muscle Insertions: Arises from the lateral epicondyle of the humerus, the lateral collateral ligament, the annular radial ligament and related fascia, and joins the common extensor tendon of the second to fifth fingers.

Innervation: The radial nerve via the posterior cord and the spinal nerves C-6, C-7, and C-8

Location: Palpate the middle of the forearm approximately three quarters of the distance between the elbow and the wrist while the patient extends his/her fingers. Place two active electrodes, 2 cm apart, over the palpable muscle mass, placing them in the direction of the muscle fibers (Figure 14–39A).

Behavioral Test: Finger extension

Tracing Comment: Figure 14–39B shows recordings from the extensor digitorum and extensor carpi radialis sites during two movements while the arm and hand are fully supported. (1) During wrist extension, recruitment from both sites is noted. (2) During finger extension, isolation at the extensor digitorum site is noted (raw sEMG).

In Figure 14–39C, three muscle sites are monitored (top down): extensor digitorum, extensor carpi radialis, and extensor carpi ulnaris. In this tracing, each finger is extended individually against resistance while the hand is supported in the neutral position in the lap. Under these conditions, the extensor digitorum placement now shows recruitment during extension of each of the four fingers. The extensor radialis and extensor carpi radialis are also active during each movement. Note that unresisted extension of the fingers yields a different pattern of recruitment (raw sEMG).

Also see tracings for extensor carpi radialis (Figure 14–38B).

Clinical Considerations: The level of support for the arm, wrist, and fingers can affect the resting tone. Wrist position (deviation) can affect the magnitude of recruitment during finger movement.

Volume Conduction: By placing the electrodes distally, one can better isolate the finger extensors from the wrist flexors. However, volume conduction from extensor digiti minimi and extensor carpi ulnaris may be a problem.

Other Sites of Interest: The finger flexors during a strong palmar grasp

Referred Pain Considerations: Trigger points in this muscle project pain down the forearm to the back of the hand and sometimes to the ring or middle finger. Projections to the lateral epicondyle are known to occur from trigger points in the ring and little finger extensors.[17]

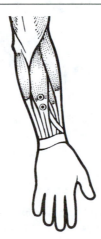

Figure 14–39A Electrode placement for the extensor digitorum site. *Source:* Copyright © Clinical Resources, Inc.

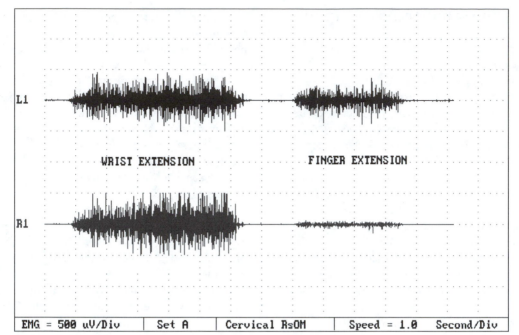

Figure 14–39B Surface EMG recordings from (**L1**) extensor digitorum and (**R1**) extensor carpi radialis during wrist extension and finger extension. *Source:* Copyright © Clinical Resources, Inc.

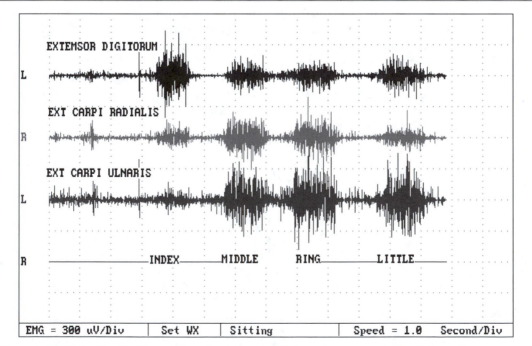

Figure 14–39C Surface EMG recordings from extensor digitorum, extensor carpi radialis, and extensor carpi ulnaris with the wrist in neutral, with resisted solitary extension of the index, middle, ring, and little fingers. *Source:* Copyright © Clinical Resources, Inc.

FLEXOR CARPI RADIALIS AND PALMARIS LONGUS PLACEMENT

Type of Placement: Quasi-specific
Action: Wrist flexion and radial deviation
Clinical Uses: Hand rehabilitation
Muscle Insertions: The flexor carpi radialis muscle arises from the medial epicondyle of the humerus and related superficial fascia, and inserts into the palmar surface of the base of the second metacarpal. The palmaris longus muscle arises from the medial epicondyle of the humerus and radiates into the palmar aponeurosis.
Innervation: The median nerve via the spinal nerves C-6 and C-7
Location: Support the arm with the fingers while palpating the ventral aspect of the forearm near the elbow on the medial (little finger) side of the arm. Ask the patient to flex the wrist. Place two active electrodes, 2 cm apart, over that muscle mass so that they run in the direction of the muscle fibers (Figure 14–40A).
Behavioral Test: Wrist flexion
Tracing Comment: In Figure 14–40B, the flexor carpi radialis and brachioradialis sites are examined while the elbow is flexed to 90 degrees and the thumb is up. First, the wrist is in radial deviation with slight flexion. A very clear separation of recordings is noted between the two sites, with the flexor carpi radialis showing a strong burst of activity. Next, the elbow flexion is resisted at the forearm. Here the brachioradialis shows a strong burst of activity, with minor activity at the flexor carpi radialis site. Finally, an isolated radial deviation is studied with resistance applied to the top of the thumb. Note the coactivation (raw sEMG).

In Figure 14–40C, both the flexor carpi radialis and flexor digitorum superficialis sites are studied. Simple wrist flexion with fingers relaxed is conducted from the neutral position. Clear separation between the wrist flexors and finger flexors is noted (raw sEMG).

In Figure 14–40D, the flexor carpi radialis and flexor carpi ulnaris sites are studied with the wrist supported in the neutral position. Flexion in midline, with ulnar deviation, and with radial deviation are studied. In the midline movement, both muscle sites activate. During the flexion with ulnar deviation, only the flexor carpi ulnaris is activated. During the flexion with radial deviation, only the flexor carpi radialis is activated (raw sEMG).

Also see tracings for flexor digitorum superficialis (Figure 14–42B).

Clinical Considerations: Support of the arm and hand may affect resting baseline levels. Deviation of the wrist can alter recruitment patterns. Interesting information regarding the compartmentalization of this muscle is available in McMahon et al.[43]

Volume Conduction: Even with closely spaced miniature electrodes, it is impossible to separate out the sEMG activity of flexor carpi radialis from palmaris longus. This placement may also record from pronator teres.

Other Sites of Interest: Flexor digitorum superficialis and flexor carpi ulnaris during wrist flexion; extensor carpi radialis (longus and brevis) during abduction of the wrist; wrist extensor muscle groups during extension

Referred Pain Considerations: Trigger points in this muscle project pain to the center of the volar wrist crease.[17]

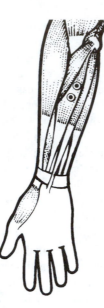

Figure 14–40A Electrode placement for the flexor carpi radialis and palmaris longus site. *Source:* Copyright © Clinical Resources, Inc.

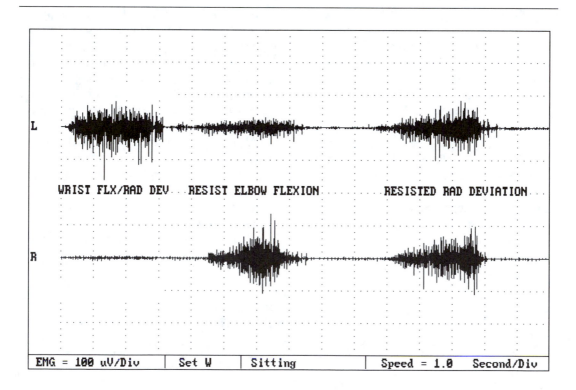

Figure 14–40B Surface EMG recordings from (**L**) flexor carpi radialis and (**R**) brachioradialis during wrist flexion and radial deviation, resisted elbow flexion, and resisted radial deviation. *Source:* Copyright © Clinical Resources, Inc.

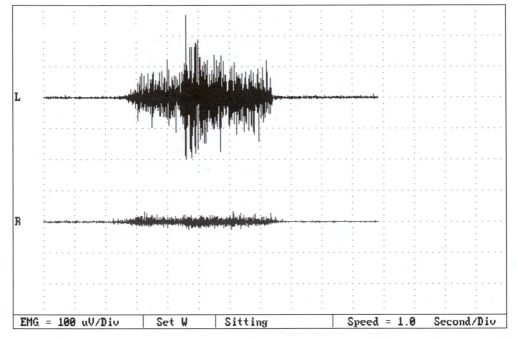

Figure 14–40C Surface EMG recordings from (**L**) flexor carpi radialis and (**R**) flexor digitorum superficialis during wrist flexion with fingers very relaxed. *Source:* Copyright © Clinical Resources, Inc.

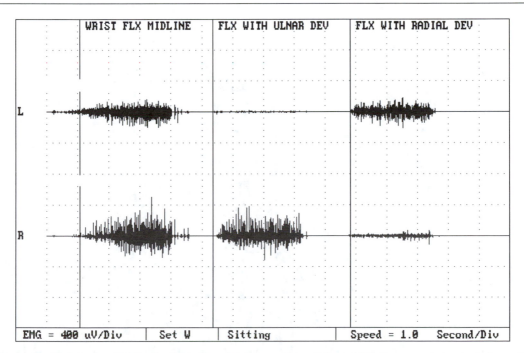

Figure 14–40D Surface EMG recordings from (**L**) flexor carpi radialis and (**R**) flexor carpi ulnaris during wrist flexion at midline, wrist flexion with ulnar deviation, and wrist flexion with radial deviation. *Source:* Copyright © Clinical Resources, Inc.

FLEXOR CARPI ULNARIS PLACEMENT

Type of Placement: Quasi-specific

Action: Flexion and adduction of the wrist

Clinical Uses: Hand rehabilitation

Muscle Insertions: This muscle arises from the medial epicondyle of the humerus and the olecranon and upper two thirds of the ulna, and inserts into the pisiform bone of the wrist and extends down to the fifth metacarpal.

Innervation: The ulnar nerve via the spinal nerves at C-8 and T-1

Location: Support the arm while palpating the medial (little finger) aspect of the forearm, approximately 2% of the distance from the elbow to the wrist. Ask the patient to deviate the hand toward the little finger side. Place two active electrodes, 2 cm apart, over the palpable muscle mass in the direction of the muscle fibers (Figure 14–41A).

Behavioral Test: Adduction and flexion of the wrist

Tracing Comment: Figure 14–41B is recorded from the flexor carpi ulnaris, flexor carpi radialis, and brachioradialis sites. Two movements are studied with the arm supported and the elbow flexed at 90 degrees with the thumb up. Radial deviation of the wrist during flexion is contrasted to resisted elbow flexion. The flexor carpi ulnaris shows a strong burst of activity during the first movement. During resisted elbow flexion, the ulnaris site shows a very strong burst pattern along with brachioradialis (raw sEMG).

Also see tracing for flexor carpi radialis (Figure 14–40D).

Clinical Considerations: Adequate support of the arm may play a role in resting sEMG levels. Wrist position affects recruitment patterns.

Volume Conduction: Flexor digitorum superficialis

Other Sites of Interest: Extensor carpi ulnaris, flexor carpi radialis, and brachioradialis sites

Referred Pain Considerations: Trigger points in this muscle project pain to the ulnar side of the volar aspect of the wrist.[17]

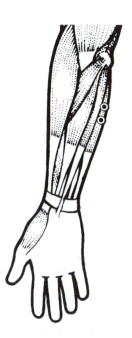

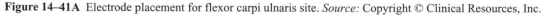

Figure 14–41A Electrode placement for flexor carpi ulnaris site. *Source:* Copyright © Clinical Resources, Inc.

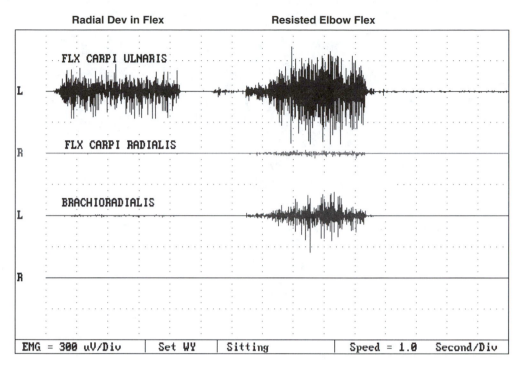

Figure 14–41B Surface EMG recordings from flexor carpi ulnaris, flexor carpi radialis, and brachioradialis during radial deviation in flexion and resisted elbow flexion. *Source:* Copyright © Clinical Resources, Inc.

FLEXOR DIGITORUM SUPERFICIALIS PLACEMENT

Type of Placement: Quasi-specific

Action: Flexor of the wrist and the second through fifth fingers

Clinical Uses: Hand rehabilitation

Muscle Insertions: This muscle arises from the medial epicondyle of the humerus, the coronoid process of the ulna, and the radius. The muscle ends in four tendons, which insert into the lateral bony crests in the center of the middle phalanges of the second to fifth digits.

Innervation: The median nerve via the spinal nerves C-7, C-8, and T-1

Location: With the wrist supported, palpate in the middle of the forearm on the ventral side, approximately three quarters of the distance from the elbow to the wrist. Ask the patient to flex only the fingers and not the wrist. Place two active electrodes, 2 cm apart, over the area where the greatest movement is felt, in the direction of the muscle fibers (Figure 14–42A).

Behavioral Test: Finger flexion, while avoiding wrist flexion

Tracing Comment: In Figure 14–42B, recordings are taken from flexor carpi radialis and flexor digitorum superficialis. The arm is supported up to the wrist, and wrist flexion is studied in the neutral position with the fingers relaxed. The fingers are then flexed without moving the wrist (raw sEMG).

Also see tracing from flexor carpi radialis (Figure 14–40C).

Clinical Considerations: Adequate support of the arm and wrist may affect resting levels.

Volume Conduction: If placed too close to flexor carpi radialis, cross-talk will occur.

Other Sites of Interest: Wrist flexors during grasping; finger extensors

Referred Pain Considerations: Trigger points in the radial head of flexor digitorum superficialis project pain down to the middle finger, while a trigger point in the humeral head projects pain into the ring and little finger.[17]

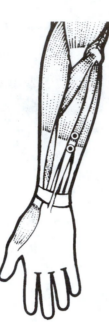

Figure 14–42A Electrode placement for the flexor digitorum superficialis site. *Source:* Copyright © Clinical Resources, Inc.

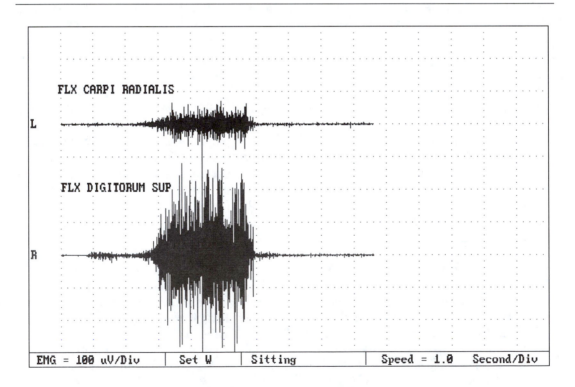

Figure 14–42B Surface EMG recordings from flexor carpi radialis and flexor digitorum superficialis during isolated flexion of the fingers. *Source:* Copyright © Clinical Resources, Inc.

ABDUCTOR POLLICIS LONGUS AND EXTENSOR POLLICIS BREVIS PLACEMENT

Type of Placement: Quasi-specific

Action: Abduct and extend the thumb

Clinical Uses: Hand rehabilitation

Muscle Insertions: The abductor pollicis longus arises from the dorsal surface of the ulna and radius, along with the interosseous membrane, and inserts onto the base of the first metacarpal. The extensor pollicis brevis arises more distally from the ulna and radius, along with the associated interosseous membrane, and inserts into the base of the proximal phalanx of the thumb.

Innervation: The radial nerve from the spinal nerves C-6, C-7, and C-8

Location: Palpate the dorsal aspect of the forearm just above the wrist on the thumb side while the patient abducts the thumb. Two active electrodes, 2 cm apart, are placed on an oblique angle approximately 4 cm above the wrist on that palpable muscle mass (Figure 14–43A).

Behavioral Test: Abduction of the thumb (thumb up)

Tracing Comment: In Figure 14–43B, four muscle sites were monitored (top to bottom): abductor pollicis longus, abductor pollicis brevis, flexor pollicis brevis, and the first dorsal interos-

seus. The hand and wrist are supported in the neutral position (thumb up). Five movements were studied. (1) With grasping a cup, the first dorsal interosseus shows a strong burst of activity with minor activity in the abductor pollicis longus and brevis. (2) With releasing the cup, a small burst of activity from abductor pollicis longus is seen. (3) When the thumb is abducted, abductor pollicis brevis and longus show a strong burst of activity with minor recruitment noted at the flexor pollicis brevis. (4) With a pincher grasp, the abductor pollicis brevis shows a strong burst of activity along with a moderate burst from flexor pollicis brevis. (5) With the final abduction of the thumb, the same pattern of recruitment is seen as during the earlier abduction (raw sEMG).

Clinical Considerations: Adequate support of the arm and wrist may affect resting levels. Without needle EMG recordings, it would be difficult to isolate specific movements of the different elements of the thumb and its joints. This sEMG recording reflects general movements of extension of the thumb.

Volume Conduction: If placed too close to extensor digitorum and extensor digiti minimi, cross-talk will occur.

Other Sites of Interest: Adductor pollicis brevis and flexor pollicis brevis

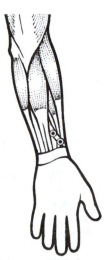

Figure 14–43A Electrode placement for the abductor pollicis longus and extensor pollicis brevis site. *Source:* Copyright © Clinical Resources, Inc.

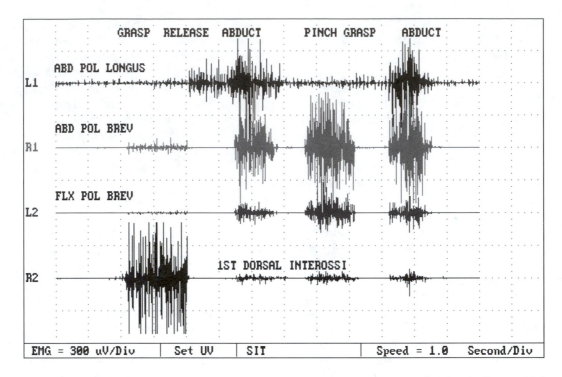

Figure 14–43B Surface EMG recordings from abductor pollicis longus, abductor pollicis brevis, flexor pollicis brevis, and the first dorsal interosseus are presented during a grasp, release, abduction, pincher grasp, and a second abduction. *Source:* Copyright © Clinical Resources, Inc.

FIRST DORSAL INTEROSSEUS PLACEMENT

Type of Placement: Specific

Action: Index finger abductor

Clinical Uses: Hand rehabilitation

Muscle Insertions: This muscle arises from the first phalanx of the thumb and index finger and inserts into the second phalanx of the index finger.

Innervation: The ulnar nerve via spinal nerves C-8 and T-1

Location: Two active electrodes are placed on the dorsal surface of the hand in the web space between the index finger and the thumb, parallel to the direction of the finger. This muscle can easily be palpated during the pincher grasp (thumb opposes index finger) (Figure 14–44).

Behavioral Test: Pincher grasp of index finger opposing the thumb

Tracing Comment: See abductor pollicis longus tracing (Figure 14–43B).

Clinical Considerations: The degree of support of the arm and hand may alter resting tone. Surface recordings from this site primarily look at gross movement of the index finger such as opposition of the thumb.

Volume Conduction: Flexor and abductor pollicis brevis

Other Sites of Interest: Thumb adductor during grasping

Referred Pain Considerations: Trigger points in the first interosseus project pain down into the index finger.[17]

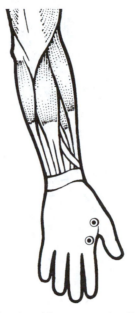

Figure 14–44 Electrode placement for the first dorsal interosseus site. *Source:* Copyright © Clinical Resources, Inc.

FLEXOR POLLICIS BREVIS PLACEMENT

Type of Placement: Quasi-specific

Action: Thumb flexion and opposition

Clinical Uses: Hand rehabilitation, pincher grasp

Muscle Insertions: The superficial aspect of this muscle arises from flexor retinaculum and inserts into the radial sesamoid bone.

Innervation: The superficial head is innervated via the median nerve via spinal nerves C-6, C-7, C-8, and T-1. The deep head of this muscle is innervated by the ulnar nerve via spinal nerves C-8 and T-1.

Location: Palpate the medial aspect of the thenar eminence while the patient abducts the thumb. Two active electrodes, 2 cm apart, are placed on the medial aspect of the thenar eminence, parallel to the direction of the thumb (Figure 14–45). Smaller, more closely spaced electrodes will provide greater specificity of recordings.

Behavioral Test: Pincher grasp, thumb oppose index finger

Tracing Comment: See abductor pollicis longus tracing (Figure 14–43B).

Clinical Considerations: The degree of support of the wrist and arm may alter resting levels. Surface recordings from this site primarily look at gross movement of the thumb (such as during opposition).

Volume Conduction: Abductor pollicis brevis, adductor pollicis

Other Sites of Interest: Adductor pollicis brevis; abductors of the thumb

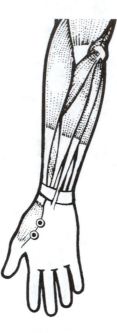

Figure 14–45 Electrode placement for flexor pollicis brevis. *Source:* Copyright © Clinical Resources, Inc.

ABDUCTOR POLLICIS BREVIS PLACEMENT

Type of Placement: Quasi-specific

Action: Abduction of the thumb

Clinical Uses: Hand rehabilitation

Muscle Insertions: This muscle arises from the scaphoid tubercle and the flexor retinaculum and inserts into the radial sesamoid bone and the proximal phalanx of the thumb.

Innervation: The median nerve via spinal nerves C-6, C-7, C-8, and T-1

Location: Two active electrodes, 2 cm apart, are placed in the center of the largest mound of the thenar eminence, running in the same direction as the thumb (Figure 14–46). Smaller, more closely spaced electrodes may provide greater specificity of recordings.

Behavioral Test: Abduct the thumb. Lay the hand palm up. Move thumb from side of index finger, out away from the fingers.

Tracing Comment: See abductor pollicis longus tracing (Figure 14–43B).

Clinical Considerations: Adequate support of the wrist and arm may alter resting levels. Initial thumb position may affect recruitment pattern.

Volume Conduction: Flexor pollicis brevis, opponens pollicis

Other Sites of Interest: Flexor pollicis brevis during abduction of the thumb; adductor muscles of the thumb

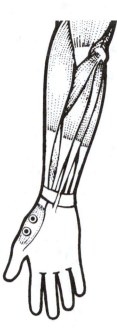

Figure 14–46 Electrode placement for abductor pollicis brevis. *Source:* Copyright © Clinical Resources, Inc.

DORSAL LUMBAR (WIDE) PLACEMENT

Type of Placement: General

Purpose: To monitor from the general region of the low back, the erector spinae

Clinical Uses: Assessing and treating back pain; teaching the patient to deactivate muscle activation patterns[13]

Location: The right and left aspects of the paraspinals are monitored separately. The active electrodes are placed, one at the T-10 and one at the L-3 level of the spine, approximately 2 cm lateral from the spine over the muscle belly (Figure 14–47A).

Behavioral Test: Walking, forward flexion, and extension

Tracing Comment: Figure 14–47B shows sEMG recordings from the right and left aspects of the dorsal lumbar site during sit-stand transitions, forward flexion and return, and walking. Note the symmetry of recruitment during the various activities. Following transitions, the recruitment patterns quiet down quickly. There is a flexion-relaxation response during forward flexion (processed sEMG).

Figure 14–47C shows an assessment and treatment technique developed by Ettare and Ettare.[13] Here, the ideal pattern is displayed during walking and quiet standing with 14 replications (processed sEMG).

Also note tracings from the cervical trapezius (Figures 14–6B, 14–6C, 14–6D) and cervical dorsal (Figures 14–18B, 14–18C) sites.

Clinical Considerations: Resting levels may be affected by the posture of sitting versus standing. Pelvic tilt may lower values. Scoliosis may be associated with asymmetry of resting values. Leg length discrepancy may play a role, as well.

Volume Conduction: Erector spinae, latissimus dorsi, quadratus lumborum

Other Sites of Interest: Cervical dorsal recordings to obtain a larger view of spinal support; gluteus maximus during walking

Artifacts: ECG, electrode slippage during forward flexion

Benchmark: Sitting 2 µV (RMS)
Standing 2 µV (RMS)
Walking: 4–6 µV (RMS)
These values are based upon a J&J M-501 EMG.[13]

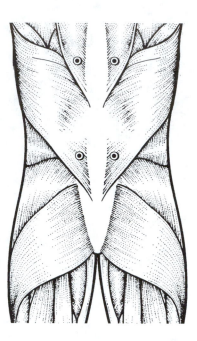

Figure 14–47A Electrode placement for the dorsal lumbar site. *Source:* Copyright © Clinical Resources, Inc.

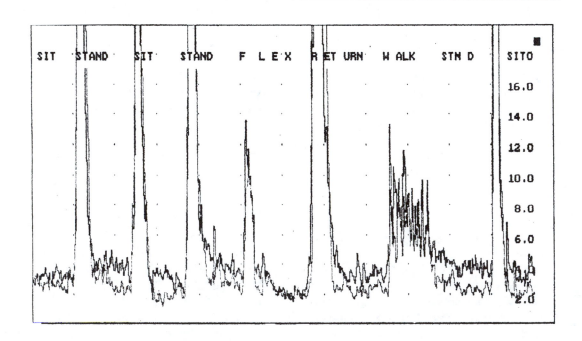

Figure 14–47B Surface EMG recordings from the right and left aspects of the dorsal lumbar site during sit-stand transitions, forward flexion, and walking. *Source:* Copyright © Clinical Resources, Inc.

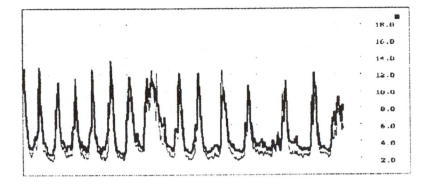

Figure 14–47C Surface EMG recordings from the right and left aspects of the dorsal lumbar site with 14 replications of standing and walking in place. The normal recordings indicate that the right and left aspects are symmetrical, and the activation pattern associated with walking quiets down quickly when the person stands. Courtesy of Biofeedback Associates of California, San Jose, California.

T-12 PARASPINAL PLACEMENT

Type of Placement: Quasi-specific

Action: To monitor the thoracic paraspinal stabilizers. These muscles are thought to be important due to the transition of the mechanical stability of the spine at T-12 level.

Clinical Uses: Assessment and treatment of back pain

Muscle Insertions: This placement is thought to monitor from the iliocostalis thoracis, longissimus thoracis, and spinalis thoracis. In general terms, it monitors from the erector spinae group.

These muscles can be anatomically separated into intersegmental muscles, acting on single and two-level joint movements (those that anchor the spine to the pelvis, the multifidus and lumbar fibers of longissimus and iliocostalis and those that span the vertebral column, the thoracic fibers of the longissimus and iliocostalis).[17] Most medial to the spinous process are the thoracic fibers of iliocostalis, the thoracic fibers of longissimus, and the multifidus. More laterally are the lumbar fibers of longissimus and the lumbar fibers of iliocostalis.

Innervation: The ventral and lateral intertransversarii receive their nerve supply from the lumbar ventral rami, while the more dorsal fibers receive their supply from the dorsal ramus.

The multifidi are innervated by the medial branch of the dorsal ramus of the spinal nerve that issues from below the particular vertebrae. The dorsal ramus separates into a medial and lateral branch, with the lateral branch innervating the more lateral and superficial muscles. It runs obliquely downward and laterally, crossing one or two segments before terminating in muscle fibers.[17]

Joint Considerations: The complex nature of the functional anatomy of the paraspinal muscle group defies easy association of muscle dysfunction to underlying articular disturbances. Certainly the spinal joints associated with the related spinal nerve should be assessed (T-10 through L-1), as should the joints and structures related to the insertions of the longer longissimus and spinalis fibers. However, this assessment should be made in the context of the posture and motion of the entire vertebral column and lower kinetic chain.

Location: To find T-12, have the patient forward flex and palpate where the lowest rib joins the spine. Going laterally from the spine approximately 2 cm, the electrodes are placed 3 cm apart, so that they run parallel to the spine over the fleshy muscle mass. It is best to place these electrodes while the patient is in a slight forward flexion. This will minimize electrode artifacts associated with skin distortions that occur during this movement (Figure 14–48A).

Behavioral Test: Prone extension, return from forward flexion of the trunk

Tracing Comment: Figure 14–48B shows sEMG recordings from C-4, T-1, T-12, and L-3 paraspinals during prone extension. Note the marked recruitment at the T-12 and L-3 sites (raw sEMG).

Figure 14–48C shows sEMG recordings from C-4, T-1, T-12, and L-3 paraspinals during side bending to the left and then right. Activity is seen all along the paraspinal muscles during this movement. At the initiation of the bend, one can see an ipsilateral contraction at the T-12 level as the patient goes to the left. Then as the patient returns to midline, both the T-12 and L-3 levels on the contralateral side show a brisk recruitment as the patient returns to midline (raw sEMG).

Clinical Considerations: Surface EMG resting and recruitment patterns may be affected by several features. Attention should be paid to scoliotic curves, rotation in the rib cage, the degree of curvature in the back, leg length discrepancies, and any antalgic postures that involve the lower and upper back.

The thoracolumbar region is of profound biomechanical significance. The floating ribs and the frontal orientation of the facet joints give the region freedom of motion that the trunk uses to flex and extend as well as to side bend. The T-11/T-12 junction provides the largest amount of vertebral rotation. In neutral standing, there is conjoined motion of side bending and ipsilateral rotation.Normal conjunct rotation of the thoracic spine in neutral involves rotation and then side bending to the same side. This is known as *rotection*. Side bending and rotation to the opposite side is termed *latection*. Both are normal movements from a neutral posture. In flexion or extension, these joined motions reverse, coupling side flexion and contralateral rotation. When the thoracolumbar spine is positioned in flexion, the ability for the region to shift from side flexion/ipsilateral rotation to side flexion/contralateral rotation is lost. The other transitional areas of the body (suboccipital; cervicothoracic, and, most significantly, the lumbosacral region) must compensate by moving more than they would otherwise.

Synergistic relationships with other trunk extensors, namely the serratus posterior and the quadratus lumborum, have been described.[17] Tightness in the region has been attributed to various muscle imbalances between the overactive erector spinae, weakened gluteus muscles, and tightened hip flexors and weakened abdominals.[44]

Volume Conduction: Latissimus dorsi, lower trapezius, erector spinae

Other Sites of Interest: Synergists with serratus posterior inferior and quadratus lumborum, and antagonists with rectus abdominis and abdominal obliques during flexion and extension; synergists to serratus posterior inferior and abdominal oblique during rotation

Referred Pain Considerations: Trigger points near the spine tend to refer pain locally. As the patient moves more laterally, trigger points in iliocostalis thoracis project pain laterally across the chest and may spill over to the anterior wall.[17]

Artifacts: Due to the degree of skin distortion experienced in the middle to lower back during certain movements, practitioners should be aware of artifact due to electrode slippage or popping during forward flexion and extension. ECG artifact is commonly seen on the left side. Respiration artifact is also possible.

Benchmark: Sitting quietly at midline ($N =$ 104): 2.0 ($\pm$ 2.0) μV (RMS)
Standing quietly at midline ($N =$ 104): 3.1 ($\pm$ 3.1) μV (RMS)
Values taken using a J&J M-501 EMG with a 100-to-200–Hz filter.[18]

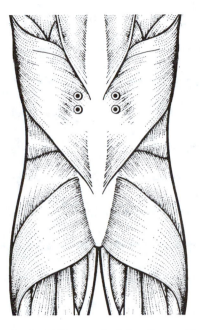

Figure 14–48A Electrode placement for the T-12 paraspinal site. *Source:* Copyright © Clinical Resources, Inc.

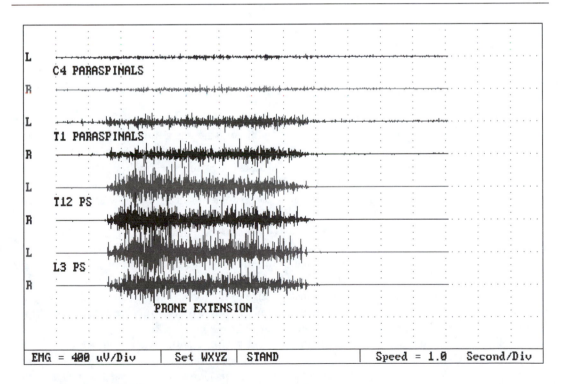

Figure 14–48B Surface EMG recordings from the cervical (C-4), T-1, T-12, and L-3 paraspinal sites during prone extension. *Source:* Copyright © Clinical Resources, Inc.

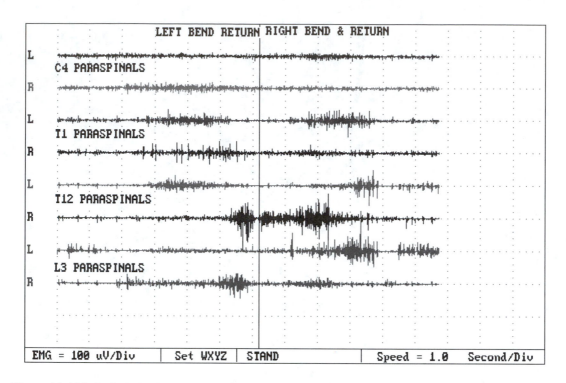

Figure 14–48C Surface EMG recordings from C-4 paraspinals, T-1, T-12, and L-3 paraspinals during side bending to the left and then right. *Source:* Copyright © Clinical Resources, Inc.

LATISSIMUS DORSI PLACEMENT

Type of Placement: Specific

Action: Medially (internally) rotates, adducts, and extends the shoulder/arm; participates in rotation, lateral bending, and extension of the torso

Clinical Uses: Shoulder and back pain

Muscle Insertions: This very broad muscle arises from the lower six thoracic vertebrae, the lumbodorsal fascia, the sacrum and crest of the ilium, and the last three or four ribs; it inserts, along with teres major, on the medial edge of the humerus.

Innervation: The thoracodorsal nerve from the posterior cord of the brachial plexus via the spinal nerves of C-6, C-7, and C-8

Joint Considerations: Related joint structures could include the spinal joints of the related motion segments (C-5/C-6, C-6/C-7, and C-7/T-1).

Additional joint structures include the shoulder complex (the scapulothoracic joint, the glenohumeral joint, and those of the clavicle) and the joints affecting the lumbodorsal fascia from which the latissimus arises (particularly the lower four ribs and thoracic vertebrae, the lumbar vertebrae, and the ilium).

Location: Palpate the scapula. Two active electrodes are placed (2 cm apart) approximately 4 cm below the inferior tip of the scapula, half the distance between the spine and the lateral edge of the torso. They are oriented in a slightly oblique angle of approximately 25 degrees (Figure 14–49A).

Behavioral Test: Extend, adduct, or medially rotate the arm.

Tracing Comment: Also see tracings from upper trapezius (Figure 14–19C), suprascapular site (Figure 14–23D), and lateral low back site

(Figure 14–51B). Figure 14–49B shows recordings from latissimus dorsi during shoulder extension (raw sEMG).

Clinical Considerations: Tightness in the latissimus dorsi is associated with increased thoracic kyphosis, rounded shoulders, and forward head posture. Leg length discrepancies, unresolved lumbar lists, or any other situation that might cause lateral bending of the trunk could lead to unilateral tightness.

Volume Conduction: Teres major, lower trapezius

Other Sites of Interest: Synergists with teres major and long head of triceps during extension, adduction, and lateral rotation; antagonist with scalene and upper trapezius during shoulder elevation

Referred Pain Considerations: Trigger points in this region project pain to the inferior angle of the scapula and may extend to the back of the shoulder and down the medial aspect of the arm and forearm.[17]

Artifacts: ECG

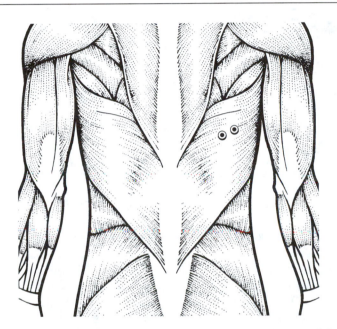

Figure 14–49A Electrode placement for latissimus dorsi site. *Source:* Copyright © Clinical Resources, Inc.

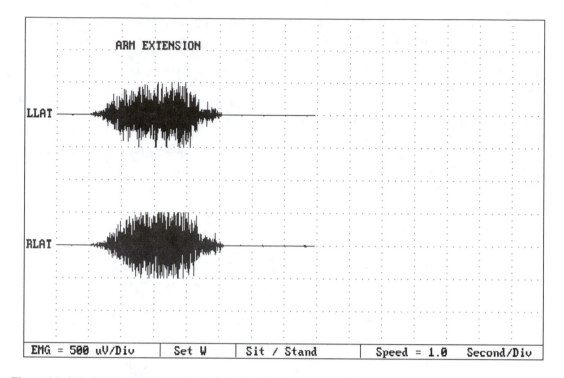

Figure 14–49B Surface EMG recordings from latissimus dorsi during shoulder extension. *Source:* Copyright © Clinical Resources, Inc.

LOW BACK (ERECTOR SPINAE) PLACEMENT AT L-3

Type of Placement: Quasi-specific

Action: To monitor the paraspinal activity of the main trunk movers and stabilizers known as the erector spinae group

Clinical Uses: Low back pain

Muscle Insertions: These electrodes are thought to record from the multifidus, rotaries, and longissimus muscle (erector spinae) groups.

Innervation: The pattern of innervation for the lumbar paraspinals is consistent with that of the thoracolumbar paraspinals. The ventral and lateral intertransversarii receive their supply from the ventral ramus of the spinal nerve; the other muscles receive their supply from the dorsal ramus of the spinal nerve. The actual muscle fibers supplied by the nerve of the given seg-

ment may be one to two segments below, as one moves more laterally from the spinous process.

Location: Palpate the iliac crest. Two active electrodes are placed parallel to the spine, 2 cm apart, approximately 2 cm from the spine over the muscle mass. The iliac crest may be used to determine the L-3 vertebra. The electrodes are best placed while the patient is in a slight forward flexion, hands resting on knees and supporting the torso (Figure 14–50A).

Behavioral Test: Forward flexion and return to midline of the torso

Tracing Comment: Figure 14–50B presents sEMG recordings from the L-3 and abdominal oblique sites during forward flexion, return to midline, and extension backward. Note the flexion-relaxation phenomenon that occurs during the hang phase of this movement. The concentric contraction that occurs during the return phase is larger than the eccentric contraction that occurs during forward flexion. Both are symmetrical. Note the stabilizing activity of abdominal obliques during extension backward (raw sEMG).

Figure 14–50C shows sEMG tracings from the C-4, T-1, T-12, and L-3 paraspinal muscles during forward flexion and return. A flexion-relaxation response occurs at the different spinal levels up the spine, and this response is displaced in time. Note the mildly abnormal asymmetry at the L-3 paraspinal site during the eccentric phase of the movement (raw sEMG).

Figure 14–50D presents tracings from the L-3 site along with tensor fasciae latae, gluteus medius and maximus, lateral and medial hamstrings, and gastrocnemius and soleus during two types of squats. The first squat entails movement primarily at the ankle and the knees, while the second squat is much deeper and entails large movements of the knee and hip. Notice how the deep squat that involves the hip strongly invokes the erector spinae at L-3.

Also see tracings for T-12 paraspinal (Figures 14–48B and 14–48C) and lateral low back placement (Figures 14–51B and 14–51C).

Clinical Considerations: Surface EMG resting and recruitment patterns may be affected by several features. Attention should be paid to scoliotic curves, rotation in the pelvis, the degree of curvature in the back, leg-length discrepancies, and any antalgic postures that involve the lower and upper back. Patterns are strongly influenced by postural elements. Surface EMG values are commonly lower in the sitting posture than in the standing posture.

The L-3 region is particularly sensitive to tightened hip flexors, often bilaterally, and tightened quadratus lumborum, often unilaterally. Posture equilibrium is a model for compensation of mechanical dysfunctions. The upper lumbar region is often found to be flexed, with restricted extension, in the presence of flattened thoracic curves and/or hyperextended lumbosacral angles. The role of the abdominal muscles, particularly the obliques, in preventing this postural dysfunction should be considered.

Volume Conduction: Quadratus lumborum, gluteus maximus, latissimus dorsi

Other Sites of Interest: Lateral low back site (quadratus lumborum), rectus abdominis, and abdominal obliques during flexion, extension, and rotation; the hamstrings and gluteus maximus during walking and trunk extension

Referred Pain Considerations: Trigger points near the spine (ie, multifidi) tend to refer pain locally and this may spill over to the anterior wall.[17]

Artifacts: Because of the degree of skin distortion experienced in the middle to lower back during certain movements, practitioners should be aware of artifact due to electrode slippage or popping during forward flexion and extension. ECG artifacts are commonly seen on the left side.

Benchmark: Sitting quietly at midline (N = 104): 1.9 ($\pm$ 2.4) µV (RMS)
Standing quietly at midline (N = 104): 3.3 ($\pm$ 3.4) µV (RMS)
Values taken using a J&J M-501 EMG with a 100-to-200–Hz filter.[18]

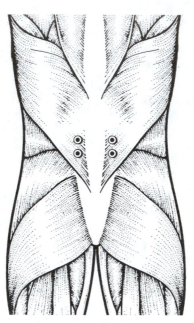

Figure 14–50A Electrode placement for the L-3 paraspinal site. *Source:* Copyright © Clinical Resources, Inc.

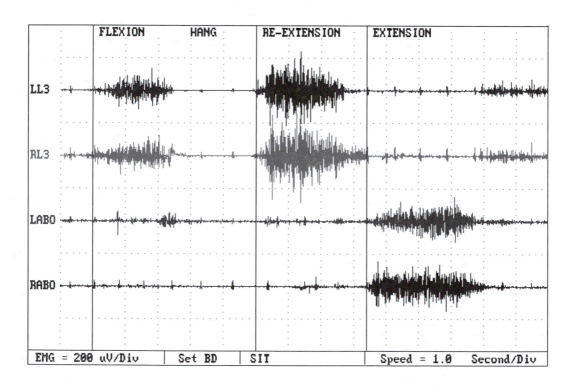

Figure 14–50B Surface EMG recordings from the L-3 paraspinal and abdominal obliques during forward flexion of the torso, return to midline, and extension of the torso. *Source:* Copyright © Clinical Resources, Inc.

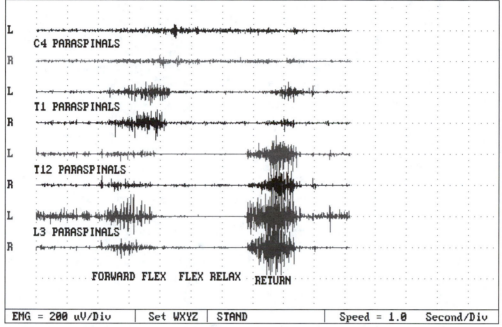

Figure 14–50C Surface EMG tracings from the C-4, T-1, T-12, and L-3 paraspinal muscles during forward flexion and return to midline. Note flexion-relaxation phenomenon at the L-3, T-12, and T-1 sites. *Source:* Copyright © Clinical Resources, Inc.

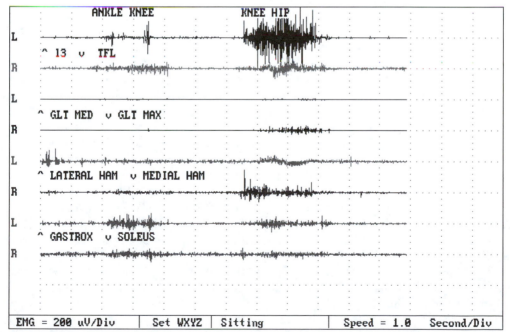

Figure 14–50D Surface EMG tracings from the L-3 site along with tensor fasciae latae, gluteus medius and maximus, lateral and medial hamstrings, and gastrocnemius and soleus during two types of squats. The first squat entails movement primarily at the ankle and the knees; the second squat is much deeper and entails large movements of the knee and hip. *Source:* Copyright © Clinical Resources, Inc.

LATERAL LOW BACK (QUADRATUS LUMBORUM AND EXTERNAL OBLIQUES) PLACEMENT

Type of Placement: Quasi-specific

Action: Stabilizing the spine in general and during side bending, rotation, extension, hip hiking, and walking in particular

Clinical Uses: Back pain

Muscle Insertions: The quadratus lumborum is a multibellied muscle that arises from the 12th rib and the transverse process of L-1 to L-4 and inserts into the posterior crest of the ilium. The external obliques arise from the 5th through 12th ribs, interdigitating with the serratus anterior on the upper ribs and with the latissimus dorsi on the lower ribs, and inserting on the iliac crest and the abdominal aponeurosis at the midline. The iliocostalis lumborum extends from the sacrum, external lip of the iliac crest, the thoracolumbar fascia, and the costal process of the upper lumbar vertebrae and inserts into the six to nine bottom ribs.

Innervation: The quadratus lumborum is innervated by the ventral rami of the 12th thoracic and upper three or four lumbar spinal nerves. The abdominal obliques are innervated by the ventral rami of the lower six thoracic spinal nerves, and, for the internal obliques, by the first lumbar spinal nerve, as well. The iliocostalis is innervated by the lateral branch of the dorsal rami of the spinal nerves of the upper lumbar segments.

Joint Considerations: The spinal joints of the lower six thoracic vertebrae, the related costovertebral joints, and the costochondral junctions should be assessed. The lumbar spinal joints as well as those affecting the lumbodorsal fascia (the sacroiliac joints and the lumbosacral junction) also could affect the function of the muscles of this site. Possibly the most important structural component is the mobility of the 11th and 12th ribs and the ilium.

Location: Palpate the 12th rib, the iliac crest, and the belly of the erector spinae muscle. Two active electrodes are placed 3 cm apart, approximately 4 cm lateral from the vertebral ridge or the belly of the erector spinae muscle, and at a slightly oblique angle at half the distance between the 12th rib and the iliac crest (Figure 14–51A).

Behavioral Test: Hip hiking on the left, then the right; lateral bending; rotation

Tracing Comment: The main muscles thought to be active in the region were monitored: the lateral low back (LLB), along with the L-3 paraspinals, latissimus dorsi, and abdominal obliques.

In Figure 14–51B, axial rotation is followed by side bending. During axial rotation, sEMG recruitment is clearly seen at all recording sites. On the ipsilateral side of the movement, the LLB site shows a large burst of recruitment, as does the latissimus dorsi and L-3 paraspinals. The abdominal obliques show a strong burst of recruitment on the side contralateral to the movement, indicating a strong rotatory component. For side-bending, a large burst of recruitment is shown at the LLB site during the concentric contraction associated with the return to midline (raw sEMG).

In Figure 14–51C, two actions were studied: lateral bending to the left and then the right, followed by hip hiking to the left and then right. During the lateral bending, notice how the LLB site contralateral to the movement provides an eccentric stabilizing function on the way down, and is a prime mover for concentric function on the way up. The contralateral abdominal oblique site also plays a role during the movement that suggests a slight axial rotation during the lateral bend. During hip hiking to the left and then right, both the L-3 and LLB sites are strongly involved. It is entirely possible that the LLB pattern is due to volume conduction from the L-3 site or the posterior fibers of the obliques. Surface recordings do not definitively demonstrate this. Minor recruitment of the abdominal obliques can also be noted (raw sEMG).

Clinical Considerations: The resting values at this site may vary dramatically as one goes from the sitting to the standing posture. The degree of pelvic tilt may also moderate the resting sEMG levels. Leg-length discrepancies or scoliosis would certainly alter the horizontal axis of the pelvis, thus providing a basis for asymmetries at this site. The practitioner should also be alert to the possibility of antalgic postures, which could affect the resting sEMG levels and alter timing issues during dynamic movement.

The quasi-specific classification noted above indicates that the muscle lies deep and thus attempted recordings at this site may reflect several muscles. One of the contributors at this site is the quadratus lumborum. Fine-wire recordings from quadratus indicate EMG activity during the five following movements: lateral flexion of the spine, hip hiking, extension of the lumbar spine, forced expiration, and trunk rotation to the same side when the pelvis is fixed (eg, sitting).[45]

The thoracolumbar junction has a tendency to become fixed into flexion. When it does so, the normal coupling of side flexion and contralateral rotation that occurs in the neutral spine becomes altered to side flexion and ipsilateral rotation. This may change the timing and amplitude of the signal seen in side flexion movements. Hyperac-

tivity in the lateral low back has been reported to be related to weakness in the gluteal muscles (Headley, personal communication). In the presence of gluteus medius weakness, lateral hip stability can be achieved via compensatory hyperactivity of the lateral low back and the tensor fascia latae.[17] Tight hip flexors on one side can participate in vertebral column rotation. The compensatory pelvic rotation creates an altered length of the lateral low back. The myofascium is lengthened on the convex side of the column.

Volume Conduction: Erector spinae, gluteus minimis, gluteus maximus, abdominals

Other Sites of Interest: External abdominal obliques, latissimus dorsi, and erector spinae

Referred Pain Considerations: Superficial trigger points at this site project pain posteriorly to the region of the sacroiliac joint and the lower buttock.[17]

Artifacts: ECG; electrode slippage and popping associated with severe skin distortions that occur as a function of forward flexion, extension, and, to a lesser extent, side bending

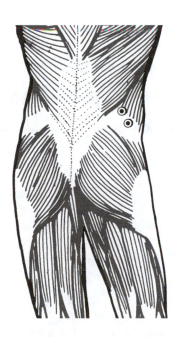

Figure 14–51A Electrode placement for the lateral low back site. *Source:* Copyright © Clinical Resources, Inc.

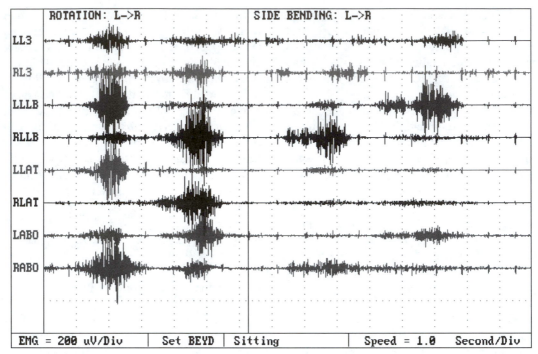

Figure 14–51B Surface EMG recordings from the L-3 paraspinals, (LLB) lateral low back, (LAT) latissimus dorsi, and (ABO) abdominal obliques sites during axial rotation and side bending. *Source:* Copyright © Clinical Resources, Inc.

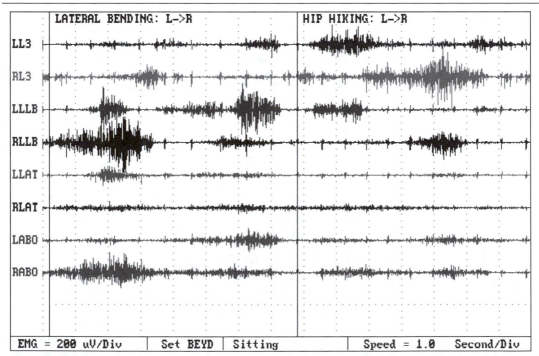

Figure 14–51C Surface EMG recordings from the L-3 paraspinals, (LLB) lateral low back, (LAT) latissimus dorsi, and (ABO) abdominal obliques sites during lateral bending and hip hiking. *Source:* Copyright © Clinical Resources, Inc.

RECTUS ABDOMINIS PLACEMENT

Type of Placement: Specific
Action: Trunk flexion, pelvic tilt
Clinical Uses: Abdominal and back pain
Muscle Insertions: This multibellied muscle arises from the 3rd through 5th ribs and the xiphoid process and inserts into the crest of the pelvic bone.
Innervation: The intercostal nerves via the ventral rami from T-5 to T-12
Location: Palpate the abdominal wall in the area close to the umbilicus. Locate the muscle mass. A thick pad of adipose tissue may be a problem. The electrodes are placed 3 cm apart and parallel to the muscle fibers of rectus so that they are located approximately 2 cm lateral and across from the umbilicus over the muscle belly (Figure 14–52A).
Behavioral Test: From the supine posture, have the patient do a curl-up. If standing, have the patient tighten the abdomen (suck it in) or do the pelvic tilt.
Tracing Comment: Figure 14–52B provides tracings from the rectus abdominis and abdominal obliques during a curl-up (partial sit-up) at midline from a supine position (raw sEMG).

Also see tracings for abdominal oblique placement (Figure 14–53B).
Clinical Considerations: This site is affected by the degree of anterior versus posterior pelvic tilt. It has its greatest level of activation when the body weight is carried on the back rather than the thighs.[16] Values may differ greatly as the patient moves from the sitting to standing posture. During a sit-up, the greatest level of activation is noted during the first 45 degrees of flexion.[46]
Volume Conduction: Abdominal obliques
Other Sites of Interest: Erector spinae muscles, latissimus dorsi
Referred Pain Considerations: Trigger points in this multibellied muscle typically project pain to the same quadrant and occasionally to the back.[17]
Artifacts: Thick pad of adipose tissue; ECG
Benchmark: Sitting quietly at midline (N = 104): 1.0 (± 2.5) µV (RMS)
Standing quietly at midline (N = 104): 1.1 (± 2.1) µV (RMS)
Values taken using a J&J M-501 EMG with a 100-to-200–Hz filter.[18]

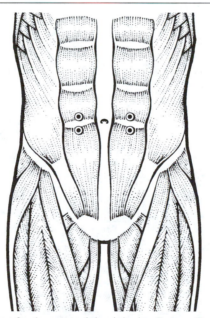

Figure 14–52A Electrode placement for the rectus abdominis site. *Source:* Copyright © Clinical Resources, Inc.

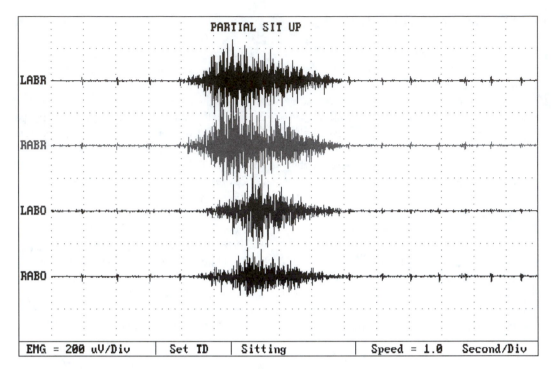

Figure 14–52B Surface EMG recordings from (ABR) rectus abdominis and (ABO) abdominal obliques during a curl-up. *Source:* Copyright © Clinical Resources, Inc.

EXTERNAL ABDOMINAL OBLIQUE PLACEMENT

Type of Placement: Quasi-specific

Action: Flexion, rotation, and side bending of the torso

Clinical Uses: Back pain and urinary incontinence

Muscle Insertions: This rather broad muscle arises from the 5th through 12th ribs, interdigitating with serratus anterior on the upper ribs and with the latissimus dorsi on the lower ribs; it passes downward and medially inserts on the iliac crest and the abdominal aponeurosis at the midline.

Innervation: The intercostal nerve via the ventral rami from T-8 to T-12

Location: Palpate the iliac crest and locate the anterior superior iliac spine. Two active electrodes are placed 2 cm apart, lateral to the rectus

abdominis directly above the anterior superior iliac spine, halfway between the crest and the ribs at a slightly oblique angle so that they run parallel to the muscle fibers (Figure 14–53A). (Note: Although this placement primarily records from the external oblique due to its superficial nature, recording from the internal obliques may be significant in some individuals and probably depends upon the depth of adipose tissue and movement strategy.)

Behavioral Test: Rotation of the torso, diagonal sit-up

Tracing Comment: Figure 14–53B provides tracings from rectus abdominis and external abdominal obliques during diagonal curl-ups to the left and then right. The rectus abdominis raises the torso, while the right and left obliques raise and rotate the torso to the left and right, respectively. The degree of separation or specificity of recruitment of the external obliques during the diagonal sit-up varies considerably from one person to another.

In Figure 14–53C, axial rotation of the trunk during standing is shown. Here, the muscles ipsilateral to the direction of the movement are activated. The degree of specificity and separation of the abdominal obliques varies greatly from one individual to another. In some individuals, there may exist a contralateral recruitment pattern for this movement (Figure 14–51B) (raw sEMG).

Also see tracings from L-3 paraspinals in Figure 14–51B and rectus abdominis (Figure 14–52B).

Clinical Considerations: The resting values at this site may vary dramatically as one goes from the sitting to the standing posture. The degree of pelvic tilt may also moderate the resting sEMG levels. Leg-length discrepancies and scoliosis would certainly alter the horizontal axis of the pelvis, thus providing a basis for asymmetries at this site. The practitioner should be alert to the possibility of antalgic postures that could affect the resting sEMG levels and alter timing issues during dynamic movement.

This site has been rated as a quasi-specific site, because the use of surface electrodes cannot differentiate between the internal and external obliques.[17] When the pelvis is fixed, the ipsilateral external obliques rotate the homolateral shoulder forward. However, most of the internal obliques rotate the homolateral shoulder backward.[29] Thus, when studying rotational movement patterns at this site, paradoxical results may be found.

Volume Conduction: Internal obliques, rectus abdominis, latissimus dorsi, and quadratus lumborum

Other Sites of Interest: The ipsilateral aspects of serratus anterior and latissimus dorsi during rotation, and the ipsilateral lateral low back (quadratus lumborum) and iliocostalis during side bending; antagonist with the contralateral homologous muscle group

Referred Pain Considerations: Trigger points at this site may project pain down into the groin or testicles.[17]

Artifacts: Thick layers of adipose tissue may attenuate the sEMG signal.

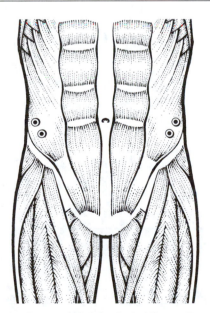

Figure 14–53A Electrode placement for external abdominal obliques. *Source:* Copyright © Clinical Resources, Inc.

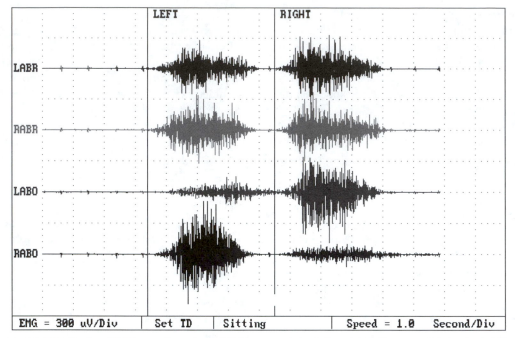

Figure 14–53B Surface EMG recordings from (ABR) rectus abdominis and (ABO) external abdominal obliques during a diagonal curl-up. *Source:* Copyright © Clinical Resources, Inc.

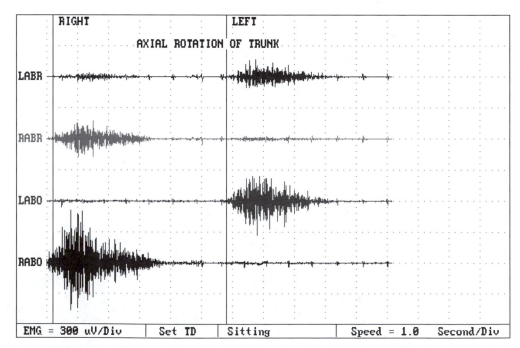

Figure 14–53C Surface EMG recordings from (ABR) rectus abdominis and (ABO) external abdominal obliques during axial rotation while standing. *Source:* Copyright © Clinical Resources, Inc.

ANKLE-TO-ANKLE (WIDE) PLACEMENT

Type of Placement: General

Purpose: To monitor the volume-conducted muscular energy from the entire lower extremity, hips, and low back

Clinical Uses: Assessment and treatment of lower extremity and low back pain

Location: The two active electrodes are placed on the right and left ankle areas. For consistency, placement near the fibular malleolus or lateral aspect of the ankle bone is desirable. However, because this is a very general recording system, exact placement is not essential (Figure 14–54A).

Behavioral Test: All of the following actions will activate the sEMG recording, with the level of activation getting smaller the farther away the activating muscle is from the recording electrodes: foot flexion; foot extension; contraction of thigh, buttocks, and low back muscles.

Tracing Comment: Figure 14–54B presents general recording from the ankle-to-ankle site, along with a wide/general recording from the rectus femoris site. Recordings on both a 100-to-200–Hz filter (narrow) and the 25-to-1000–Hz filter (wide) are displayed during systematic activation of various muscle groups in the lower extremities. The subject first tensed the foot, then the calf, then the thigh, and finally the buttocks. As the activated muscle gets farther and farther away from the recording site, its amplitude gets smaller. But isometric contractions of the buttocks may be seen using this electrode placement. Also note that the ECG artifact usually seen under the conditions of the widely spaced electrodes and filters that go below 30 Hz is not seen in this tracing because of the extremely high resting levels (around 40 microvolts RMS). Recordings from the rectus femoris are always the smaller of the recruitment patterns (processed sEMG).

Clinical Considerations: Values are strongly affected by seated versus standing posture. Weight distribution and foot and toe position during standing, and subtle changes in limb position during sitting may affect the resting sEMG levels.

One can easily demonstrate how this site monitors all the muscles of both lower extremities and lower torso by systematically asking the patient to tense and release each major muscle group of the left extremity, the gluteus maximus, erector spinae, and the muscles of the right lower extremity.

Volume Conduction: From all of the muscles of the lower extremity, hip, and low back

Artifacts: ECG

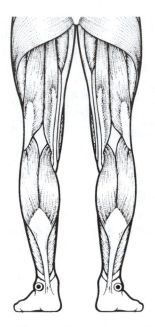

Figure 14–54A Electrode placement for ankle-to-ankle site. *Source:* Copyright © Clinical Resources, Inc.

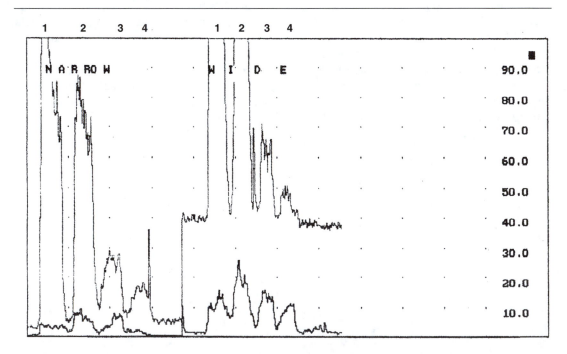

Figure 14–54B Surface EMG recordings from ankle-to-ankle site, along with rectus femoris (wide) during right-sided (**1**) dorsiflexion, (**2**) knee flexion, (**3**) hip flexion, and (**4**) unilateral gluteal squeeze. The left side of the tracing (narrow) is done with the 100-to-200–Hz band-pass filter, while the right side of the tracing is done using the 25-to-1000–Hz band-pass filter. *Source:* Copyright © Clinical Resources, Inc.

GLUTEUS MAXIMUS PLACEMENT

Type of Placement: Specific

Action: Hip extender and lateral rotator

Clinical Uses: Commonly used in assessment and treatment of low back pain, this muscle site is often observed to be overly inhibited (Headley, personal communication). This is also found to be true in hip dysfunction.

Muscle Insertions: This very large and broad muscle arises from the iliac crest, the ala of the ilium, the posterior superior iliac spine, the sacrum, and the coccyx; three quarters of this muscle inserts into the iliotibial tract, while one quarter inserts into the gluteal tuberosity of the femur.

Innervation: The inferior gluteal nerve with fibers from the ventral rami of L-5 and S-1 through the dorsal division of the sacral plexus

Joint Considerations: The spinal joints of L-4/L-5 and L-5/S-1 should be cleared of any dysfunction, if dysfunction persists at this site. The sacroiliac joint and the hip should also be assessed. Because of the contribution of the gluteus maximus to the iliotibial band, the [obscured] the superior tibulofibular articulation [obscured] the implications for lower kinetic chai[obscured] lationships) also may play a role in the [obscured] tion of the gluteus maximus.

Location: Two possible locations a[obscured] For the upper gluteus maximus, two act[obscured] trodes (3 cm apart) are placed half the [obscured] between the trochanter (hip) and the sacr[obscured] brae in the middle of the muscle on an oblique angle at the level of the trochanter or slightly above. For the lower gluteus maximus, placement resides in the middle of the muscle clearly below the level of the trochanter, one to two inches above the gluteal fold (Figure 14–55A).

Behavioral Test: While the patient is in the prone posture, or when he/she is standing and supported with hands on the wall, ask him/her to extend the leg back. Alternative movements include stair stepping, sit to stand, and external rotation of the thigh.

Tracing Comment: In Figure 14–55B, tracings for the right aspect of the L-3 (erector spinae), gluteus maximus for the upper site, and medial hamstring muscles are presented during prone hip extension. All three muscle groups work synergistically, with only a slightly larger recruitment pattern noted when the knee is flexed during this movement.

In Figure 14–55C, the upper and lower gluteus maximus sites are studied along with gluteus medius and tensor fasciae latae during the prone leg extension. The lower gluteus maximus site reflects a larger recruitment pattern than the upper gluteus site. This may reflect differences in muscle mass, thickness of adipose tissue, or level of muscle recruitment for this individual. Whether to use upper or lower placement depends on which site provides the best window to observe gluteal activity.

In Figure 14–55D, tracings for several of the major hip movers and stabilizers are presented while the individual is seated. Other muscle groups are known to participate in the movements described, but they are probably too deep to isolate and label. The more superficial muscles were monitored during external lateral [obscured] exion abduction and inter[obscured] on of the hip. The recruit[obscured]ht aspect of gluteus maxi[obscured]ius, tensor fasciae latae, [obscured] presented. The flat lines [obscured]flect no sEMG input to [obscured]s maximus shows a burst [obscured]nsion and lateral rotation [obscured] medius appears to be active in all movements but hip flexion. Tensor fasciae latae is least active during external/lateral rotation, as is rectus femoris. Rectus femoris is most active during hip flexion.

Also see tracings for hamstrings (Figures 14–64B, 14–64C, and 14–64D).

Clinical Considerations: Activity of the gluteus maximus is probably best studied during prone extension or standing postures. Leg-length discrepancy may contribute to asymmetrical patterns. It may be useful to study this muscle during walking patterns, because it has been reported to fatigue easily or become easily inhibited during walking. Pronation of the foot

[handwritten note on sticky: See Behavioral Test – Clinic Consid's – prone ext std posture walking]

and instability of the foot in stance and early push-off would contribute to hypoactivity of this site. Inhibited gluteus maximus is also seen in patients who stand/walk/run with pelvis pushed forward onto the "Y" ligaments. One can facilitate recruitment of gluteus maximus during leg extension by having the patient engage in a pelvic tilt first.

Substitution of the trunk extensors and biceps femoris for the gluteus maximus in prone hip extension has been described[47] but not confirmed.[48] Quadratus lumborum has been proposed as a synergist capable of substituting for a hypoactive gluteus maximus. In the presence of limited hip extension, the tensor fasciae latae and gluteus maximus lose balance with the tensor fasciae latae dominating hip motion.

Volume Conduction: Usually not a problem

Other Sites of Interest: Erector spinae and hamstrings during extension of the trunk, particularly from the forward flexed position; the hamstrings, gluteus medius, and gluteus minimis during extension of the thigh; the rectus femoris during flexion; and the tensor fasciae latae during medial rotation

Referred Pain Considerations: Trigger points in this muscle typically project pain locally into the buttocks.[17]

Artifacts: Thick adipose fat pad may attenuate the signal. Electrode slippage and movement artifact during walking may be a problem.

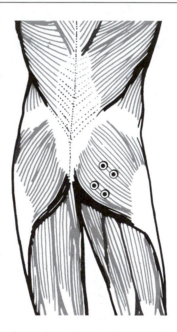

Figure 14–55A Electrode placement for the upper and lower gluteus maximus sites. *Source:* Copyright © Clinical Resources, Inc.

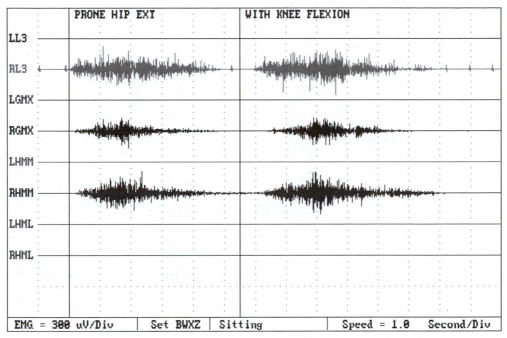

Figure 14–55B Surface EMG recordings from the right aspect of the L-3 (erector spinae), (GMX) gluteus maximus for the upper site, and (HMM) medial hamstring muscles are presented during prone hip extension with and without knee flexion. *Source:* Copyright © Clinical Resources, Inc.

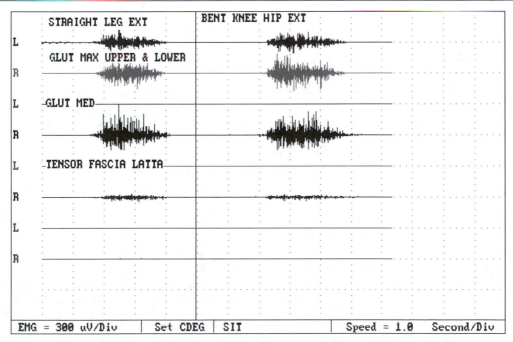

Figure 14–55C Surface EMG recordings from the upper and lower gluteus maximus sites are studied along with gluteus medius and tensor fasciae latae during the straight leg extension and bent knee hip extension in the prone posture. *Source:* Copyright © Clinical Resources, Inc.

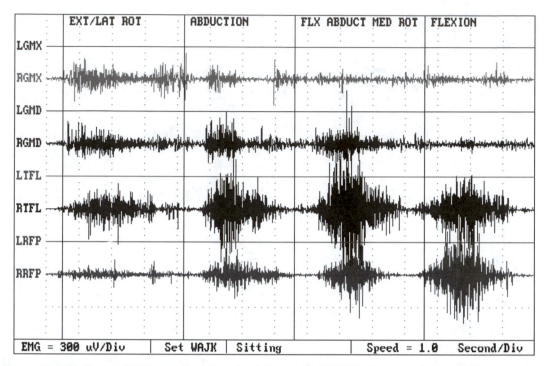

Figure 14–55D Surface EMG recordings from the right aspect of (GMX) gluteus maximus and (GMD) gluteus medius, (TFL) tensor fasciae latae, and (RFP) rectus femoris are presented during external/lateral rotation; abduction; flexion, abduction, and internal rotation of the hip; and flexion of the hip. The flat lines for the left aspects of these sites reflect no sEMG input to those leads. *Source:* Copyright © Clinical Resources, Inc.

GLUTEUS MEDIUS PLACEMENT

Type of Placement: Specific

Action: Hip abductor and stabilizer

Clinical Uses: Low back pain and hip rehabilitation

Muscle Insertions: This muscle arises from the gluteal surface of the ilium and inserts onto the trochanter.

Innervation: The superior gluteal nerve with fibers from L-5 and S-1 via their ventral rami and then via the dorsal branches of the sacral plexus

Joint Considerations: The spinal joints of segments L-4 to L-5 and L-5 to S-1 could be source of dysfunction for their myotomes, which include the gluteus medius.

The joints of origin/insertion of the gluteus medius could also create altered muscle function. These include the ilium in relation to the sacroiliac joint complex and the hip joint. Indirect contributions to gluteus medius dysfunction might include lower kinetic chain problems, particularly laxity of the longitudinal axis of the midfoot.[49] Piriformis spasm or hypertrophy might create problems at the greater sciatic foramen.

Location: Palpate the iliac crest. Two active electrodes 2 cm apart are placed parallel to the muscle fibers over the proximal third of the distance between the iliac crest and the greater trochanter. It is important to be anterior to the gluteus maximus to minimize cross-talk (Figure 14–56A).

Behavioral Test: While patient is side lying or standing sideways while supporting self against a wall, have the patient abduct the leg; have patient walk.

Tracing Comment: In Figure 14–56B, the upper and lower gluteus maximus, the gluteus medius, and the tensor fasciae latae are shown for the right side only. The subject is asked to stand, supporting his/her body with the left hand against a wall. Abduction of the leg is conducted in three ways: with extension, movement in the sagittal plane, and with flexion. Note that recruitment from gluteus medius is much smaller when abduction is conducted with flexion. To find recruitment of gluteus medius, one must conduct this activity either in the sagittal plane or with extension.

Figure 14–56C is conducted using the same recording sites and in the same posture. The subject is then asked to abduct the leg in the sagittal plane first in the neutral position, then again with internal rotation, and finally with external rotation. Here we see a clear synergy pattern, in which tensor fasciae latae activates during internal rotation while the recruitment from gluteus medius is augmented during external rotation.

Also see tracings for Figure 14–55D, Figure 14–57B, and Figure 14–57C.

Clinical Considerations: Activity of the gluteus medius is probably best studied during standing postures. Leg-length discrepancy may contribute to asymmetrical patterns. It may also be useful to study this muscle during walking patterns.

Indwelling electromyographic studies[16] have clearly demonstrated gluteus medius to be the prime abductor of the thigh. The anterior portion of the gluteus medius has been demonstrated to be active during internal (medial) rotation and ambulation.[50] Carrying a load on the ipsilateral side reduced EMG recruitment, while carrying the load on the contralateral side increased EMG recruitment.[51]

Gluteus medius is prone to inhibition, particularly after injury or procedure. Typical substitution patterns include tensor fasciae latae and/or gait substitutions that overwork the quadratus lumborum.

Volume Conduction: Gluteus maximus, erector spinae

Other Sites of Interest: Gluteus minimus, tensor fasciae latae during abduction

Referred Pain Considerations: Trigger points at this site commonly project pain and tenderness along the posterior crest of the ilium, to the sacrum, and to the posterior and lateral aspects of the buttocks.[17]

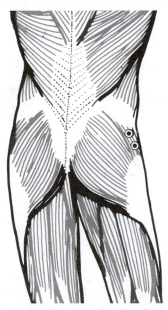

Figure 14–56A Electrode placement for the gluteus medius site. *Source:* Copyright © Clinical Resources, Inc.

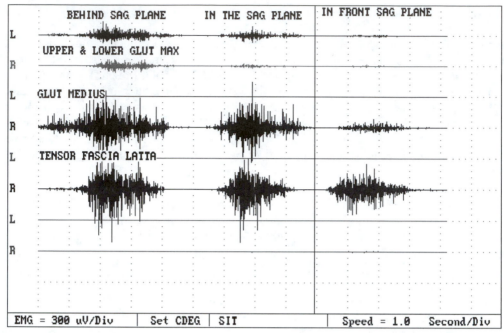

Figure 14–56B Surface EMG recordings from the upper and lower gluteus maximus, the gluteus medius, and the tensor fasciae latae are shown for the right side only. The subject is asked to stand, supporting his/her body with the left hand against a wall. The movement pattern of abduction of the leg is conducted in three ways: with extension, in the sagittal plane, and with flexion. *Source:* Copyright © Clinical Resources, Inc.

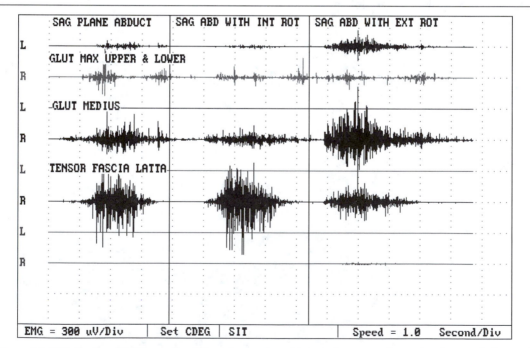

Figure 14–56C Surface EMG recordings from the upper and lower gluteus maximus, the gluteus medius, and the tensor fasciae latae are shown for the right side only. The subject is asked to stand, supporting his/her body with the left hand against a wall. Abduction of the leg is conducted in three ways: in neutral foot position, with internal rotation, and with external rotation. *Source:* Copyright © Clinical Resources, Inc.

TENSOR FASCIAE LATAE PLACEMENT

Type of Placement: Specific

Action: Hip flexor, abductor, medial rotator, and knee extensor

Clinical Uses: Hip rehabilitation

Muscle Insertions: This muscle arises from the anterior superior iliac spine and inserts into the iliotibial tract.

Innervation: The superior gluteal nerve carrying fibers from L-4 and L-5 via their ventral rami and then via the dorsal branches of the sacral plexus

Joint Considerations: The spinal joints of L-3 to L-4 and L-4 to L-5 should be suspected in the case of dysfunction of the tensor fasciae latae muscle. The ilium and its articulations, the sacroiliac complex and the pubic symphysis, should also be checked. The distal insertions of the iliotibial tract should also be considered when ruling out articular contributions to the dysfunction seen at this site. These include the distal femur, the lateral patella, and the lateral retinaculum of the knee. The most distal insertion includes the anterolateral tibia and the head of the fibula.

Location: Palpate just below the anterior superior iliac spine of the iliac crest while the leg is extended. Two active electrodes, 2 cm apart, are placed parallel to the muscle fibers approximately 2 cm below the anterior superior iliac spine (Figure 14–57A).

Behavioral Test: Standing on one leg; abduction of leg with internal rotation; walking

Tracing Comment: Figure 14–57B represents recordings from the right side of the body only during unilateral stance on the right leg for gluteus maximus, gluteus medius, tensor fasciae latae, and rectus femoris (proximal). The tensor fasciae latae shows the predicted burst pattern that stabilizes the hip and knee. The slight activation at the gluteus medius site could represent cross-talk or a minimal synergistic contraction.

In Figure 14–57C, abduction of the leg is conducted behind the sagittal plane, in the sagittal plane, and behind the sagittal plane while side lying. This tracing differs from tracings from the same movements during standing (Figure 14–56B) in that the tensor fasciae latae is more clearly active in all three planes of movement, while the gluteus medius shows most of its activation during abduction with extension.

Also see tracings for gluteus maximus (Figures 14–55C, 14–55D) and gluteus medius (Figures 14–56B, 14–56C).

Clinical Considerations: Activity of the tensor fasciae latae is probably best studied during standing or side lying postures. Leg-length discrepancy may contribute to asymmetrical patterns. It may be useful to study this muscle during walking patterns.

Fine-wire studies of this muscle demonstrate that different aspects of it are active during different aspects of lower extremity use (ie, anteromedial fibers are always active during flexion and abduction of the thigh; and posterolateral fibers are always active during medial rotation[52]). Using surface electrodes, one would not be able to separate out these different sections and movements. Instead, one would expect to see tensor fasciae latae to be active across the entire range of motion noted using fine-wire techniques. It has been observed that tensor fasciae latae is active during hip flexion, abduction, and unilateral stance.

Pelvic inclination as compensation for the limited hip extension from tight tensor fasciae latae and/or tight hip flexors has been proposed[53,54] but also refuted.[55] Economy in gait may also be affected by tight hip flexors.[54] Inability to get the center of the body over the middle of the foot in stance will allow the tensor fasciae latae to remain tight.[49] An ipsilateral long leg can increase the tension on the iliotibial band and presumably the stretch on the tensor muscle. External tibial torsion, rearfoot eversion, and forefoot pronation can also be related to iliotibial band tightness.[56]

The lateral line of body that incorporates the quadratus lumborum, the origin of the oblique abdominals, and the latissimus dorsi, can carry fascial restrictions that hide dysfunctions in multiple layers of compensatory adaptations. The substitution of the tensor fasciae latae for weak gluteus medius is common. A lifestyle that includes excessive sitting can perpetuate tightness in the tensor fasciae latae and weakness in the gluteus medius. Trochanteric bursitis, as well as problems with lateral migration of the patella, is frequently associated with this condition.

Volume Conduction: If electrodes are placed too far lateral, volume conduction from gluteus medius may be a problem.

Other Sites of Interest: Rectus femoris and sartorius during flexion of the hip; gluteus maximus

Referred Pain Considerations: Trigger points at this site project pain to the anterolateral thigh over the greater trochanter and extending down the thigh toward the knee.[17]

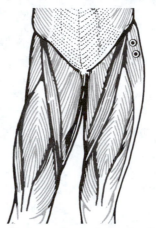

Figure 14–57A Electrode placement for the tensor fasciae latae site. *Source:* Copyright © Clinical Resources, Inc.

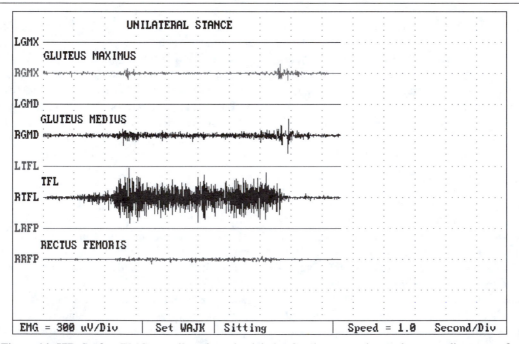

Figure 14–57B Surface EMG recordings from the right leg for gluteus maximus, gluteus medius, tensor fasciae latae, and rectus femoris (proximal) during unilateral stance on the right leg. *Source:* Copyright © Clinical Resources, Inc.

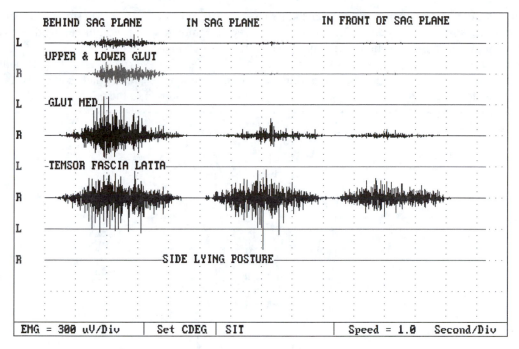

Figure 14–57C Surface EMG recordings from the upper and lower gluteus maximus, the gluteus medius, and the tensor fasciae latae are shown for the right side only while in the side lying position. The movements are abduction with extension, abduction, and abduction with flexion. *Source:* Copyright © Clinical Resources, Inc.

FEMORAL TRIANGLE (ILIOPSOAS) PLACEMENT

Type of Placement: Quasi-specific

Action: Hip flexion

Clinical Uses: Hip rehabilitation

Muscle Insertions: The iliopsoas arises from the first to fifth lumbar and the inner surface of the ilium and inserts on the lesser trochanter of the femur.

Innervation: The lumbar plexus via spinal nerves at L-1 to L-4

Location: Palpate the proximal/medial/anterior aspect of the thigh just below the pelvis for the femoral triangle. Locate the femoral pulse. Go lateral to this, yet medial to the quadriceps femoris and inferior to the inguinal ligament. Two active electrodes, 2 cm apart, are placed parallel to the muscle fibers. It is important to stay proximal to avoid cross-talk with rectus femoris (Figure 14–58A).

Behavioral Test: In quadrupedal stance (on hands and knees), flex hip

Tracing Comment: Figure 14–58B shows sEMG recordings from the right aspect of tensor fasciae latae, iliopsoas, rectus femoris, and sartorius sites during hip flexion. Hip flexion was conducted in the three postures of standing, sitting, and quadrupedal stance. Hip flexion recruitment patterns are not clearly seen at the iliopsoas site in the two postures of standing and sitting. Only during the quadrupedal stance, where the rectus femoris is in the shortened position, is there robust flexor action at this site. The tensor fasciae latae site is active during all three positions of hip flexion.

Clinical Considerations: This site is considered a quasi-specific site because of the depth of this muscle. Without fine-wire recordings, it is difficult to know with certainty that the iliopsoas muscle is making the major contribution to the surface EMG signal. However, the iliopsoas is well known for hip flexion,[16] and this site is a good one to study hip flexion activities. Hip flexion studies may be done in many positions: supine, sitting, standing, or quadrupedal stance.

The recruitment pattern may differ, depending upon the position. In addition, studies done with an open versus closed kinetic chain may affect the recording.

Volume Conduction: Sartorius, rectus femoris, adductor magnus

Other Sites of Interest: Tensor fasciae latae, rectus femoris, sartorius, gluteus medius, and gluteus maximus

Referred Pain Considerations: Trigger points at this site tend to project pain downward onto the anterior portion of the thigh.[17]

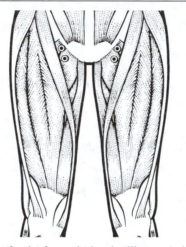

Figure 14–58A Electrode placement for the femoral triangle (iliopsoas) site. *Source:* Copyright © Clinical Resources, Inc.

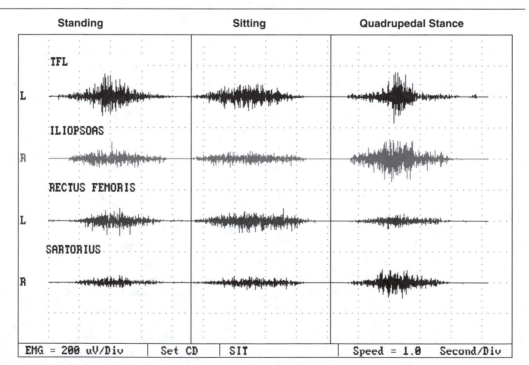

Figure 14–58B Surface EMG recordings from the right aspect of tensor fasciae latae, iliopsoas, rectus femoris, and sartorius sites are presented during hip flexion. *Source:* Copyright © Clinical Resources, Inc.

HIP FLEXOR (SARTORIUS) PLACEMENT

Type of Placement: Quasi-specific

Action: Hip flexion and external (lateral) rotation during flexion of the knee

Clinical Uses: Rehabilitation

Muscle Insertions: This muscle arises from the superior aspect of the iliac spine and inserts distally on the medial surface of the upper tibia.

Innervation: The femoral nerve via spinal nerves at L-2 and L-3

Location: Palpate the proximal aspect of the thigh. Two active electrodes, 2 cm apart, are placed parallel to the muscle fibers, approximately 4 cm distal from the anterior superior iliac spine, obliquely on the anterior surface of the thigh. It is important to stay proximal in an attempt to minimize cross-talk with rectus femoris (Figure 14–59A).

Behavioral Test: From the supine posture, flex and externally rotate the thigh while flexing the knee.

Tracing Comment: Figure 14–59B shows sEMG recording from the right aspect of tensor fasciae latae, iliopsoas, rectus femoris, and sartorius sites during tailor (cross-legged) sitting and external rotation of the hip while in a quadrupedal stance (on hands and knees). While activity is noted at the sartorius site, it is difficult to see any isolation of recruitment during the above movements.

Clinical Considerations: This site is considered a quasi-specific site due to the potential cross-talk using surface electrodes. Like the femoral triangle (iliopsoas) site, this site is a good one to monitor hip flexion and hip flexion with external rotation, even though it is difficult to identify the specific muscle contributing to the sEMG signal. Hip flexion and external rotation studies may be done in many positions: supine, sitting, standing, or quadrupedal stance. The recruitment pattern may differ, depending upon the position.

Volume Conduction: Rectus femoris, iliopsoas, adductor magnus

Other Sites of Interest: Rectus femoris, femoral triangle (iliopsoas), and tensor fasciae latae in hip flexion; gluteus maximus and hamstrings

Referred Pain Considerations: Trigger points at this site project pain locally along the course of the muscle itself.[17]

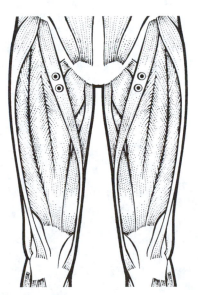

Figure 14–59A Electrode placement for the hip flexor (sartorius) site. *Source:* Copyright © Clinical Resources, Inc.

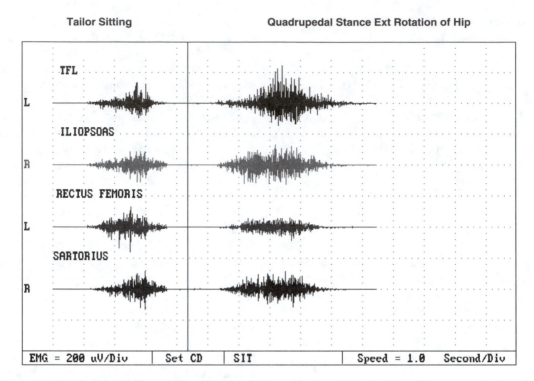

Figure 14–59B Surface EMG recordings from the right aspect of tensor fasciae latae, iliopsoas, rectus femoris, and sartorius sites during tailor (cross-legged) sitting and external rotation of the hip while in a quadrupedal stance. *Source:* Copyright © Clinical Resources, Inc.

RECTUS FEMORIS PLACEMENT

Type of Placement: Specific
Action: Knee extensor and hip flexor
Clinical Uses: Hip and knee rehabilitation
Muscle Insertions: This muscle arises from the anterior ridge of the iliac crest and inserts into the upper border of the patella via the quadriceps tendon.

Location: This muscle is located on the center of the anterior surface of the thigh, approximately half the distance between the knee and the iliac spine. The two active electrodes are placed 2 cm apart, parallel to the muscle fibers (Figure 14–60A, right leg). *Variations:* The electrodes may be placed with a wide spacing (10 to 15 cm apart) to monitor from the quadriceps in general (Figure 14–60A, left leg).

Behavioral Test: While the patient is seated ask him/her to extend the knee. While the patient is standing, ask him/her to squat slightly.

Tracing Comment: In Figure 14–60B, the rectus femoris is presented during hip flexion and knee extension, along with straight leg raising. As can be seen, a strong burst pattern is present for both hip flexion and knee extension. Supine straight leg raising, however, brings about the largest level of recruitment.

In Figure 14–60C, the vastus medialis oblique, the vastus lateralis, the rectus femoris are compared to the medial hamstring and lateral hamstring during isometric flexion and extension of the knee. Note the strong and isolated contractions of the anterior and posterior compartments of the thigh during these efforts (raw sEMG).

Also see tracings from gluteus maximus (Figure 14–55D), tensor fasciae latae (Figure 14–57B), femoral triangle (Figure 14–58B), and hip flexor (Figure 14–59B).

Clinical Considerations: Recordings of resting tone and recruitment patterns at this site are affected by isometric efforts versus weight-bearing movements. Surface EMG monitoring and feedback training for rectus femoris have been used in the rehabilitation of patients with anterior cruciate ligament dysfunctions and repair.[57,58]

Volume Conduction: Vastus lateralis, vastus medialis, vastus intermedius, sartorius, adductor longus, and adductor brevis

Other Sites of Interest: Vastus lateralis and vastus medialis during knee extension, sartorius and tensor fasciae latae during hip flexion, hamstring

Referred Pain Considerations: Trigger points in the proximal aspect of this muscle project pain down to the knee.[17]

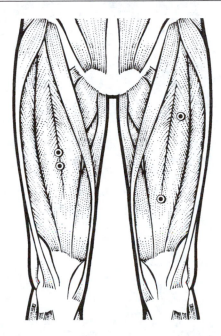

Figure 14–60A Electrode placement for the rectus femoris site (left side) and quadriceps muscles in general (right side). *Source:* Copyright © Clinical Resources, Inc.

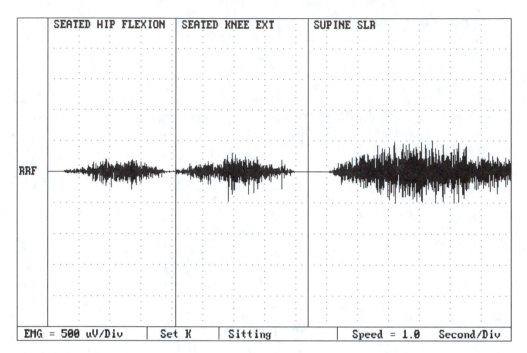

Figure 14–60B Surface EMG recordings from the rectus femoris site during hip flexion, knee extension, and supine straight leg raising. *Source:* Copyright © Clinical Resources, Inc.

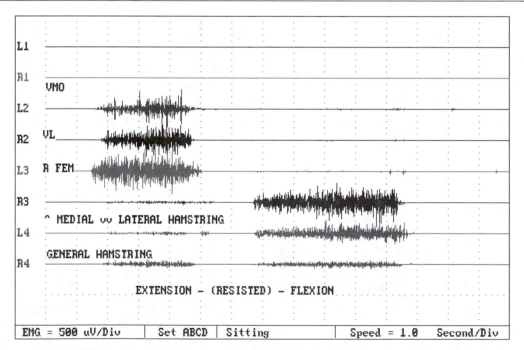

Figure 14–60C Surface recordings from the (VMO) vastus medialis oblique, the (VL) vastus lateralis, the (R FEM) rectus femoris are compared to the medial hamstring and lateral hamstring during isometric flexion and extension of the knee. *Source:* Copyright © Clinical Resources, Inc.

VASTUS LATERALIS PLACEMENT

Type of Placement: Specific

Action: Extensor muscles of the knee

Clinical Uses: General knee rehabilitation; patellofemoral pain

Muscle Insertions: This muscle arises from the lateral surface of the greater trochanter, the intertrochanteric line, the gluteal tuberosity, and the lateral lip of the linea aspera. It inserts into the superior rim of the patella via the patella tendon.

Innervation: The muscle is innervated via the femoral nerve carrying fibers from the L-2, L-3, and L-4 spinal nerves. The femoral nerve is formed by the ventral rami of the spinal nerves as they pass down along and through psoas major, then pass under the inguinal ligament where it separates into anterior and posterior branches. The vastus lateralis receives its innervation in the distal portion of the muscle.

Joint Considerations: The L-2/L-3 and L-3/L-4 joints need to be cleared of problems in the presence of abnormal activity in this region. The patellofemoral joint is central to the role of the vastus lateralis. It is usually symptomatic in the presence of quadriceps imbalance/dysfunction. A symptomatic patellofemoral joint can be the cause of quadriceps dysfunction; at other times it can be the result of quadriceps dysfunction.

Location: Two active electrodes, 2 cm apart, are placed approximately 3 to 5 cm above the patella, on an oblique angle just lateral to midline (Figure 14–61A).

Behavioral Test: Have the patient extend the knee while seated, or squat while standing.

Tracing Comment: Figure 14–61B presents tensor fasciae latae, adductor magnus, rectus femoris, vastus medialis oblique, vastus lateralis, medial hamstring, and the long head and lateral hamstring for the right leg during two squats. Note the strong recruitment in vastus lateralis and vastus medialis oblique as they stabilize the knee in both movements, and in rectus femoris during its eccentric contractions. Hamstrings are quiet in this individual, but this may not always be the case (raw sEMG).

Also see tracings for Figure 14–60C.

Clinical Considerations: Recordings of resting tone and recruitment patterns at this site are affected by isometric efforts versus weight-bearing movements. The relationship between vastus lateralis and vastus medialis oblique has been studied extensively; these muscles are relatively balanced in timing and magnitude during knee extension.[16,59] The ratio of vastus medialis oblique to vastus lateralis has been found to be 1.10 (± 0.27) for normalized sEMG.[60]

Femoral anteversion or tibial torsion can change the orientation of the fibers. Poor functional alignment of the lower extremity can create chronic excitation of the vastus lateralis secondary to the dysfunctional pull such alignment causes the muscle to exert upon the path of the patella.

Tightness in the iliotibial band as a result of ilial torsion or as a result of conditions related to lower kinetic chain dysfunction can alter the line of pull of the lateral quadriceps or the length tension of the muscle and affect vastus lateralis function.

Gait is a fundamental function of the quadriceps muscle. Idiosyncratic gaits can mask weakness in the hip flexors and/or hip stabilizers, placing more burden upon the quadriceps for preventing collapse at heel strike through midstance. Collapse of the longitudinal arch at mid- to late-stance limits the lateral sway of the pelvis and keeps the lateral structures from thoroughly stretching. It could be that iliotibial band tightness from this or other sources creates patellar tracking problems that lead to vastus medialis oblique dysfunction and vastus lateralis hyperactivity. However, it could be that vastus medialis oblique dysfunction leads to iliotibial band tightness.

Volume Conduction: Rectus femoris and vastus intermedius

Other Sites of Interest: Rectus femoris and vastus medialis oblique during extension of the knee; hamstrings

Referred Pain Considerations: Trigger points at this site tend to project pain along the lateral aspect of the thigh and knee.[17]

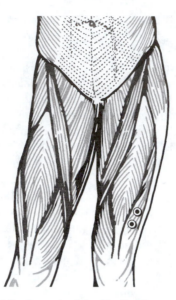

Figure 14–61A Electrode placement for the vastus lateralis site. *Source:* Copyright © Clinical Resources, Inc.

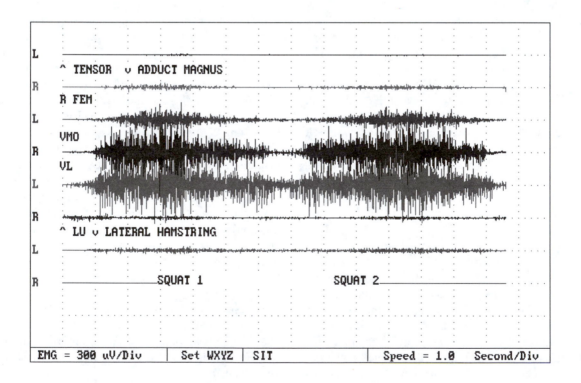

Figure 14–61B Surface EMG recordings from tensor fasciae latae, adductor magnus, (R FEM) rectus femoris, (VMO) vastus medialis oblique, (VL) vastus lateralis, medial hamstring, and lateral hamstring for the right leg only during two bilateral squats. *Source:* Copyright © Clinical Resources, Inc.

VASTUS MEDIALIS (OBLIQUE) PLACEMENT

Type of Placement: Specific

Action: Assists in the medial tracking of the patella by stabilizing the patella in the trochlear groove

Clinical Uses: General knee rehabilitation, patellofemoral pain

Muscle Insertions: The vastus medialis arises from the entire length of the posteromedial aspect of the shaft of the femur, to the lower half of the intertrochanteric line, the medial lip of the linea aspera, and the tendons of the adductor longus and magnus. It inserts into the patella via the tendon. The oblique aspect of the vastus medialis also inserts into the medial patella retinaculum.

Innervation: The muscle is innervated by the femoral nerve, carrying fibers from the L-2, L-3, and L-4 spinal nerves. The femoral nerve is formed by the ventral rami of the spinal nerves as they pass down along and through psoas major, then passing under the inguinal ligament where it separates into anterior and posterior branches. The vastus medialis receives its innervation by a portion of the deep branch of the femoral nerve after it passes through the adductor tunnel, and goes to the middle portion of the muscle.

Joint Considerations: The L-2/L-3 and L-3/L-4 joints need to be cleared of problems in the presence of abnormal activity in this region. The patellofemoral joint has a strong influence on the vastus medialis. It is usually symptomatic in the presence of quadriceps imbalance/dysfunction. A symptomatic patellofemoral joint can be the cause of quadriceps dysfunction; at other times it can be the result of quadriceps dysfunction. Additionally the pubic symphysis should be checked, as dysfunctions there can negatively affect the adductor origins of the vastus medialis.

Location: The placement for vastus medialis oblique is done using 2-cm spacing with the electrodes placed at oblique angle (55 degrees), 2 cm medially from the superior rim of the patella. Palpate for the muscle during extension of the knee. It is somewhat easier to palpate toward the end of range of motion. The electrodes are placed on the distal third of the vastus medialis (Figure 14–62).

Behavioral Test: Ask the patient to extend his/her knee while seated, or partially squat during standing.

Tracing Comment: Refer to tracing for the vastus lateralis site (Figure 14–61B).

Clinical Considerations: Recordings of resting tone and recruitment patterns at this site are affected by isometric efforts versus weight-bearing movements. The relationship between vastus lateralis and vastus medialis oblique has been studied extensively; these muscles are relatively balanced in timing and magnitude during knee extension.[16,59] The ratio of vastus medialis to vastus lateralis has been found to be 1.10 ($\pm$0.27) for normalized sEMG.[60] It is probably best to study these relationships in a closed kinetic chain (ie, squats and isometrics). Several authors have suggested the use of sEMG feedback therapy in the treatment of patellofemoral pain.[61,62] In general, the sEMG biofeedback therapies attempt to selectively recruit and uptrain the vastus medialis oblique. For a review of the research in this area, see *Clinical Applications in Surface Electromyography* by Kasman et al.[63]

Femoral anteversion or tibial torsion can change the orientation of the fibers. Poor functional alignment of the lower extremity can create chronic excitation of the vastus medialis secondary to the dysfunctional stretch such alignment causes on the muscle. Tightness in the iliotibial band as a result of ilial torsion or as a result of conditions related to lower kinetic chain dysfunction can alter the line of pull of the lateral quadriceps or the length-tension of the muscle and can affect the medial portion's functional efficiency.

Gait is a fundamental function of the quadriceps muscle. Idiosyncratic gaits can mask weakness in the hip flexors, hip stabilizers, and/or the hip adductors, placing more burden upon the lateral quadriceps for preventing collapse at heel strike through midstance. This can lead to tightness and imbalance between the lateral and medial quadriceps functions.

Collapse of the longitudinal arch at mid- to late stance limits the lateral sway, and keeps the lateral structures from thoroughly stretching. Iliotibial band tightness from this or other sources can create patellar tracking problems and lead to medial quadriceps dysfunction and appear as relative vastus medialis hypoactivity.

Volume Conduction: Rectus femoris, adductor longus and magnus

Other Sites of Interest: Vastus lateralis and rectus femoris; hamstring and adductor magnus

Referred Pain Considerations: Trigger points at this site refer pain to the medial and anterior aspects of the knee.[17]

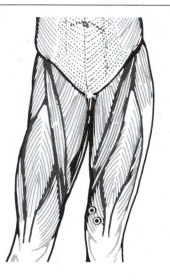

Figure 14–62 Electrode placement for vastus medialis oblique site. *Source:* Copyright © Clinical Resources, Inc.

HIP ADDUCTOR (ADDUCTOR LONGUS/ GRACILIS) PLACEMENT

Type of Placement: Quasi-specific

Action: Adduction of the leg

Clinical Uses: Rehabilitation of cerebral palsy scissor gait

Muscle Insertions: The adductor longus muscle arises from the superior ramus of the pubis and inserts into the middle third of the medial lip of the linea aspera. The gracilis originates from the inferior half of the symphysis pubis and the medial margin of the inferior ramus of the pubic bone. It inserts in the proximal part of the medial surface of the tibia.

Innervation: The obturator nerve via the spinal nerves at L-2 to L-4

Location: Two active electrodes 2 cm apart are placed on the medial aspect of the thigh in an oblique direction 4 cm from the pubis. Palpate the area while the patient conducts an isometric adduction. Avoid placing electrodes close to the midline of the thigh so as to avoid cross-talk from rectus femoris (Figure 14–63A).

Behavioral Test: Pressing the knees together to adduct the legs; walking

Tracing Comment: Figure 14–63B presents tensor fasciae latae, adductor magnus, rectus femoris, vastus medialis oblique, vastus lateralis, long head, and medial hamstrings during an isometric adduction and abduction of the leg. The largest recruitment patterns occur at the tensor fasciae latae and adductor magnus sites.

Clinical Considerations: Recordings of resting tone and recruitment patterns at this site are affected by isometric efforts versus weight-bearing movements. This muscle is active during ambulation, and fine-wire studies have demonstrated that it is most active before, during, and slightly after toe off.[50,64,65]

Volume Conduction: Rectus femoris, vastus medialis, and adductor magnus

Other Sites of Interest: Adductor brevis and magnus, gracilis, gluteus medius, gluteus minimis, and tensor fasciae latae muscles

Referred Pain Considerations: Trigger points at this site project pain upward toward the groin and downward to the knee and shin.[17]

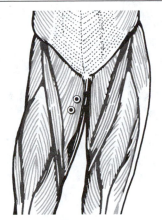

Figure 14–63A EMG electrode placement for adductor longus site. *Source:* Copyright © Clinical Resources, Inc.

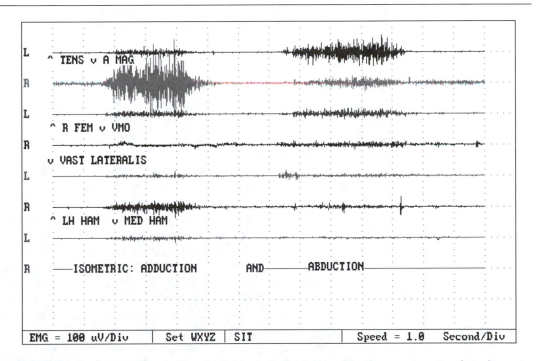

Figure 14–63B Surface EMG recordings from tensor fasciae latae, adductor magnus, rectus femoris, vastus medialis, vastus lateralis, and long head and medial aspects of the hamstrings during isometric adduction and abduction of the leg. *Source:* Copyright © Clinical Resources, Inc.

MEDIAL AND LATERAL HAMSTRING PLACEMENT

Type of Placement: Specific and general

Action: Flexion of the knee, medial or lateral rotation and extension of the hip

Clinical Uses: Knee, hip, and back pain

Muscle Insertions: Two muscles, the biceps femoris (lateral), and semitendinosus (medial) arise from the ischial tuberosity and insert on the lateral and medial heads of the tibia, respectively. The semimembranosus arises from the ischial tuberosity and inserts into the posterior medial tibial condyle.

Innervation: The tibial nerve via L-4, L-5, and S-1

Location: For general recordings, two electrodes 3 to 4 cm apart may be placed parallel to the muscle in the center of the back of the thigh, approximately half the distance from the gluteal fold to the back of the leg (Figure 14–64A, right leg).

For specific recording of biceps femoris, the two active electrodes are placed 2 cm apart parallel to the muscle fibers on the lateral aspect of the thigh two thirds the distance between the trochanter and the back of the knee. Palpate for the muscle while manually muscle testing with the knee at 90 degrees and the thigh in a slight lateral rotation. Semitendinosus may be monitored by placing electrode on the medial aspect of the thigh, located approximately 3 cm in from the lateral border of the thigh and approximately half the distance from the gluteal fold to the back of the knee. Palpate this area while manually muscle testing with the knee at 90 degrees and the thigh in the midline position (Figure 14–64A, left leg).

Behavioral Test: With the patient prone, ask patient to flex the knee against resistance. In standing, have patient flex his/her knee.

Tracing Comment: In Figure 14–64B, the L-3 paraspinals, tensor fasciae latae, gluteus medius and maximus, lateral and medial hamstrings, and gastrocnemius and soleus are monitored during forward flexion of the torso. The L-3 site shows the flexion-relaxation response. However, the hamstring and soleus are placed on stretch and become quite active. The medial aspect of the hamstring in this patient is abnormally active (raw sEMG).

In Figure 14–64C, the L-3 paraspinals, tensor fasciae latae, gluteus medius and maximus, and lateral and medial hamstrings are monitored during flexion, abduction, and extension of the hip while standing. Hip flexion brought about a strong recruitment pattern for the tensor fasciae latae. Abduction also strongly activated the tensor fasciae latae. Extension activated all of the muscle groups; it was the only movement that activated the hamstrings (raw sEMG).

In Figure 14–64D, the same muscles are monitored as in Figure 14–64C, but this time the posture is prone, and the movements are all extensions with different angles of rotation to the leg. This is a particularly interesting recording, in that it shows that the tensor fasciae latae no longer participates in extension when the leg is laterally rotated. The lumbar paraspinals, on the other hand, become more active when the leg is laterally rotated during extension. And, of course, the lateral hamstring becomes more active during extension as the leg is laterally rotated.

Also see tracings for rectus femoris (Figure 14–60C).

Clinical Considerations: Recordings of resting tone and recruitment patterns at this site are affected by isometric efforts versus weight-bearing movements, along with the initial angle of the knee.

The hamstrings are known to be electrically silent when standing in neutral,[16] but active when the trunk is flexed while standing or when the arms are extended.[44] In walking, hamstrings are most active just before or at heel strike.[16] The long head of biceps femoris shows activity beginning at midswing and lasting through the period of heel strike.[66] The tendency for the hamstring muscle to become tight and hyperactive is associated with a corresponding tendency for the gluteus maximus to become laxed and inhibited. Finally, there is an interesting review of the firing pattern of hip muscles during prone extension by Pierce and Lee.[48]

Volume Conduction: Lateral and medial hamstrings, quadriceps

Other Sites of Interest: Gluteus maximus for hip extension; sartorius, gastrocnemius, and plantaris during knee flexion; femoral triangle (iliopsoas), tensor fasciae latae, rectus femoris during extension of the hip; knee flexion for quadriceps femoris

Referred Pain Considerations: Trigger points in semitendinosus project pain up to the gluteal fold, while biceps femoris projects pain down to the back of the knee.[17]

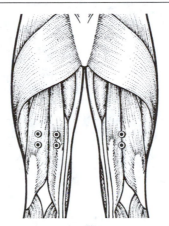

Figure 14–64A Electrode placement for lateral and medial hamstrings (left) and a general placement (right). *Source:* Copyright © Clinical Resources, Inc.

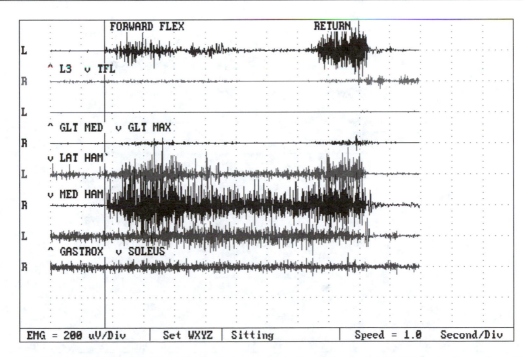

Figure 14–64B Surface EMG readings for the L-3 paraspinals, tensor fasciae latae, gluteus medius and maximus, lateral and medial hamstrings, and gastrocnemius and soleus during forward flexion of the torso. *Source:* Copyright © Clinical Resources, Inc.

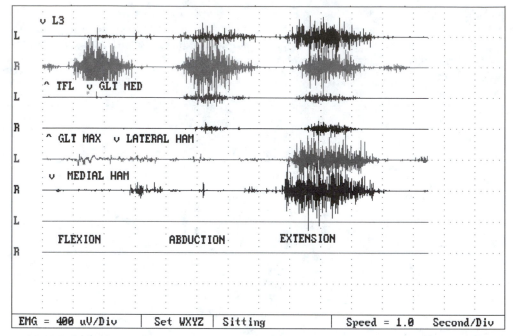

Figure 14–64C Surface EMG readings for the L-3 paraspinals, tensor fasciae latae, gluteus medius and maximus, and lateral and medial hamstrings during flexion, abduction, and extension of the hip while standing. *Source:* Copyright © Clinical Resources, Inc.

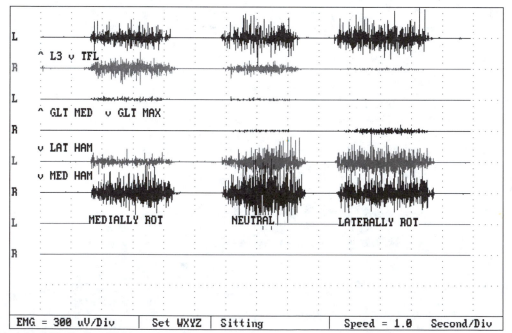

Figure 14–64D Surface EMG readings for the L-3 paraspinals, tensor fasciae latae, gluteus medius and maximus, and lateral and medial hamstrings during prone extension of the leg while it is medially rotated, neutral, and laterally rotated. *Source:* Copyright © Clinical Resources, Inc.

ANKLE DORSIFLEXOR (TIBIALIS ANTERIOR) PLACEMENT

Type of Placement: Quasi-specific

Action: Dorsiflexors of the foot

Clinical Uses: Used in the treatment of the swing-through phase of gait training for stroke

Muscle Insertions: Several different muscle groups are potentially monitored from this site: tibialis anterior, extensor hallucis longus, and extensor digitorum longus. The tibialis anterior is the largest and most superficial muscle group and contributes most heavily to the sEMG signal.

Location: Two active electrodes, 2 cm apart, are placed parallel to and just lateral to the medial shaft of the tibia (shin), at approximately one quarter to one third the distance between the knee and the ankle. Palpate the area while the patient dorsiflexes the foot. Place electrode over the largest muscle mass (Figure 14–65A).

Behavioral Test: Dorsiflex the foot

Tracing Comment: Two tracings are presented. Figure 14–65B reflects recordings from soleus, gastrocnemius, anterior tibialis, and rectus femoris for the left leg. The right aspect was not monitored and the flat lines represent no input. With the patient supported in some way and both feet flat on the ground, the patient is asked to lean or sway forward and then backward. The soleus and gastrocnemius stabilize the individual during the forward sway, while the anterior tibialis and rectus femoris stabilize the patient during the backward sway. The rectus femoris comes into play only as a hip flexor, and as the patient sways far enough back to invoke this action.

In Figure 14–65C, recordings from the anterior tibialis, general gastrocnemius, medial gastrocnemius, lateral gastrocnemius, lateral soleus, and medial soleus of the right leg during standing on toes (plantar flexion) versus standing on heels (dorsiflexion). All aspects of the posterior compartment are active during toe standing, while only the anterior compartment is active during heel standing.

Clinical Considerations: This site is rated as quasi-specific because of the close proximity of and potential cross-talk from surrounding muscles. It is an excellent site, however, to study and give feedback for dorsiflexion. It serves different functions when weighted versus not weighted. When not weight bearing, it dorsiflexes the foot; when weight bearing, it shifts the postural weight back.[16]

During walking, it is most active at heel strike and primarily serves to prevent "foot slap." It also assists the toes in clearing the floor during swing phase of gait.[16] For this reason, it is a useful site in rehabilitation of foot drop.

This site is also used to monitor the tibialis anterior while retraining foot position. The tibialis posterior is necessary to create the arch/neutral foot position. But often, people cheat and use the tibialis anterior in an attempt to lift the arch. Surface EMG monitoring of the tibialis anterior can be used to downtrain unnecessary substitution patterns.

This site is also used to examine the tibialis anterior for excessive recruitment in patients with shin splints. Often, insufficient dorsiflexion is noted in these patients' range of motion, and downtraining can be nicely coupled with a stretching program.

With maximal squatting with the heels flat on the floor, the tibialis anterior was found to be at 60% of its maximum voluntary contraction.[67]

Volume Conduction: Potential contributions from extensor hallucis, extensor digitorum longus, and soleus

Other Sites of Interest: Gastrocnemius, soleus, rectus femoris, medial hamstrings

Referred Pain Considerations: Trigger points in tibialis anterior tend to project pain downward to the great toe.[17]

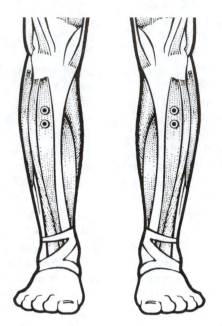

Figure 14–65A Electrode placement for the ankle dorsiflexor (tibialis anterior) site. *Source:* Copyright © Clinical Resources, Inc.

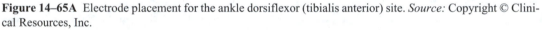

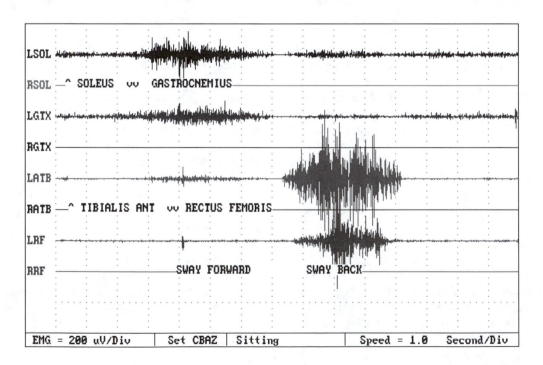

Figure 14–65B Surface EMG recordings from soleus, gastrocnemius, anterior tibialis, and rectus femoris for the left leg during an anterior sway and posterior sway. The right aspect was not monitored and the flat lines represent no input. *Source:* Copyright © Clinical Resources, Inc.

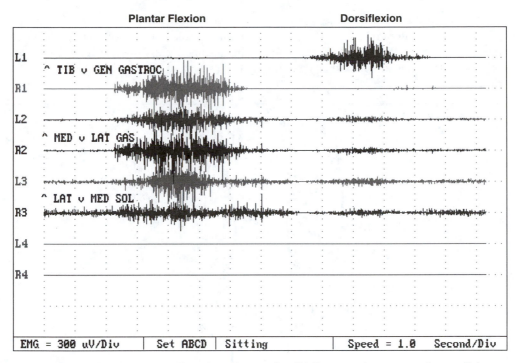

Figure 14–65C Surface EMG recordings from the anterior tibialis, general gastrocnemius, medial gastrocnemius, lateral gastrocnemius, lateral soleus, and medial soleus of the right leg during standing on toes (plantar flexion) versus standing on heels (dorsiflexion). *Source:* Copyright © Clinical Resources, Inc.

GASTROCNEMIUS PLACEMENT

Type of Placement: Specific and general

Action: Plantar flexor (of the foot); knee flexion

Clinical Uses: Gait retraining

Muscle Insertions: The muscle crosses two joints, with the medial and lateral heads of this muscle arising from just above the femoral condyles. It inserts into the calcaneus via the Achilles tendon (heel).

Innervation: Tibial nerve via S-1 and S-2

Location: General recordings from this muscle may be obtained by placing the two active electrodes proximally so that one electrode resides on each muscle. See Figure 14–66, right leg. Cross-talk from the dorsiflexors would be expected.

Specific recordings from the medial or lateral aspect may be obtained by placing active electrodes 2 cm apart, running parallel to the muscle fibers, just distal from the knee and 2 cm medial or lateral to midline. See Figure 14–66, left leg.

Behavioral Test: While standing, lean forward. In an open kinetic chain, plantar flex the foot, (point the toe), and in a closed kinetic chain, stand on toes.

Tracing Comment: See tracings for hamstrings (Figure 14–64B) and tibialis anterior (Figure 14–65B) for postural sway off the central axis of gravity and (Figure 14–65C) for dorsiflexion and plantar flexion.

Clinical Considerations: This muscle assists in plantar flexion in the controlling of the forward movement of the leg over the fixed foot during ambulation.[17]

This site is affected by the position of the body over the center of gravity. It is quiet in the neutral posture, but the more forward it is over its axis, the more active it becomes. It is most active when one is standing on the toes.[67] Knee position changes the strength of the recording. As the knee becomes flexed, it becomes less effective as a plantar flexor.

Volume Conduction: Soleus, extensor hallucis, and extensor digitorum longus

Other Sites of Interest: Soleus for plantar flexion; tibialis anterior; hamstring for knee flexion; quadriceps

Referred Pain Considerations: Trigger points in this muscle may project pain to the insole of the foot and locally to the calf area.[17]

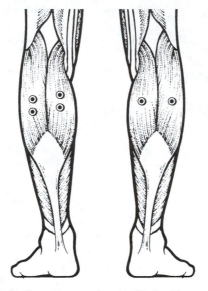

Figure 14–66 Electrode placement for the gastrocnemius site. Right side represents the general placement. Left side represents the more specific placement. *Source:* Copyright © Clinical Resources, Inc.

SOLEUS PLACEMENT

Type of Placement: Quasi-specific

Action: Plantar flexor and inverter of the foot

Clinical Uses: Gait training

Muscle Insertions: This muscle arises from the posterior head and upper third of the fibula, the middle of the tibia, and the tendinous arch, and joins the gastrocnemius to insert into the Achilles tendon.

Innervation: The tibial nerve via L-5, S-1, and S-2

Location: Two electrodes, 2 cm apart, are placed parallel to the muscle fibers on the inferior and lateral aspects of the leg, clearly below the belly of gastrocnemius (Figure 14–67A).

Behavioral Test: Forward leaning while standing or dorsiflexion of the foot

Tracing Comment: Figure 14–67B shows recordings from the anterior tibialis site, general gastrocnemius site, medial gastrocnemius site, lateral gastrocnemius site, lateral soleus site, and medial soleus site of the right leg during inversion and eversion of the foot. The possibility of cross-talk from peroneus and tibialis posterior entering the sEMG signal must be considered (raw sEMG).

Also see tracings from Figure 14–65B for postural sway off the central axis of gravity and Figure 14–65C for dorsiflexion and plantar flexion.

Clinical Considerations: This site was rated in the quasi-specific category because Perry et al's systematic study of the selectivity of surface sensors indicated that only 36% of the amplified signal came from the soleus.[68] The remaining

64% of the amplified signal represented cross-talk from neighboring muscles (primarily gastrocnemius).

The soleus muscle is commonly studied during ambulation. Its primary purpose is thought to be stabilizing the knee during the stance phase of gait.[16] It is also known to provide ankle stability and restrain the forward movement of the tibia over the fixed foot.

The soleus, along with tibialis anterior, is well known for its role in maintaining upright posture.[16] As the body sways forward over the center of gravity, the soleus becomes more active. High heels tend to activate the soleus group.[69]

Volume Conduction: Gastrocnemius, peroneus longus, posterior tibialis, flexor hallicus longus, and flexor digitorum longus

Other Sites of Interest: Gastrocnemius during planter flexion; tibialis anterior

Referred Pain Considerations: Trigger points at this site tend to project pain down to the heel or up into the calf. They are also known to project pain up to the sacroiliac joint.[17]

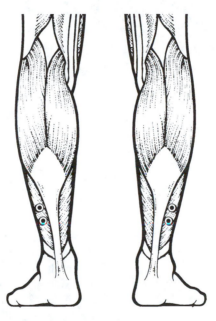

Figure 14–67A Electrode placement for the soleus site. *Source:* Copyright © Clinical Resources, Inc.

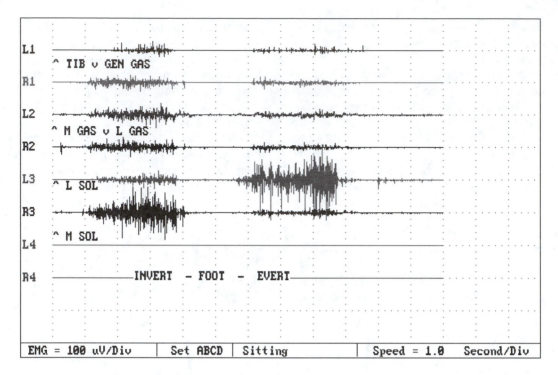

Figure 14–67B Surface EMG recordings from the anterior tibialis, general gastrocnemius, medial gastrocnemius, lateral gastrocnemius, lateral soleus, and medial soleus of the right leg during inversion and eversion of the foot. *Source:* Copyright © Clinical Resources, Inc.

EXTENSOR DIGITORUM BREVIS PLACEMENT

Type of Placement: Specific

Action: Dorsiflexion of the toes and eversion of the foot

Clinical Uses: Neurologic rehabilitation, gait training

Muscle Insertions: These muscles arise from the calcaneus and insert into the tendons of the dorsal aponeurosis of the second to fourth digits.

Innervation: The peroneal nerve via the spinal nerves at L-5 and S-1

Location: Two active electrodes, 2 cm apart, are placed parallel to the muscle fibers (same direction of the metatarsal bones) on the dorsal, lateral aspect of the foot, half the distance from the ankle to the base of the toes (Figure 14–68A).

Behavioral Test: Dorsiflexion of the toes

Tracing Comment: In Figure 14–68B, the extensor digitorum brevis is presented during dorsiflexion of the toes (raw sEMG).

Clinical Considerations: The primary function of this muscle is to extend the second, third, and fourth toes, and it is usually not included in a discussion regarding gait. However, a novel use of this site is to monitor and provide feedback during the swing phase of gait to assist the patient in dorsiflexion.[70]

Volume Conduction: Extensor hallucis brevis

Other Sites of Interest: Extensor digitorum longus, extensor hallucis longus, and abductor hallucis during gait

Referred Pain Considerations: Trigger points at this site project pain locally over the dorsum of the foot.[17]

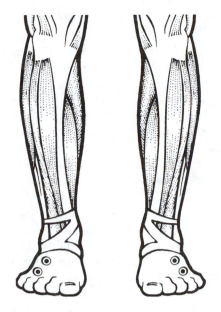

Figure 14–68A Electrode placement for extensor digitorum brevis site. *Source:* Copyright © Clinical Resources, Inc.

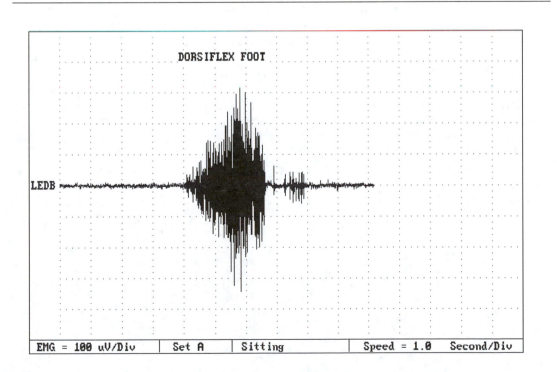

Figure 14–68B Surface EMG recording from the extensor digitorum brevis site during dorsiflexion of the toes and foot. *Source:* Copyright © Clinical Resources, Inc.

PERIVAGINAL AND PERIRECTAL PLACEMENT

Type of Placement: Quasi-specific

Purpose: Monitors from the levator ani and transversus perinei profundus. It is thought that the sphincter ani externus contributes heavily to recordings using the rectal sensor. It is thought that the bulbospongiosus contributes heavily to recordings using the vaginal sensor. These placement sites monitor the general support offered by the pelvic floor.

Clinical Uses: Urinary and fecal incontinence, urogenital pain (vestibulitus/vulvodynia and prostatitis)

Muscle Insertions: The levator ani arises from the pubic bone, the tendinous arch of the levator ani muscle and ischial spine. Its fibers are divisible into the puborectalis, the prerectal, pubococcygeal, and iliococcygeal muscles. The deeper iliococcygeal muscle of the levator ani forms a hammock across the pelvic floor. The sphincter ani externus encircles the anus. The bulbospongiosus muscle in the male arises from the perineal body and inserts into the corpus spongiosis and corpus cavernosus that it encloses. In the female, the bulbospongiosus muscle also arises from the perineal body and then surrounds the vagina on its way to the corpora cavernosa clitoridis.

Location: The vaginal sensor is inserted into the vagina, and the rectal sensor is inserted into the rectum. A cross-sectional view of this electrode placement may be seen in Figure 14–69A. Comparison of recordings from this type of sensor and fine-wire EMG recording has shown very high correlations.[71,72]

In addition, surface electrodes may be placed near or on the labia of the vagina as shown in Figure 14–69B. This electrode placement is found to correlate quite well ($r > 0.95$) (Jantos, personal communication). An example of this correlation is seen in the simultaneous recording from a vaginal sensor and an external surface electrode in Figure 14–69D. Finally, external perianal surface recordings may be conducted using the placement shown in Figure 14–69E.[73]

Behavioral Test: Kegel exercise; tense or flick pelvic floor

Tracing Comment: Figure 14–69C presents an intravaginal sEMG recording. Its normalcy is reflected by (1) the low resting baseline; (2) good recruitment with clear demarcation between rest and contraction; (3) strong contraction without any fatigue; (4) abrupt fall from contraction to resting baseline; and (5) a low resting baseline with good muscle stability (ie, low variance) postcontraction.

Clinical Considerations: Effects may change as a function of prone, sitting, or standing postures. May be affected by squats, coughs, sneezes, and exertional lifts.

Volume Conduction: Gluteus maximus, abdominals, adductors of the thigh

Referred Pain Considerations: Trigger points in the levator ani can refer pain to the sacral region.[17]

Benchmark: Resting baseline: 2.0 ($\pm$ 0.2) μV (RMS)

Strong contraction: 17.5 μV (RMS)

Values taken using a Thought Technology EMG with a 25-to-1000–Hz filter.

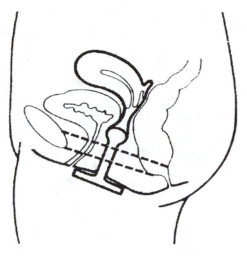

Figure 14–69A Cross-sectional view of an sEMG sensor inserted into the vagina. *Source:* Copyright © Marek Jantos, PhD.

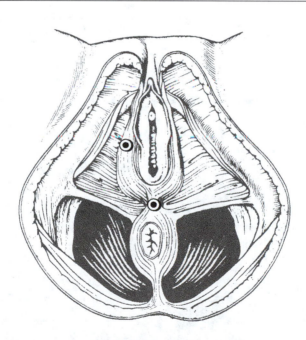

Figure 14–69B. Electrode placement for the perivaginal and perirectal sites are in the vagina and anus, respectively. *Source:* Reprinted with permission from Kahle, Leonhardt, and Plaatzer, *Color Atlas and Textbook of Human Anatomy*, Vol 1, © 1978, Georg Thieme Verlag.

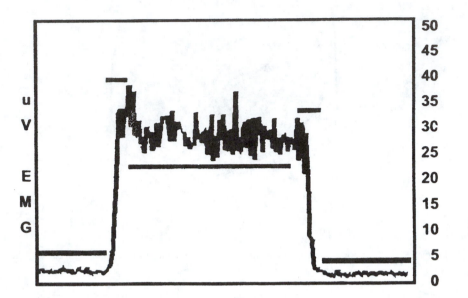

Figure 14–69C Intravaginal sEMG recording with a baseline, contraction, and return to baseline. *Source:* Copyright © Marek Jantos, PhD.

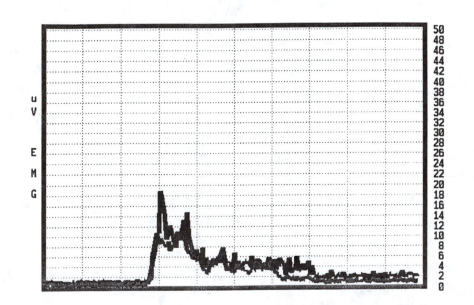

Figure 14–69D Simultaneous time series recordings from (Figure 14–69A) intravaginal and (Figure 14–69B) external electrode placement. Note the high correlation between the two. *Source:* Copyright © Marek Jantos, PhD.

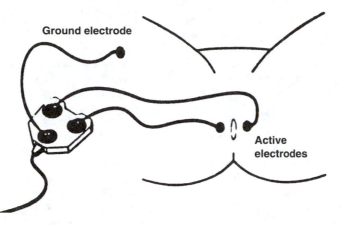

Ground electrode

Active electrodes

Figure 14–69E Electrode placement for perianal recordings using an external placement strategy. *Source:* Reprinted with permission from J Corocos, S Drew, and L West, Urinary and Fecal Incontinence, *Electromyography: Applications in Physical Therapy*, © 1992, Thought Technology.

REFERENCES

1. Lader MH, Mathews AM. A physiological model of phobic anxiety and desensitization. *Behav Res Ther*. 1968;6:411–421.

2. Malmo RB, Shagass C. Physiologic studies of reaction to stress in anxiety and early schizophrenia. *Psychosomatic Med*. 1949;11:9–24.

3. Goldstein B. Electromyography: A measure of skeletal muscle response. In: Greenfield S, Sternbach R, eds. *Handbook of Psychophysiology*. New York: Holt, Rinehart & Winston; 1972.

4. Munro RR. Electromyography of the muscles of mastication. In: Griffin CJ, Harris R, eds. *The Temporomandibular Joint Syndrome*. Basel, Switzerland: S Darger; 1975. Monographs in Oral Sciences, vol 4.

5. Schwartz M, ed. *Biofeedback: A Practitioner's Guide*. New York: Guilford; 1987.

6. Andrasik F, Blanchard EB. Biofeedback treatment of muscle contraction headache. In: Hatch JP, Fischer JG, Rugh J, eds. *Biofeedback: Studies in Clinical Efficacy*. New York: Plenum Press; 1987.

7. Donaldson S, Skubick D, Donaldson M. *Electromyography, Trigger Points and Myofascial Syndromes*. Calgary, Alberta: Behavioral Health Consultants; 1991.

8. Hudzynski L, Lawrence G. Significance of EMG surface electrode placement models and headache findings. *Headache*. 1988;28:30–35.

9. Zemach-Berson D, Zemach-Berson K, Reese M. *Relaxercise*. San Francisco: Harper; 1990.

10. Schneider C, Wilson E. Special considerations for EMG biofeedback training. In: *Foundations of Biofeedback Practice*. Wheat Ridge, CO: Biofeedback Society of America; 1985.

11. Bryant M. Biofeedback in the treatment of selected dysphagic patients. *Dysphagia*. 1991;6:140–144.

12. Curtis D, Braham SL, Karr S, Holborow G, Worman D. Identification of unopposed intact muscle pair actions affecting swallowing: potential for rehabilitation. *Dysphagia*. 1987;3:57–64.

13. Ettare D, Ettare R. Muscle learning therapy: A treatment protocol. In: Cram JR, ed. *Clinical EMG for Surface Recordings, II*. Nevada City, CA: Clinical Resources; 1990:197–234.

14. Cahn T, Cram JR. Muscle scanning: support for the back. *Perceptual and Motor Skills*. 1990;70:851–857.

15. Peper E, Wilson V, Taylor W et al. Repetitive strain injury. *Phys Ther Prod*. September 1994:17–22.

16. Basmajian JV, DeLuca C. *Muscles Alive*. 5th ed. Baltimore: Williams & Wilkins; 1985.

17. Travell J, Simons D. *Myofascial Pain and Dysfunction: A Trigger Point Manual, I and II*. Baltimore: Williams & Wilkins; 1983.

18. Cram JR. EMG muscle scanning and diagnostic manual for surface recordings. In: Cram JR, ed. *Clinical EMG for Surface Recordings, II*. Nevada City, CA: Clinical Resources; 1990:1–142.

19. Staling LM, Fetcher P, Vorro J. Premature occlusal contact influence on mandibular kinesiology. In: Komi PV, ed. *Biomechanics, V-A*. Baltimore: University Park Press; 1976.

20. Cacioppo JT, Tassinary G, Fridlund AJ. The skeletalmotor system. In: Cacioppo JT, Tassinary G, eds. *Principles of Psychophysiology*. New York: Cambridge University Press; 1990.

21. Bennett H, Kornhauser S. Assessment of general anesthesia by facial muscle electromyography (FACE). *Am J Electromed*. June 1995:94–97.

22. Ekman P, Friesen WV. *Unmasking the Human Face*. Englewood Cliffs, NJ: Prentice Hall; 1972.

23. Sackeim HA, Gur RC, Saucy MC. Emotions are expressed more intensely on the left side of the face. *Science*. 1978;202:434–436.

24. Worth DR. Movements of the cervical spine in modern manual therapy of the vertebral column. In: Grieve G, ed. *Modern Manual Therapy of the Vertebral Column*. New York: Churchill Livingstone; 1986.

25. Carstensen B. Indications and contraindications for manual therapy for temporomandibular joint dysfunction. In: Grieve G, ed. *Modern Manual Therapy of the Vertebral Column*. New York: Churchill Livingstone; 1986.

26. Upledger J, Vredevoogd JD. *CranioSacral Therapy*. Seattle, WA: Eastland Press; 1983.

27. Campbell EJM. Accessory muscles. In: Campbell EJM, Agostioni E, Davis JN, eds. *The Respiratory Muscles: Mechanics and Neural Control*. Philadelphia: WB Saunders; 1970.

28. Kendall FP, Kendall E, McCreary BA. *Muscles, Testing and Function*. 3rd ed. Baltimore: Williams & Wilkins; 1983.

29. Gray H. *Anatomy of the Human Body*. 29th ed. Goss CM, ed. Philadelphia: Lea & Febiger; 1973.

30. Cook EE, Gray, VL, Savinar-Nogue E, Madeiros J. Shoulder antagonistic strength ratios: a comparison between college-level baseball pitchers and non-pitchers. *J Orthop Sports Phys Ther*. March 1987:451–461.

31. Duchenne GB. *Physiologie des Mouvement*. Kaplan EB, trans. Philadelphia: WB Saunders; 1949.

32. Rasch PJ, Burke RK. *Kinesiology and Applied Anatomy*. Philadelphia: Lea & Febiger; 1978.

33. Taylor W. Dynamic EMG biofeedback in assessment and treatment using a neuromuscular re-education model. In: Cram JR, ed. *Clinical EMG for Surface Recordings, Volume 2*. Nevada City, CA: Clinical Resources; 1990:175–196.

34. Hollingshead WH. *Functional Anatomy of the Limbs and Back*. Philadelphia: WB Saunders; 1976.

35. Bao S, Mathiassen SE, Winkel J. Normalizing upper trapezius EMG amplitude: comparison of different procedures. *J Electromyogr Kinesiol*. 1995;5:251–257.

36. McConnell JS. *Treatment of the Unstable Shoulder: Course Manual*. Marina Del Rey, CA: McConnell Seminars; 1993.

37. Lundervold AJS. Electromyographic investigations of position and manner of working in typewriting. *Acta Physiol Scand*. 1951;24:84.

38. Skubick D, Clasby R, Donaldson CCS, Marshall W. Carpal tunnel syndrome as an expression of muscular dysfunction in the neck. *J Occup Rehab*. 1993;3:31–43.

39. Singh M, Karpovich PV. Isotonic and isometric forces of forearm flexors and extensors. *J Applied Physiol*. 1966;21:1435.

40. Sullivan WE, Mortensen OA, Miles M, Green LS. Electromyographic studies of m. biceps brachii during normal voluntary movement at the elbow. *Anat Rec*. 1950;107:243–251.

41. Travill AA. Electromyographic study of the extensor apparatus of the forearm. *Anat Rec*. 1962;144:373–376.

42. Mortimer JT, Kerstein MD, Magnusson R, Petersen H. Muscle blood flow in the human biceps as a function of developed muscle force. *Arch Surg*. 1971;103:376–377.

43. McMahon T, Pianta R, Couch L, Wolf S, Segal R, Mason L. Normalized electromyographic activity patterns in human extensor carpi radialis longus and flexor carpi radialis muscles: differential activity. In: Anderson PA, Hobart DJ, Danoff JV, eds. *Electromyographical Kinesiology*. Amsterdam: Elsevier; 1991:39–42.

44. Joseph J, Williams PL. Electromyography of certain hip muscles. *J Anat*. 1957;91:286–294.

45. Simons D. Functions of the quadratus lumborum muscle and relation of its myofascial trigger points to low back pain. *Pain Abstracts, I*. Montreal: Second World Congress on Pain; August 1978.

46. Flint MM. An electromyographic comparison of the function of the iliacus and rectus abdominis muscles. *J Am Phys Ther Assoc*. 1965;45:248–253.

47. Jull G, Janda V. Muscles and motor control in low back pain: Assessment and management. In: Twomey L, Taylor J, eds. *Physical Therapy of the Low Back*. New York: Churchill Livingstone; 1987.

48. Pierce M, Lee W. Muscle firing order during active prone hip extension. *J Orthop Sports Phys Ther*. 1990; 12:2–9.

49. Jackson R. Functional relations of the lower half. Unpublished data, 1996.

50. Greenlaw RK. *Function of Muscles about the Hip during Normal Level Walking*. Kingston, Ont: Queen's University. Thesis.

51. Neumann DA, Cook TM. Effect of load and carrying position on the electromyographic activity of the gluteus medius muscle during walking. *Phys Ther*. 1985; 65:305–311.

52. Pere EB, Stern JT, Schwartz JM. Functional differentiation within the tensor fasciae latae. *J Bone Joint Surg Am.* 1981;63:1457–1471.

53. Godges J et al. The effects of two stretching procedures on hip range of motion and gait economy. *J Orthop Sports Phys Ther.* March 1989:350–357.

54. Godges J, McRae P, Engelkey K. Effects of exercise on hip range of motion, trunk muscle performance and gait economy. *Phys Ther.* 1993;73:468–477.

55. Godges J, Heino J, Carter C. Relationship between hip extension range of motion and postural alignment. *J Orthop Sports Phys Ther.* 1990;12:243–247.

56. Gose J, Schweizer P. Iliotibial band tightness. *J Orthop Sports Phys Ther.* April 1989:399–407.

57. Draper V. Electromyographic biofeedback and recovery of quadriceps femoris muscle function following anterior cruciate ligament reconstruction. *Phys Ther.* 1990;69:11–17.

58. Draper V, Ballard L. Electrical stimulation versus electromyographic biofeedback in the recovery of quadriceps femoris muscle function following anterior cruciate ligament surgery. *Phys Ther.* 1991;71:455–463.

59. Basmajian JV, Harden TP, Regenos EM. Integrated action of the four heads of the quadriceps femoris: an electromyographic study. *Anat Rec.* 1972;172:15–20.

60. Souza DR, Gross MT. Comparison of vastus medialis oblique: vastus lateralis muscle integrated electromyographic ratios between healthy subjects and patients with patellofemoral pain. *Phys Ther.* 1991;71:310–320.

61. Felder CR, Lesson MA. The use of electromyographic biofeedback for training the vastus medialis oblique in patients with patellofemoral pain. *Physical Ther Prod.* March 1990:49–52.

62. McConnell JS. *McConnell Patellofemoral Treatment Plan: Course Manual.* Marina Del Rey, CA: McConnell Seminars; 1991.

63. Kasman G, Cram J, Wolf S. *Clinical Applications in Surface Electromyography.* Gaithersburg, MD: Aspen Publishers; 1997.

64. Close JR. *Motor Function in the Lower Extremity.* Springfield, IL: Charles C Thomas; 1964.

65. Green DL, Morris JM. Role of adductor longus and adductor magnus in postural movements and in ambulation. *Am J Phys Med.* 1970;49:223–240.

66. Murray MP, Mollinger LA, Gardner GM, et al. Kinematic and EMG patterns during slow, free and fast walking. *J Orthop Res.* 1984;2:272–280.

67. Okada M. An electromyographic estimation of the relative muscular load in different human postures. *J Hum Ergol.* 1972;1:75–93.

68. Perry J, Easterday CS, Antonelli DJ. Surface versus intramuscular electrodes for electromyography of superficial and deep muscles. *Phys Ther.* 1981;61:7–15.

69. Campbell KM, Biggs NL, Blanton PL, et al. Electromyographic investigation of the relative activity among four components of the triceps surae. *Am J Phys Med.* 1973;52:30–41.

70. Wolf S. *Anatomy and Electrode Placement: Upper Extremities; Face and Back; Lower Extremities* [video]. Nevada City, CA: Clinical Resources; 1991.

71. Maizels M, Pirlit CF. Pediatric urodynamics: a clinical comparison for surface versus needle pelvic floor/external sphincter electromyography. *J Urol.* 1979;122:518–522.

72. Nygaard I et al. Exercise and incontinence. *Obstet Gynecol.* 1983;75:848–851.

73. Corocos J, Drew S, West L. *Urinary and Fecal Incontinence: Electromyography Applications in Physical Therapy.* Montreal: Thought Technology; 1992.

Chapter Questions

1. As a general rule, the depth of an sEMG recording is directly proportionate to:
   a. the size of the muscle below
   b. the type of the muscle fiber below
   c. the interelectrode distance
   d. the shape of the electrode

2. The quasi-specific site designation is offered when:
   a. the intended muscle for recording lies beneath another muscle
   b. the intended muscle for recording is superficial
   c. the intended muscle for recording lies close to other muscles
   d. a or c

3. The location for an electrode placement needs to be verified by:
   a. muscle testing with electrode attached
   b. knowledge of muscle origin and insertions
   c. knowledge of muscle function
   d. all of the above

4. The sEMG tracings presented in the atlas are:
   a. based on normative groups
   b. samples reflecting one individual subject's performance
   c. examples of an ideal recruitment pattern
   d. none of the above

5. Benchmark values presented in the atlas:
   a. are based on normative data
   b. are useful for resting baseline comparisons only
   c. are useful for resting tone and dynamic movement peaks
   d. are based on normalized values
   e. a and b

6. Abduction reflects:
   a. movement toward the body
   b. movement away from the body
   c. movement of an upward nature
   d. movement of a downward nature

7. In the upper extremities, *supination* is:
   a. palm-up position
   b. palm-down position
   c. the neutral position
   d. none of the above

8. Which of the following is not one of the attributes of the lower extremities?
   a. side bending
   b. flexion
   c. extension
   d. abduction
   e. adduction

9. The frontal (wide) placement is best used:
   a. to monitor stress
   b. to reach general relaxation
   c. to monitor negative emotions
   d. both a and b
   e. a, b, and c

10. Using the temporal mastoid (wide) placement, it is possible to observe recruitment during:
    a. eyebrow flashes
    b. head rotation
    c. ear wiggling
    d. a and b
    e. a, b, and c

11. If sEMG recruitment at the temporalis site is associated with elevation of the mandible, which site would you monitor to see jaw opening?
    a. zygomaticus
    b. suprahyoid
    c. masseter
    d. none of the above

12. When using the cervical trapezius placement, ECG artifact:
    a. will contaminate the left lead
    b. will contaminate the right lead
    c. will contaminate both leads
    d. is only a problem if you are using the 100-to-200–Hz filter

13. Which pattern of muscle recruitment would one expect to see during cervical rotation to the left?
    a. right sternocleidomastoid, right C-4 paraspinals
    b. right sternocleidomastoid, left C-4 paraspinals
    c. left sternocleidomastoid, right C-4 paraspinals
    d. left sternocleidomastoid, left C-4 paraspinals

14. During a deep inspiration, one would expect to see the scalene muscles:
    a. show a symmetrical recruitment pattern
    b. show an asymmetrical recruitment pattern
    c. not be involved in respiratory patterns
    d. recruit four times more than upper trapezius

15. The posterior deltoid should recruit most heavily during:
    a. shoulder elevation
    b. external rotation
    c. extension of the arm
    d. a, b, and c tend to recruit at the same level

16. The ratio of the peak contraction between upper and lower trapezius during abduction of the arms to 90 degrees should be approximately:
    a. 3:1
    b. 1:1
    c. 1:3
    d. 10:1

17. Recruitment patterns for serratus anterior are greatest during:
    a. wall push-up
    b. kneeling push-up
    c. floor push-up
    d. forward flexion of the arms

18. Which of the deltoids is most heavily recruited during forward flexion of the arms?
    a. anterior deltoid
    b. middle deltoid
    c. posterior deltoid
    d. both b and c

19. The widely spaced extensor-flexor site on the forearm will show activation during:
    a. extension
    b. flexion
    c. making a fist
    d. a and c
    e. a, b, and c

20. During elbow flexion in the pronated position, one would expect the biceps:
    a. to fire briskly along with brachioradialis
    b. not to recruit
    c. to fire briskly without brachioradialis
    d. to fire only during the first 30 degrees of arc

21. When placing electrodes on the triceps, the arm:
    a. should be flexed at 90 degrees
    b. should be fully extended
    c. should be in the position the practitioner plans to train in
    d. can be in any convenient position

22. The extensor carpi ulnaris tends to show the least amount of recruitment during:
    a. resisted radial deviation
    b. resisted ulnar deviation
    c. resisted wrist extension
    d. none of the above

23. Placement for extensor digitorum should be:
    a. over the belly of the muscle
    b. at the distal end of the muscle belly
    c. at the proximal end of the muscle
    d. none of the above

24. During forward flexion of the torso, a flexion-relaxation response should be seen:
    a. at the L-3 site only
    b. at the L-3 and T-12 sites only
    c. at the L-3, T-12, and T-1 sites only
    d. at the L-3, T-12, T-1, and C-4 sites

25. During axial rotation of the trunk, do the abdominal muscles play a role?
    a. definitely yes
    b. definitely no
    c. only during extreme end range of motion
    d. only during the first 15 degrees of arc

26. During a diagonal sit-up to the left, which electrode placements on the abdominal muscles seem to recruit heavily?
    a. right rectus and left oblique
    b. left rectus and right oblique
    c. left and right rectus and left oblique
    d. left and right rectus and right oblique

27. Which action would you expect to recruit the gluteus medius most heavily?
    a. abduction of the leg with internal rotation
    b. abduction of the leg with external rotation
    c. abduction of the leg in the neutral position
    d. a, b, and c would recruit equally

28. Which action would you expect to recruit the tensor fasciae latae the least?
    a. abduction of the leg with internal rotation
    b. abduction of the leg with external rotation
    c. abduction of the leg in the neutral position
    d. a, b, and c would recruit equally

29. What can be said about the flexors of the hip (femoral triangle site and hip flexor site/sartorius and iliopsoas) sites?
    a. They are easily isolated.
    b. They are quasi-specific sites.
    c. They are specific sites.
    d. They are general sites.

30. The relative balance between vastus lateralis (VL) and vastus medialis oblique (VMO) has been indicated in patellofemoral pain. What should the normal ratio of the peak VMO:VL be?
    a. 1:3
    b. 3:1
    c. a little over 1:1
    d. a little under 1:1

31. The level of recruitment during prone leg extension of the tensor fasciae latae is reduced when the leg is laterally rotated. Which position would reduce the recruitment of lateral hamstrings during leg extension?
    a. medial rotation
    b. neutral position
    c. lateral rotation
    d. a, b, and c would recruit about the same

32. The tibialis anterior placement site is:
    a. a specific site
    b. a quasi-specific site
    c. a general site
    d. a linear site

33. Which of the following characteristics of the recruitment pattern for the pelvic floor is not one of its normal attributes?

    a. low resting baseline
    b. good demarcation between rest and contraction
    c. strong contraction with minimal fatigue
    d. high variance during postcontraction period

Glossary of Terms

abduction: Movement away from midline of the sagittal plane.

abrasion of the skin: A procedure by which the oils and horny layer of skin are removed by rubbing the skin with a rough texture. It is used to reduce impedance and to improve recording quality.

active electrode: An electrode design that incorporates the EMG preamplifier in an adjacent housing directly at the recording site. It commonly uses a very high input impedance, rendering it less sensitive to the impedance of the electrode interface.

active range of motion: Joint motion produced by muscle contraction.

adduction: Movement toward the midline of the sagittal plane.

adipose tissue: The subcutaneous fat layer between the surface of the skin and the muscle. This tissue is known to attenuate the source EMG as it travels to the surface. The greater the thickness of the adipose, the greater the attenuation. It is recommended that the thickness be measured prior to sEMG recordings.

agonist muscle group: The muscle group that initiates a contraction of movement.

alpha motor system: The part of the central nervous system that activates the extrafusal muscle fibers.

amplitude probability distribution function: A graphical representation of the variability of sEMG activity. Here the amplitude of the sEMG signal for a specified epoch of time is plotted as a histogram, with amplitude plotted along the X axis and the frequency of a given amplitude plotted along the Y axis. This may be used to inspect for the presence of interspersed rest during a work task.

ankle-to-ankle recordings: A procedure in which the recording electrodes are placed on the right and left ankle. This procedure is used to teach systemic relaxation to the lower extremities, hips, and low back region.

antagonist muscle group: A muscle group that provides a negative, stabilizing force during a contraction or movement.

antalgic posture: Adoption of a postural stance that occurs in response to pain.

ballistic contraction: Movement that is executed in the fastest possible speed.

band-pass filter: This defines the lower and upper frequency limits (expressed in Hertz) of the energy of the sEMG signal that is passed on for further amplification. Some sEMG amplifiers use a very narrow 100-to-200–Hz band-pass filter, allowing only about 20% of the EMG spectrum to be processed. Others use a wider 15-to-500–Hz band-pass filter, allowing 98% of the sEMG to be processed.

bilateral electrode placement: A technique in which each of the recording electrodes from a differential amplifier is placed on the right and left aspects of a muscle group.

bracing: The habitual and inappropriate use of postural muscles.

cocontraction: The tendency of agonist and antagonist muscle groups to activate simultaneously. This is commonly expressed as a percent asymmetry for normalized sEMG.

common mode rejection: A characteristic of a differential amplifier, in which the signal that is common to both recording electrodes in reference to ground is eliminated from further amplification. This reduces the environmental noise that might otherwise contaminate the signal. It is mathematically defined as a common mode rejection ratio (CMRR) and should be at 90 dB or better.

concentric contraction: The activation of a muscle that is associated with the shortening of its length.

contracture: An electrically silent, involuntary state of maintained muscle shortness due to decreased extensibility (ie, increased stiffness) of the passive elastic properties of the connective tissue. The elasticity of the muscle should be concurrently determined through palpation, and the muscle length and joint angle should be reported along with the sEMG levels.

derecruitment: Training in the reduction of sEMG activity. This is commonly associated with teaching the patient to turn off a recruitment pattern once the movement is completed.

differential amplification: A characteristic of the sEMG amplifier, in which the biological potential reaching both recording electrodes is compared to that of the reference electrode, and only the energy that is different is passed on for further amplification. Also see *common mode rejection*.

direct contact electrode: Surface EMG that makes contact with the skin.

discrimination training: Surface EMG biofeedback training procedure in which the subject learns to associate a specific RMS microvolt level with proprioceptive sensations. Extrinsic feedback is withdrawn as the subject comes to discriminate different levels of muscle tension.

downtraining: Training in the reduction of sEMG activity. This is commonly associated with relaxation training.

dynamic sEMG evaluation: The use of single or multisite sEMG recordings for the study of recruitment patterns of muscles during movement. The record is examined for stereotypic sEMG events as a function of the range of motion arc—such as symmetry of recruitment, cocontractions, synergies, substitution patterns, and irritability (differentiated from needle EMG findings).

dysponesis: Literally "bad effort." In the context of sEMG, it implies inappropriate site or intensity of muscle activation.

eccentric contraction: Muscle contraction generated as a muscle increases in length.

EMG: The sum of the energy from all muscle action potentials detected by the recording electrode.

fascia: A sheet of fibrous tissue that encapsulates muscles and groups of muscles and separates muscle layers or groups.

flexion cross-extension reflex: This is a polysynaptic reflex that excites the flexor group and inhibits the extensor group on the ipsilateral side of pain, while simultaneously exciting the extensor group and inhibiting the flexor group on the contralateral side.

flexion-relaxation: A phenomenon commonly seen in the lumbar paraspinal during forward flexion of the neck or torso. At the end range of motion, there is a reduction in signal amplitude of sEMG as the body moves out onto ligament support.

floating electrode: Surface EMG electrode that is recessed above the skin and uses an electrolytic medium to bridge between the electrode and the skin.

free nerve ending: The sensory apparatus in the muscle that is sensitive to pain. It senses pain when the internal environment is too acidotic or when there is swelling and edema.

frontal EMG: Surface EMG biofeedback procedure where the recording electrodes are placed on the frontalis muscle directly above each eye. This is used for systemic relaxation training.

gain: How much larger an amplifier makes the biological signal. The amount of gain or amplification determines how large or small the sEMG appears on the visual display.

gamma motor system: The part of the central nervous system that is known to activate the intrafusal muscle fibers associated with the muscle spindle.

Golgi tendon organ: Part of the sensory system of muscle, this tissue is located at the tendon/muscle junction, is in series with the muscle, and informs the central nervous system of the strength of contraction or effort made by the muscle.

integral average (μV/sec): A method for quantifying sEMG in which the absolute value of each sEMG data point is obtained and then the data are simply summed and then averaged. The following formula is used:

$$I\{|m(t)|\} = 1/T\int_t^{t+T} |m(t)| \, dt$$

interelectrode distance: The distance between the two recording electrodes (differential amplification). The closer the electrodes are spaced, the more circumscribed is the area of effective recording. The further apart the electrodes, the more general the sEMG recording.

isometric contraction: A muscle contraction in which the muscle length, and thus joint angle, is kept constant.

isotonic contraction: A muscle contraction in which the tension of the muscle is kept constant through regulation of external forces.

kinetic chain: Movement in which the distal segment is fixed, such as during weight bearing of the lower limb. Movement at one joint induces movement at another joint.

ligament: A band or sheet of fibrous tissue connecting bones, cartilage, or other structures.

maximum voluntary contraction (MVC): The greatest amount of effort an individual can put forth with volitional activation of a particular muscle or muscle group.

motor unit: The alpha motor neuron, its axon, the neuromuscular junction, and the muscle fibers it innervates (from 3 to 2000). It is the smallest motor unit under voluntary control.

muscle action potential (MAP): The transmembrane voltage wave associated with the depolarization of muscle fibers. MAPs of a single motor unit may be detected by nearby electrodes residing in the muscle. Populations of MAPs may be detected by sEMG electrodes.

muscle irritability: The persistence of sEMG activity following the cessation of voluntary contraction of a muscle (differentiated from irritability seen with needle EMG findings).

muscle scanning: A clinical procedure in which multiple sites are evaluated using surface electrodes set at a fixed distance and held in place by hand.

muscle spasm: Reflexive increase in sEMG activity in muscle (with or without shortening). The activity cannot be stopped voluntarily.

muscle spindle: Part of the sensory system of muscle, this tissue is located in the muscle itself, is parallel to the muscle fibers, and informs the central nervous system of the instantaneous length and velocity of change of muscle fibers. It also represents the "stretch receptor," and when the muscle is stretched the output of the muscle spindle provides an excitatory influence on the lower motor neuron that innervates the muscle of origin.

myofascial trigger point: A hyperirritable spot, usually with a taut band of skeletal muscle or in the muscle fascia, that is painful on compression and gives rise to characteristic referred pain patterns, tenderness, and autonomic phenomena.

myotatic unit: A group of agonist and antagonist muscles that function together as a unit because they share a common spinal reflex response.

normative data: Quantitative description of the behavior of the muscles under controlled conditions for a representative sample of healthy subjects. It may include means and standard deviations of raw data or consist of standardized/normalized scores.

passive range of motion: Joint motion produced by external force and without voluntary assistance by the subject.

peak to peak: The unit of measurement associated with raw sEMG recordings.

processed sEMG: This represents a mathematically derived presentation of the sEMG signal. Common methods include integral, root mean square (RMS), and spectral analysis representations.

protective guarding: The learned motor response in which the individual favors an injured area by substituting other muscle groups. For example, the patient may learn to redistribute weight-bearing load toward the side opposite the injury. At the same segmental level, typically the sEMG activation pattern is located on the side opposite that of the reported pain.

raw sEMG: This represents a peak-to-peak oscilloscopic display of the sEMG signal. The signal is not processed; there is no rectification, no time constants, no conversions or transformations of the sEMG data.

root mean square (RMS): A method for quantifying sEMG in which each sEMG value is first squared, then summed and averaged, and finally the root of the product is derived. The following formula is used:

$$RMS\{|m(t)|\} = 1/T <\int_t^{t+T} m^2(t)\ dt>^{1/2}$$

sarcomere: The basic anatomical unit of muscle fiber, consisting of a single unit of overlapping myosin and actin filaments extending from one Z line to the next Z line.

scratch reflex: A polysynaptic suprasegmental reflex, where the stimulus evokes a motor response several segments away, whose action is directed toward eradicating the stimulation of the original segment.

spectral analysis: The sEMG signal is recorded and submitted for a decomposition of the energy into its frequency components, typically using a fast fourier transformation (FFT). This may be used to verify that the sEMG is "clean" of 60-Hz noise, and to assess muscle fatigue.

splinting: The phenomenon where muscles reflexively contract around an injured joint to provide a protective stability (immobility) to that joint. These activation patterns are found on the same side of the injury and are associated with increased sEMG activity for the muscles that cross that joint. Also referred to as *acute reflexive spasm*.

static sEMG evaluation: The use of multisite sEMG recordings at rest (neutral postures), for the study of patterns of muscle activity. The record is examined for: splinting, protective guarding, antalgia, chronic bracing.

substitution patterns: When the muscle action of a primary mover or stabilizer is replaced by a muscle that would not normally perform that action.

surface electromyography (sEMG): The use of surface electrodes for the recording of electrical potentials from the underlying musculature. It is used in the study of posture, movement, and emotional expression. The record is typically inspected for evidence of the following: emotional lability, antalgic postures, splinting, guarding, cocontractions, symmetries and asymmetries, flexion-relaxation, and other recruitment patterns.

symmetry: The degree of parity between the right and left aspects of a given muscle group. This may be assessed during rest, or the peak activity may be assessed for symmetry during the eccentric or concentric phase of a contraction.

synergistic muscle: A muscle group that participates in an additive fashion with other muscles to create a smooth, coordinated movement.

systemic relaxation training: Surface EMG biofeedback training procedure in which feedback is given from the frontal region or other larger regions.

time constant: A characteristic of a resistor compactor (RC) circuit used in amplifiers to smooth out the sEMG signal. The larger the time constant, the smoother the variations of recording from the sEMG signal.

unilateral electrode placement: A technique in which the recording electrodes of a differential amplifier are placed on one side (right or left) of a homologous muscle pair.

uptraining: Surface EMG biofeedback training procedure in which feedback is used to increase the recruitment of a specific muscle group.

withdrawal reflex: A fixed action pattern in which the muscles automatically move a body part away from the source of a painful stimulus.

wrist-to-wrist recordings: A procedure in which the recording electrodes of a differential amplifier are placed on the right and left wrists. This procedure is used to teach systemic relaxation of the upper extremities, torso, neck, and head.

Answers to Chapter Questions

Chapter 2. Anatomy and Physiology
1a, 2b, 3d, 4c, 5b, 6b, 7a, 8b, 9c, 10a, 11b, 12a, 13b, 14b, 15c, 16c, 17a, 18d, 19a, 20b, 21d, 22d, 23a, 24d, 25b, 26b, 27c, 28a, 29b, 30c, 31a, 32a, 33d, 34b, 35b.

Chapter 3. Instrumentation
1b, 2d, 3b,4c, 5c, 6c, 7c, 8c, 9b, 10a, 11b, 12a, 13b, 14b, 15c, 16a, 17d, 18c.

Chapter 4. Electrode and Site Selection Strategies
1b, 2c, 3c, 4d, 5a, 6a, 7b, 8e, 9a, 10d, 11e, 12d.

Chapter 5. General Assessment Considerations
1c, 2b, 3b, 4a, 5b, 6b, 7d.

Chapter 6. Static Assessment and Clinical Protocol
1e, 2b, 3d, 4d, 5b, 6d, 7d, 8e.

Chapter 7. Emotional Assessment and Clinical Protocol
1a, 2b, 3a, 4d, 5c, 6d.

Chapter 8. Dynamic Assessment
1d, 2b, 3b, 4d, 5b, 6a, 7c, 8d, 9b, 10c, 11b, 12a, 13e.

Chapter 9. Treatment Considerations and Protocols
1c, 2a, 3d, 4b, 5a, 6a, 7b, 8c, 9b, 10a, 11d, 12c, 13a, 14e, 15c, 16c, 17d, 18a.

Chapter 10. Documentation
1b, 2b, 3a, 4b.

Chapter 14. Electrode Placements
1c, 2d, 3d, 4b, 5e, 6b, 7a, 8a, 9e, 10e, 11b, 12a, 13b, 14c, 15c, 16b, 17c, 18a, 19e, 20b, 21c, 22b, 23b, 24d, 25a, 26d, 27b, 28b, 29b, 30c, 31a, 32b, 33d.

Index